Lynn Fitzgerald Macksey, MSN, RN, CRNA

To Keith, Kevin, and Kimberly,
my greatest teachers

Pediatric Anesthesia and Emergency Drug Guide SECOND EDITION

Lynn Fitzgerald Macksey, MSN, RN, CRNA

Department of Anesthesiology
University of North Carolina at Chapel Hill School of Medicine
Chapel Hill, North Carolina

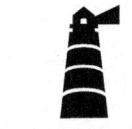

JONES & BARTLETT
LEARNING

World Headquarters
Jones & Bartlett Learning
25 Mall Road
Burlington, MA 01803
978-443-5000
info@jblearning.com
www.jblearning.com

Jones & Bartlett books and products are available through most bookstores and online booksellers. To contact Jones & Bartlett Learning directly, call 800-832-0034, fax 978-443-8000, or visit our website, www.jblearning.com.

Substantial discounts on bulk quantities of Jones & Bartlett Learning publications are available to corporations, professional associations, and other qualified organizations. For details and specific discount information, contact the special sales department at Jones & Bartlett Learning via the above contact information or send an email to specialsales@jblearning.com.

The content, statements, views, and opinions herein are the sole expression of the respective authors and not that of Jones & Bartlett Learning, LLC. Reference herein to any specific commercial product, process, or service by trade name, trademark, manufacturer, or otherwise does not constitute or imply its endorsement or recommendation by Jones & Bartlett Learning, LLC and such reference shall not be used for advertising or product endorsement purposes. All trademarks displayed are the trademarks of the parties noted herein. *Pediatric Anesthesia and Emergency Drug Guide, Second Edition* is an independent publication and has not been authorized, sponsored, or otherwise approved by the owners of the trademarks or service marks referenced in this product.

There may be images in this book that feature models; these models do not necessarily endorse, represent, or participate in the activities represented in the images. Any screenshots in this product are for educational and instructive purposes only. Any individuals and scenarios featured in the case studies throughout this product may be real or fictitious, but are used for instructional purposes only.

Production Credits	
VP, Executive Publisher: David D. Cella	Composition: CAE Solutions Corp.
Executive Editor: Amanda Martin	Cover Design: Kristin E. Parker
Acquisitions Editor: Teresa Reilly	Rights & Media Specialist: Wes DeShano
Editorial Assistant: Lauren Vaughn	Media Development Editor: Shannon Sheehan
Senior Production Editor: Amanda Clerkin	Cover Image: © Lamella/Shutterstock
Marketing Communications Manager: Katie Hennessy	Printing and Binding: Gasch Printing
VP, Manufacturing and Inventory Control: Therese Connell	Cover Printing: Gasch Printing

Library of Congress Cataloging-in-Publication Data
Names: Macksey, Lynn Fitzgerald, author.
Title: Pediatric anesthesia and emergency drug guide / Lynn Fitzgerald Macksey.
Other titles: Pediatric anesthetic and emergency drug guide
Description: Second edition. | Burlington, Massachusetts : Jones & Bartlett Learning, [2017] | Preceded by Pediatric anesthetic and emergency drug guide / Lynn Fitzgerald Macksey c2009. | Includes bibliographical references.
Identifiers: LCCN 2015503830 | ISBN 9781284090987
Subjects: | MESH: Anesthesia—methods—Nurses' Instruction. | Anesthetics—administration & dosage—Nurses' Instruction. | Emergencies—Nurses' Instruction. | Pediatrics—methods—Nurses' Instruction.
Classification: LCC RD139 | NLM WO 440 | DDC 617.9/6083—dc23
LC record available at http://lccn.loc.gov/2015503830

6048

Printed in the United States of America
26 25   10 9 8 7

Contents

Contents

Contents

Disclaimer

The author, editor, and publisher have made every effort to provide accurate information. However, they are not responsible for errors, omissions, or for any outcomes related to the use of the contents of this book and take no responsibility for the use of the products and procedures described. Treatments and side effects described in this book may not be applicable to all people; likewise, some people may require a dose or experience a side effect that is not described herein. Drugs and medical devices are discussed that may have limited availability controlled by the Food and Drug Administration (FDA) for use only in a research study or clinical trial. Research, clinical practice, and government regulations often change the accepted standard in this field. When consideration is being given to use of any drug in the clinical setting, the health care provider or reader is responsible for determining FDA status of the drug, reading the package insert, and reviewing prescribing information for the most up-to-date recommendations on dose, precautions, and contraindications, and determining the appropriate usage for the product. This is especially important in the case of drugs that are new or seldom used.

SECTION

1

Introduction

All calculated medications listed in this text are given in their **average or best dose**. This is different from the first edition of the *Pediatric Anesthesia and Emergency Drug Guide*, in which the maximum dose was listed for the precalculated drugs.

Many commonly used anesthetics, antibiotics, and emergency bolus drugs are included in the "precalculated drug" pages. Precalculated drugs are grouped into sections but do not necessarily appear in alphabetical order.

Important: Some medication routes or dosages may be inappropriate for an individual of a given age. *Make sure to check the Drug Dosages and Ranges Chart regarding recommended dosing information.*

Some drugs listed require mixing with a dilutent. For example, remifentanil can be mixed 1 mg/20 mL (to equal 50 mcg/mL) or 1 mg/40 mL (to equal 25 mcg/mL), but I have listed the supplied mg/mL as 50 mcg/mL, the most common ratio we use in our practice. Several drugs are listed in this fashion.

In the emergency drug precalculated pages, dantrolene is mixed in several different percent solutions. The dosage per kilogram is listed but the milliliter amount to be given could not be calculated.

A complete list of commonly used drugs for the pediatric patient is provided in the "Drugs Dosages and Ranges Listed Alphabetically" section, along with their usual drug dosing and ranges, if applicable. There are many more drugs listed here than are in the precalculated pages. Drug categories listed are as follows:

- Antisialagogue premedication
- Sedation premedication
- Induction
- Opioids IV
- Opioids PO
- Nonopioid analgesics
- Muscle relaxants
- Reversal agents

- Antibiotics
- Nausea prophylaxis
- Antihistamines
- Anticonvulsants
- Diuretics
- Miscellaneous medications
- Common local anesthetics
- Local anesthetic maximums
- Epidural agents
- Emergency drugs
  - Antihypertensives IV push
  - Emergency medications: bolus
  - Emergency medications: infusions

2

Normal Vital Signs, Weight, and H&H

■ Normal vital signs per age

	Premature	0-3 mo	3-6 mo	6 mo-1 y	1-3 y	3-6 y	6-12 y	> 12 y
kg	1.5-3	3-7	4.5-9.5	6.5-12.5	9-15	15-21	21-40	40+
SBP	55-75/ 35-45	65-85/ 45-55	70-90/ 50-65	80-100/ 55-65	90-105/ 55-70	95-110/ 60-75	100-120/ 60-75	110-135/ 65-85
HR	120-170	100-150	90-120	80-110	70-110	65-110	60-95	55-85
RESP	55-60	30-60	30-60	30-50	24-40	22-34	18-30	12-16

Goal of median systolic blood pressure: **(age in years × 2) + 90 mm Hg**

Goal of lowest systolic blood pressure: **(age in years × 2) + 70 mm Hg**

■ Pediatric estimated weight and BSA formulas

Estimated weight in kilograms: $2 \times$ age in years $+ 9 = $ kg

Estimated body surface area (BSA): $\dfrac{4 \times kg + 7}{90 + kg}$

■ Pediatric normal weights per age

Months	General kg Weight	Girl kg Weight	Boy kg Weight
Birth	3.0	3	3.9
1 month	3.3-5		
2 months	4-6		
3 months	4.5-7		
4 months	5.5-8		
5 months	6-9		
6 months	6.5-9.5		
7 months	7-10		
8 months	7.5-10.5		
9-11 months	8-11.5		
12 months	9-12.5	10	10
2 years		12	13
3 years		15	15
4 years		16	17
5 years		19	19
6 years		21	21
7 years		24	23
8 years		26	25
9 years		29	28
10 years		32	31
11 years		36	35
12 years		40	40
13 years		45	45
14 years		49	51
15 years		52	57
16 years		53	62
17 years		54	63
18 years		59	69

■ Normal Hgb/Hct at specific ages

Age	Hgb (Gm/dL)	Hct (%)
1-3 d	14-20	45-61
4-9 d	13-19	42-60
10-14 d	12-18	39-57
15-30 d	10-16	31-49
1-6 mo	9.5-12.9	29-42
7-24 mo	10.5-12.5	33-38
25-60 mo	11.5-13.0	34-39
6-8 y	11.5-14.5	35-42
9-18 y	12-15	36-42

Normal Hct: (usually 3 times the hemoglobin value)
Lowest acceptable Hct for neonates: 38–40%
Lowest acceptable Hct for 12-year-old: 28%

3

Pediatric NPO Guidelines, Fluids, Colloids, and Blood Products

■ NPO guidelines prior to surgery

Solids 6–8 hours
Formula 6 hours
Breast milk 4 hours
Clears 2 hours

■ IV fluids

Maintenance

0–10 kg: 4 mL/kg/hr
10–20 kg: 2 mL/kg/hr
>20 kg: 1 mL/kg/hr
IVF < 1 y: D_5.2NS via syringe pump or buratrol drip
chamber IV tubing
IVF > 1 y: lactated Ringer's 500 mL bag with microdrip
tubing

Deficit Replacement

Maintenance rate × hours NPO = deficit fluid need

IVF for deficit replacement: lactated Ringer's (replacement
for third-space and insensible losses).

Note: Pediatric patients have 3 times greater surface area to weight ratio = greater insensible fluid loss.

Formula to Find IV mL/hr

$$\frac{\text{Dose} \times 60 \text{ (min)} \times \text{kg}}{\text{mcg/mL}} = \text{mL/hr}$$

Formula to Find Dose Being Given at Certain mL Rate

$$\frac{\text{(mcg/mL)} \times \text{mL running}}{\text{kg} \times 60 \text{ (min)}} = \text{mcg/kg/min}$$

■ Colloid/Blood products

Estimates of circulating blood volume in children (EBV):

Premature newborn EBV: 90–100 mL/kg

Full-term newborn EBV: 80–90 mL/kg

3 mo–3 y EBV: 75–80 mL/kg

3–6 y EBV: 70–75 mL/kg

>6 y EBV: 65–70 mL/kg

Systemic Responses to Blood Loss

Organ System	<25% Blood Loss	25-40% Blood Loss	>45% Blood Loss
Cardiac	Weak, thready pulse	Increased heart rate	Hypotension, tachycardia
			Bradycardia indicates severe blood loss and impending circulatory collapse
CNS	Lethargic, irritable, confused	Change in level of consciousness, dulled response to pain	Comatose
Skin	Cool, clammy	Cyanotic, decreased capillary refill, cold extremities	Pale, cold
Kidneys	Decreased urinary output, increased specific gravity	Minimal urinary output	Minimal urinary output

Allowable Blood Loss

Allowable blood loss (ABL): $EBV \times (Hct_1 - Hct_2)/avg\ Hct$

The decision to transfuse blood products depends on preoperative hemoglobin levels, surgical loss, and the patient's cardiovascular response.

Blood Loss Replacement

Albumin	4.5–6.8 mL/kg of 5% albumin solution for shock states
PRBCs	10–15 mL/kg (increases hemoglobin by 2–3 g/dL)
Platelets	10 mL/kg (a dose of 5–10 mL/kg or 1 unit/10 kg increases platelet count by 50,000 mm^3)
Fresh frozen plasma	10–15 mL/kg (increases clotting factor levels by 15% and fibrinogen rises by 40 mg/dL)
Cryoprecipitate	0.17 unit cryo/1 kg (increases fibrinogen by 100 mg/dL)

4
Pediatric Circuits, Intubation Equipment, Mac, and Volatile Inhaled Anesthetics

■ Pediatric circuits

Circle and Bain Circuit Comparisons

Circuit	Advantages	Disadvantages
Circle	Inspired concentration of gases is constant; minimal pollution of volatile gases into environment; conserves moisture and heat; lower fresh gas flows reduce volatile agent used	Unidirectional valves; infants < 10 kg have increased work of breathing to overcome resistance to valves
Bain	The Bain circuit is a non-rebreathing circuit, but the fresh gas flow tubing is directed within the inspiratory limb, with fresh gas entering the circuit near the mask.	Anesthesia gas machine requires special equipment for Bain circuit.
	Mainly used to warm and humidify air-warming of inspired fresh gases by the exhaled gas present in the outer tubing, which adds warmth and humidity to inspired gases; it has the ability to scavenge exhaled gases. The Bain circuit allows for spontaneous or controlled ventilation with minimal resistance in circuit because there are no valves. Minimum fresh gas flow in spontaneous breathing: 100-150 mL/kg; minimum fresh gas flow in controlled ventilation is 70 mL/kg.	Any disconnection of inner fresh gas flows could cause hypercarbia.
		Inner tubing can kink; if the inner tube leaks or becomes detached from the fresh gas port, a significant increase in dead space can occur.
	Make sure $ETCO_2$ waveform returns to zero. If not, then baby is rebreathing CO_2 and needs higher total gas flows.	Requires higher gas flows to decrease hypercarbia.
	Bypasses CO_2 absorber, so there is no rebreathing.	
	Lightweight, reusable, easily sterilized.	

Intubation Equipment per Weight

kg	Approximate Age	ETT ID mm	LMA Classic	Cuff Volume	Largest ETT Fit Through LMA	DLEBT	Univent	Bronchial Blocker
1–2.5	Preemie	2.5–3.0						
2.5–3.5	Newborn	3.0–3.5						
3.5–5.0	4 mo	3.5	1					
5–8	9 mo	3.5–4.0	1	Up to 4 mL	3.5			
8–10	10–12 mo	4.0–4.5	1.5	Up to 7 mL	4.0			
10–20	2–5 y	4.5–5.0	2	Up to 10 mL	4.5			ETT 4.5–5.5 = 5F
20–30	5–9 y	5.0–6.0	2.5	Up to 14 mL	5.0	>8yo: 26 Fr	3.5 uncuffed	
30–50	10–15 y	6.0–7.0	3	Up to 20 mL	6.0	26–28	4.5 cuffed	ETT 6–7.0 = 7F
50–70	>15 y	7.0–7.5	4	Up to 30 mL	6.0	32	6 cuffed	
70–100	16–18 y	7.5	5	Up to 40 mL	7.0	35	7 cuffed	>7.5 ETT = 9F

Additional Information on Intubation

Uncuffed endotracheal tube (ETT) size: age + 16/4

(e.g., 2 year old: 2 + 16/4 = 18 ÷ 4 = 4.5)

Alternative formula for uncuffed tubes: age/4 + 4

(e.g., 2 year old: 2/4 + 4 = 0.5 + 4 = 4.5)

If using a cuffed ETT, choose 0.5 to 1 full mm size smaller than an appropriate-sized uncuffed tube; the cuff increases the outer diameter of the tube by 0.5 mm.

These formulas help to estimate ETT size based on age but are not foolproof. Another option is to look at the little finger of the child—this is an estimate to the size of ETT to use.

Carina should be at approximately T5.

Depth ETT to lip: ETT size $\times$ 3 = cm to tape and secure tube

Distance with nasal: ETT $\times$ 4

DLEBT: 4 $\times$ ETT in mm + 2

Air leak with endotracheal tube:

- Less than 10 cm H_2O suggests an inappropriately small ETT.
- Greater than 40 cm H_2O suggests an inappropriately large ETT.
- 10–25 cm H_2O is appropriate for cases without a need for high airway pressures.
- 25–35 cm H_2O is appropriate when higher peak inspiratory pressures are needed.
- Inflate ETT cuff cautiously to the "just seal" point and check the cuff during the case, but especially when nitrous oxide is used.

Cuffed versus uncuffed ETTs

Uncuffed tubes are often used to prevent trauma to the cricoid cartilage (the narrowest portion of the pediatric airway, just below the vocal cords) and allow a larger mm ETT, which results in a decrease in the work of breathing. Many practitioners, however, will place a cuffed ETT in infants > 3–4 months old for the following reasons:

- The work of breathing is not an issue when infants are mechanically ventilated.
- Placing a cuffed ETT decreases the number of intubation passes.
- A cuffed ETT uses lower fresh gas flows.
- There is less air leakage and operating room pollution from volatile anesthetics.

■ Blade and vent bag per weight

Age	Blade and Size	Ventilator Bag
Birth-6 mo	0 Miller	0.5 L
<1 y	0-1 Miller	
6 mo-2 y		
>1 y	1 Miller	
	1 Wis Hipple	1 L
	1.5 Wis Hipple	
2-3 y	1 Mac	
	1 Miller	
2-6 y		2 L
6 y and older		
5-7 y	1.5 Miller	
	2 Mac	
8-10 y	1-2 Phillips	3 L
	2 Miller	
	MAC 3	
>10 y	2 Phillips	
	2 Miller	

■ Pediatric syndromes associated with difficult airway

Angioneurotic edema
Apert's syndrome
Beckwith-Widermann syndrome
Carpenter's syndrome
Cherubism
Collagen diseases
Congenital neck masses
Cri du chat syndrome
Croup
Cruzon's syndrome
Cystic syndrome
Down syndrome
Edwards syndrome
Epiglottis
Facial trauma/burns
Farber syndrome
Freeman-Sheldon syndrome
Gangrenous stomatitis

Goldenhar syndrome
Hemangioma
Klippel-Feil syndrome
Laryngeal trauma
Meckel's syndrome
Myocitis ossificans
Orofacial-digital syndrome
Peritonsillar abscess
Pierre Robin syndrome
Retropharyngeal abscess
Russell-silver syndrome
Rheumatoid diseases
Schwatz-Jampel syndrome
Scleroderma
Silver's syndrome
Smith-Lemli-Opitz syndrome
Treacher Collins syndrome
Turner's syndrome

■ MAC of volatile inhaled anesthetics

Agent	Neonate	Infant	Child
Isoflurane	1.3%	1.7%	1.6%
Sevoflurane: Low solubility; time to reach alveolar levels is 1/10 than with isoflurane. Best for inhaled induction.	3.3%	3.2%	2.5%
Desflurane: Do not use for induction due to laryngospasm risk.	5.0	7.0	6.6

- MAC is decreased in neonates up to 1 month old: There is an increased uptake and distribution of volatile anesthetics, with an increased potential for volatile overdose. MAC increases in the first 6 months of life and decreases thereafter. MAC is increased in adolescents.

■ Inhaled induction with volatile anesthetics

- In a quiet, cooperative child: 30% oxygen, 70% nitrous oxide; increase sevoflurane in small increments every 2–3 seconds. Once IV is started, turn N_2O off and run 100% FiO_2 and volatile agent. Once Stage 3 anesthesia is achieved and heart rate decreases, sevoflurane can be decreased.

- Rapid induction is necessary in an uncooperative child: 30% oxygen, 70% nitrous oxide with 8% sevoflurane. Hold face mask gently but tightly to child's face to avoid loss of seal and subsequent decrease in volatile. Once Stage 3 anesthesia is achieved and heart rate decreases, sevoflurane can be decreased.

■ General information: inhaled anesthetics

- The uptake of volatile anesthetic is affected by the solubility of the gas in blood.
- Higher incidence of bradycardia, hypotension, and cardiac arrest are noted during inhaled induction with infants.
- Desflurane and sevoflurane cause a higher incidence of emergence delirium in pediatrics as compared to isoflurane.

- Right-to-left shunt (e.g., tetralogy of Fallot, transposition of great vessels, etc.) slows uptake of volatile agents slightly. *Slow on and slow off.* Uptake is slower with more soluble gases. *R-L shunt shortens the onset time of IV induction agents.*
- Left-to-right shunt (ASD, VSD, PDA, BT shunt) leads to volume overload of the right heart and pulmonary circulation, which in turn causes uptake of volatile agents to be slightly faster. The increase depends on the size of the shunt. *L-R shunt slightly prolongs the onset time of IV induction agents.*

■ Pediatric uptake and distribution

Uptake of inhaled anesthetics is more rapid in infants and children than adults. This is related to the following factors:

- High alveolar ventilation (especially in relation to functional residual capacity [FRC]—the "alveolar/ventilation to FRC ratio" in infants is about 5:1, whereas that in adults is 1.4:1).

- Increased minute ventilation.
- Cardiac output—a high cardiac output removes the anesthetic agent so quickly from the alveoli that the partial pressure in the alveoli does not have time to increase, nor does the partial pressure in the blood.
- Body composition (small body mass).
- B:G solubility coefficients.
- Tissue solubility coefficients.

5
Pediatric Anesthesia Equipment and Drug Setup

- Change monitor to neonatal or pediatric settings
- Pediatric cart
- Portable pulse oximeter for saturation monitoring during transfer to recovery room, if appropriate
- **Suction**
- Yankauer and appropriate-sized soft catheter for mouth and ETT suction
- Circuit with appropriate-sized vent bag
- Masks
- Pediatric laryngoscope handles
- Laryngoscope blades × 2 (multiple types and sizes)
- Uncuffed and cuffed tubes: 1 size smaller and larger than calculated
- Stylets for ETT
- Oral airways
- Tongue depressor
- Warming blanket
- Temp probe/patch
- Pedi BP cuffs—different sizes
- Three-lead EKG

5 Pediatric Anesthesia Equipment and Drug Setup   33

- IV start pack
- Buratrol-type of drip chamber that holds limited quantities of IV fluids
- IV extension sets

■ Nasal intubations

- Tracheal accordion tubes
- Magill forceps
- Hot sterile water bottle (to soak NTT)
- Oxymetazoline nasal spray (*Afrin*)
- Lubricant
- Soft rubber obturators

■ Emergency drugs

For every pediatric case, emergency drugs should be drawn up and precalculated *before taking a child to the OR*. Some providers write the calculations for atropine and succinylcholine at the very top of the anesthesia record in case of emergency. **Figure 5-1** shows succinylcholine and atropine emergency dosages calculated and written out.

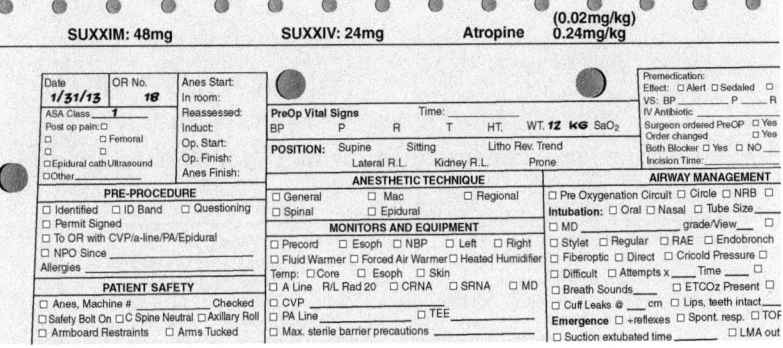

FIGURE 5-1

Emergency Drugs Set Up for Pediatrics

3 mL syringe succinylcholine for IV dose in case of laryngospasm

IV dose: Succinylcholine 2 mg/kg IV

5 mL syringe succinylcholine with IM needle for IM injection in case of laryngospasm

IM dose: Succinylcholine 4 mg/kg IM

5 Pediatric Anesthesia Equipment and Drug Setup   35

TB syringe *Robinul*

IV dose: *Robinul* 0.01 mg/kg

TB syringe atropine—with IM needle in case IV line is lost

IV dose: Atropine 0.02 mg/kg

Note: Atropine stock is usually supplied in 0.4 mg vials or 1 mg vials.

1 mg vial = 1,000 mcg: 0.1 mL = 0.1 mg
0.2 mg vial = 200 mcg: 0.1 mL = 20 mcg

Atropine vials supplied in 0.4 mg
Example: If child is 12 kg and atropine dose is 0.02 mg/kg
0.4 mg/vial : 1 mL :: 0.24 mg : x mL
x = 0.6 mL

Atropine vials supplied in 1 mg
Example: If child is 12 kg and atropine dose is 0.02 mg/kg
1 mg/vial : 1 mL :: 0.24 mg : x mL
x = 0.24 mL

---

10 mL syringe for IV dose epinephrine: 10 mcg/mL

Epinephrine for pulseless arrest or bradycardia:

IV dose: 0.01 mg/kg IV/IO

Can repeat every 3–5 min

Maximum 1 mg

ETT dose of epinephrine is 2–3 times the IV/IO dose.

How to mix: Take two 10 mL vials of normal saline and label one vial with an epinephrine sticker. Take 1 mL out of the stickered vial; add 1 mL of 1:1,000 epinephrine to stickered vial. Now you have a mixture of epinephrine 100 mcg/mL. Take a 10 mL syringe, draw up 1 mL of the 100 mcg/mL mixture, and then add 9 mL of normal saline. Now you have epinephrine 10 mcg/mL. (Put the 100 mcg/mL away so it isn't accidentally mistaken for the 10 mcg/mL.)

■ Pediatric induction-maintenance drugs setup for pediatrics

- TB syringe **fentanyl** 50 mcg (total 1 mL)
- 5 mL or 10 mL syringe of **propofol**
- 3 mL syringe **succinylcholine** for IV (see the discussion of emergency drugs)
- 10 mL syringe of **0.9% normal saline** (for flush)
- 2 mL **rocuronium** (or other nondepolarizing muscle relaxant, if needed)

6

Pediatric Pharmacology: Perioperative and Emergency Drugs

■ Synopsis

- Postnatal age is important in determining maturity of drug metabolism.
- The neonate has a qualitative and quantitative reduction in protein binding. This causes an apparently larger volume of distribution (compared to adults) and leads to higher drug requirements.
- Premature infants and neonates have limited baroreceptor reflexes; anesthetics exacerbate these limits.
- Infants < 44 weeks post-conceptual age have extremely high incidence of apnea and bradycardia after GETA or heavy sedation; they need to spend the night through the whole sleep cycle. Children < 60 weeks old should stay at least 8 hours.
- Infants have a period of anemia at 3–6 months with the destruction of fetal hemoglobin and the concurrent but slow production of RBCs.
- Opioids should be used carefully in children < 1 year old because they are more sensitive to respiratory depression.
- The blood–brain barrier is immature in children, so lipid-soluble drugs diffuse easily.

- The hepatic enzyme systems are incompletely developed or absent at birth. Phase I and II processes develop within a few days of birth, and conjugation reactions develop by 3 months. Immature hepatic processes affect the metabolism of drugs before the child is 3 months old, such that the duration of action of a drug is usually longer.

- Renal clearance of most drugs reaches adult values by 3 months of age. Before the child is 3 months old, however, the elimination of drugs is affected by its immature renal function and the duration of action of a drug is usually longer.

- Maturation of the neuromuscular junction is not complete until the child is about 2 months of age. However, the initial dose of the nondepolarizing muscle relaxant is not different from that of an adult because of the relatively large volume of distribution. The neonate and infant require more succinylcholine on a body weight basis than do older children because of the increased volume of distribution.

- The first sign of LA toxicity in infants and children may be dysrhythmias or CV collapse.

■ Top considerations of anesthetic selection in pediatrics

1. Protect cardiac output and hemodynamic control.
2. Balance postoperative pain control with adequate respiratory function.

PALS Guidelines

- Lipid-soluble drugs can be given via ETT: lidocaine, epinephrine, atropine, and naloxone.
- Vasopressin can be given via ETT but human studies regarding dosing are limited.
- The recommended ETT dose of epinephrine is 10 times the IV/IO dose; for other ETT-approved drugs the dose is 2–3 times the IV/IO dose.

■ **Drug dosages and ranges listed alphabetically**

ANTISIALAGOGUE PREMEDICATION

atropine	<5 kg: **0.02** mg/kg IV/IM/SQ 30-60 min preop >5 kg: 0.01-**0.02** mg/kg IV/IM/SQ 30-60 min preop Minimum dose: 0.1 mg; max single dose: 0.5 mg
glycopyrrolate *Robinul*	0.004 mg/kg IM 30-60 min preop up to 0.009 mg/kg
scopolamine	4-7 mo: 100 mcg IM × 1; give 45-60 min preop 7 mo-3 y: 150 mcg IM × 1; give 45-60 min preop 3-8 y: 200 mcg IM × 1; give 45-60 min preop 8-12 y: 300 mcg IM × 1; give 45-60 min preop

SEDATION PREMEDICATION

chloral hydrate	50-75 mg/kg PO or PR max 1 Gm in divided doses
clonidine *Catapres*	Preop: 2.5 mcg/kg PO

dexmedetomidine *Precedex*

Loading dose: 0.5-1 mcg/kg over 10 minutes

Pt weight in kg _____ (#1) × 1 mcg/kg = _____ (#2)
_____ mcg (#2) ÷ 4 mcg/mL = _____ (#3)
_____ mL (#3) × 3 _____ mL/hour (#4)
Set IV pump rate at #4 with volume limit at #3

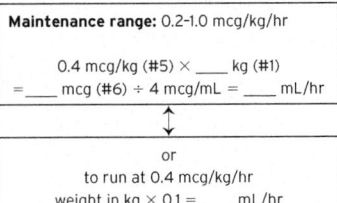

Maintenance range: 0.2-1.0 mcg/kg/hr

0.4 mcg/kg (#5) × _____ kg (#1)
= _____ mcg (#6) ÷ 4 mcg/mL = _____ mL/hr

↕

or
to run at 0.4 mcg/kg/hr
weight in kg × 0.1 = _____ mL/hr

Mix 400 mcg in 96 mL normal saline = 4 mcg/mL
Caution: Do not use *Precedex* in a patient with second- or third-degree heart block.

meperidine *Demerol* *Safety in pediatric patients has not been established*	Preop: 1.0-2.2 mg/kg SQ/IM × 1 Start: 30-90 min before anesthesia; max: 100 mg/dose
midazolam *Versed*	0.05-0.1 mg/kg IV/IO slowly; max: 0.6 mg/kg 0.25-0.5 mg/kg PO; max: 20 mg total 0.1-0.15 mg/kg IM; max: 0.5 mg/kg 0.2 mg/kg IN; max: 10 mg total

INDUCTION

atropine vagolytic	0.02 mg/kg IM/IV/IO 0.04-0.06 mg/kg ETT Minimal dose 0.1 mg; max single dose 0.5 mg
etomidate *Amidate*	>10 y: 0.3-0.6 mg/kg over 30-60 sec Usual dose 0.3 mg/kg
glycopyrrolate *Robinul* vagolytic	0.004 mg/kg IV; max: 0.009 mg

ketamine *Ketalar*	1-2 mg/kg IV slowly; usual dose 2 mg/kg
Consider concurrent midazolam	4-5 mg/kg IM stun dose × 1; usual dose 5 mg/kg
	6-10 mg/kg PO × 1 (mix with beverage)
	4-8 mg/kg PR; usual dose 5 mg/kg
methohexital *Brevital*	6.6-10 mg/kg slow IM (5% sol)
IV route not recommended in children	25 mg/kg PR (1% sol)
propofol *Diprivan*	Induction: 2-3 mg/kg IV slowly; usual dose 3 mg/kg
	Infusion: 50-300 mcg/kg/min IV

OPIOIDS IV

Comparative Potencies

Meperidine	0.1
Morphine	1
Methadone	1
Alfentanil	40
Fentanyl	150
Sufentanil	1,500

alfentanil *Alfenta*	Pain: 5-10 mcg/kg slow IV
	Induction: 10-50 mcg/kg slow IV
clonidine *Catapres*	Analgesia: 0.3 mcg/kg/**hr** IV/infusion
fentanyl *Sublimaze*	0.5-3.0 mcg/kg IV slowly; avg 1 mcg/kg
	2 mcg/kg IN
	0.5-2 mcg/kg/**hr** infusion
	High dose: 4-10 mcg/kg IV slowly; avg 5 mcg/kg
	Cardiac: 10-50 mcg/kg IV slowly
hydromorphone *Dilaudid*	<6 mo: 0.005 mg/kg slow IV/SQ
	>6 mo <50 kg: 0.015-0.02 mg/kg slow IV/SQ
	Start 0.015 mg/kg
	0.03-0.08 mg/kg PO
	>50 kg: 1-2 mg IV/SQ; start 1 mg

meperidine *Demerol*
   *Safety in pediatric patients has not
   been established*
	1.0–1.75 mg/kg PO/SQ/IM; start 1 mg/kg
	Max: adult dose 100 mg/dose

methadone *Dolophine*	0.1 mg/kg IV/dose slowly q 4 hr × 2–3 doses; max: 10 mg/dose
morphine	<6 mo: 0.05–0.2 mg/kg slow IV/IM/SQ Start 0.05 mg/kg; max: 15 mg >6 mo: 0.1–0.2 mg/kg IV/IM/SQ Usual 0.1 mg/kg; max: 15 mg

remifentanil *Ultiva*
For 50 mcg/mL → mix
   1 mg in 20 mL
   5 mg in 100 mL
For 25 mcg/mL → mix
   1 mg in 40 mL
   5 mg in 200 mL
Mix in 0.9% NS, sterile water, D_5W
	Induction: 0.5–1.0 mcg/kg IV over 30–60 sec
	Avg 0.5 mcg/kg
	Maintenance with volatile anesthetic: 0.05–1.3 mcg/kg/min
	infusion; avg 0.25 mcg/kg/min
	Maintenance with 70% nitrous oxide: 0.4–1.0 mcg/kg/min
	infusion; avg 0.7 mcg/kg/min

sufentanil *Sufenta*	0.5–2 mcg/kg IV; start 0.5 mcg/kg Intranasal: 0.5–0.7 mcg/kg Total dose: 10–20 mcg/kg

OPIOIDS PO

acetaminophen with codeine *Percocet*
   *Many mixtures for elixir, suspension,
   tablets, or capsules*
	<12 y: 0.5–1 mg/kg PO

codeine	0.5–1 mg/kg PO; max: 60 mg/dose q 6 hr
oxycodone	0.05–0.15 mg/kg PO

NONOPIOID ANALGESICS

acetaminophen *Tylenol*	<12 y: 15 mg/kg PO 10-20 mg/kg PR; usual dose 20 mg/kg >12 y: 325-650 mg PO
acetaminophen IV *Ofirmev* Only for children >2 y old	2-12 y: 15 mg/kg slow IV; max: 750 mg Administer over 15 min in syringe pump
ibuprofen	10 mg/kg PO

toradol *Ketorolac*
  Only for children >2 y old
  (may decrease prostaglandins)
	<50 kg: 0.5 mg/kg slow IV
	Max IV dose: 15 mg
	1 mg/kg IM; max IM dose: 30 mg

MUSCLE RELAXANTS (INTUBATING DOSES)

atracurium *Tracrium*	*>1 mo −2 y*: 0.3-0.4 mg/kg slow IV with volatile *>2 y:* Initial: 0.5 mg/kg IV over 60 sec Repeat: 0.08-0.1 mg/kg q 20-45 min If follows succinylcholine: 0.2-0.4 mg/kg slow IV
cisatracurium *Nimbex*	0.1-0.2 mg/kg slowly; usual 0.1 mg/kg
pancuronium *Pavulon*	<1 mo: 0.02 mg/kg slow IV >1 mo: 0.1 mg/kg slow IV
rocuronium *Zemuron* *Range: 0.6-1.2 mg/kg*	0.6 mg/kg IV slowly RSI: 1.2 mg/kg IV
succinylcholine *Anectine* Consider giving atropine first	2 mg/kg IV slowly 4 mg/kg IM; max: 5 mL (20 mg/mL) at injection site Laryngospasm: 0.5 mg/kg IV
vecuronium *Norcuron*	0.1 mg/kg IV slowly

REVERSAL AGENTS

atropine	0.01-0.02 mg/kg slow IV (10-20 mcg/kg IV) Usual 0.02 mg/kg For each 0.007 mg/kg neostigmine Minimum dose: 0.1 mg; max single dose: 0.5 mg
edrophonium *Tensilon*	Neonates: 0.1 mg single dose Infants/children: 0.04 mg/kg/dose IV slowly × 1 No response after 1 min: 0.16 mg/kg/dose Total max dose: 5 mg for <34 kg; 10 mg for >34 kg Preceded by (usually) atropine or glycopyrrolate
flumazenil *Romazicon* *Caution: Variable elimination half-life in pediatrics; observe child 2 hr after reversal agent is given*	0.01 mg/kg/dose IV over 15 sec; max: 0.2 mg/dose × 1-5 doses Then 0.05-1 mg/kg up to 1 mg total dose
glycopyrrolate *Robinul*	0.007 mg/kg IV per 0.07 mg of neostigmine; max: 1 mg
naloxone *Narcan* *Caution: Naloxone has a relatively short duration of action compared to many opioids, and continued monitoring of the patient with repeat dosing of naloxone (q 20-60 min) may be necessary.*	<5 y or <20 kg: 0.1 mg/kg slow IV/IO/IM/SQ >5 y or >20 kg: 2 mg/dose slow IV/IO/IM/SQ q 2-3 min; max total dose: 2 mg Via ETT: optimal endotracheal dose unknown; current expert recommendations are 2 × IV dose
neostigmine *Prostigmin, Bloxiverz*	0.03-0.07 mg/kg IV slowly; usual: 0.07 mg/kg; max: 5 mg/dose Preceded by atropine or (usually) glycopyrrolate
pyridostigmine	0.1-0.25 mg/kg/dose slow IV; preceded by atropine or glycopyrrolate

ANTIBIOTICS

ampicillin	50 mg/kg IV slowly; potential toxic dose <6 y old: 300 mg/kg Max dose >6 y old: 2,000 mg
ampicillin and sulbactam *Unasyn*	1 mo-1 y: 50-75 mg/kg ampicillin slow IV Usual start dose 50 mg/kg >1 y: 50-100 mg/kg ampicillin slow IV Usual start dose 50 mg/kg Max: 3.1 Gm
cefazolin *Ancef*	25 mg/kg IV slowly; max: 1 Gm
ceftriaxone *Rocephin*	25 mg/kg IV slowly; max: 2,000 mg
cefuroxime *Zinacef, Ceftin*	50 mg/kg IV slowly max: 1,500 mg
clindamycin *Cleocin*	10 mg/kg IV slowly; max single dose: 900 mg
ertapenem *Invanz*	3 mo-12 y: 15 mg/kg IV slowly; max: 1,000 mg >12 y: 1 Gm slow IV or IM
gentamicin	2 mg/kg IV slowly; no max dose
levofloxacin *Levaquin*	10 mg/kg IV slowly; max: 750 mg
metronidazole *Flagyl*	10 mg/kg IV over 60 min; max: 500 mg
piperacillin and tazobactam *Zosyn*	<40 kg and 2-9 mo: 80 mg (piperacillin component)/kg IV over 30 min q 6 hr; max: 3.375 Gm <40 kg and >9 mo: 100 mg (piperacillin component)/kg IV over 30 min q 8 hr; max: 3.375 Gm 40 kg: 3.375 Gm IV over 30 min q 6 hr
vancomycin	15 mg/kg IV slowly; max: 1,000 mg

NAUSEA PROPHYLAXIS

dexamethasone *Decadron*	0.25 mg/kg IV slowly; max: 10 mg
diphenhydramine *Benadryl*	1.25 mg/kg IV/IM q 6 hr; max: 300 mg/day
dolasetron *Anzemet*	Contraindicated in children <18 y (due to cardiac conduction defects)
droperidol	0.01-0.015 mg/kg IV slowly; max: 1.25 mg
granisetron *Kytril >2 y old*	2-16 y: 10 mcg/kg IV slowly
metoclopramide *Reglan* *Caution: extrapyramidal signs*	0.1-0.2 mg/kg/dose IV slowly; usual 0.2 mg/kg/dose
ondansetron *Zofran*	0.15 mg/kg IV slowly; max: 4 mg/dose
palonosetron *Aloxi*	1 mo-17 y: 20 mcg/kg IV over 15 min; max: 1.5 mg
promethazine *Phenergan* *Caution: extrapyramidal signs*	>2 y: 0.5 mg/kg/dose slow IV/IM/PO; max: 25 mg/dose
scopolamine	6 mcg/kg/dose slow IV/IM/SQ; max: 0.3 mg/dose

ANTIHISTAMINES

diphenhydramine *Benadryl*	0.5 mg/kg/dose slow IV/PO q 6 hr
famotidine *Pepcid*	1 mg/kg/day IV slowly, divided BID 1 mg/kg/day PO, divided BID Max: 40 mg BID
ranitidine *Zantac*	>1 mo: 1 mg/kg/dose IV slowly q 8 hr Max: 50 mg/day

ANTICONVULSANTS

diazepam	*Valium*	1 mo-5 y: 0.1-0.3 mg/kg IV slowly q 5-10 min over 3-5 min; max: 5 mg
		5-12 y: 0.1-0.3 mg/kg IV slowly q 5-10 min; max: 10 mg
		>12 y: 5-10 mg IV slowly q 10-15 min; max: 30 mg
keppra		50 mg/kg IV over 15 min
lorazepam	*Ativan*	0.05-0.1 mg/kg IV slowly × 1
		May repeat 0.05 mg/kg IV × 1 after 10-15 min
midazolam	*Versed*	0.15 mg/kg IV slowly × 1, then 0.06-1.1 mg/kg/hr IV infusion
phenytoin	*Dilantin*	Load: 15-20 mg/kg IV slowly over 30 min; max: 1.5 Gm
		Maintenance: 3 mg/kg IV q 12 hr

DIURETICS

furosemide	*Lasix* (edema)	1 mg/kg/dose slow IV/IM; max: 20 mg
mannitol (cerebral edema)		0.25-1 Gm/kg IV over 30 min

MISCELLANEOUS MEDICATIONS

albuterol *Ventolin/Proventil* (inhalation)		4-8 puffs q 20 min PRN with spacer
		<20 kg: 2.5 mg/dose q 20 min in NS via nebulizer
		>20 kg: 5 mg/dose q 20 min in NS via nebulizer
aminocaproic acid *Amicar* *Supplied as 5 Gm in 20 mL = 250 mg/mL; antifibrinolytic*		100-200 mg/kg IV × 1, then 100 mg/kg q 4-6 hr; max: 30 Gm/day
caffeine citrate *Cafcit* (apnea)		20 mg/kg IV over 30 min

desmopressin *DDAVP*	*Diabetes Insipidus:*
Supplied as 4 mcg/mL = 16 IU;	3 mo–12 y:
1 mcg of DDAVP is equivalent to	Intranasal: 5–30 mcg/day
4 IU (international units)	Slow IV/SQ: 0.1–1 mcg/day
	>12 y: 2–4 mcg/day divided q 12 hr slow IV/SQ
	Hemophilia (DDAVP increases FVIII levels):
	0.3 mcg/kg in 50 mL NS over 15–30 min
dexamethasone *Decadron* (edema/croup)	0.6 mg/kg IV slowly; max: 16 mg
epinephrine racemic nebulizer	<20 kg: 0.25 mL of 2.25% into 4 mL NS 20–40 kg: 0.5 mL of 2.25% into 4 mL NS >40 kg: 0.75 mL of 2.25% into 4 mL NS Administer over 10–15 min; may repeat q 1–2 hr
glucagon	Neonate: 0.02–0.2 mg/kg SQ/IM/IV; max: 1 mg <20 kg: 0.5 mg IM/SQ/IV (0.5 unit) >20 kg: 1 mg IM/SQ/IV (1 unit)
glucose dextrose	0.5–1 **Gm**/kg IV slowly
D_5NS = 5 Gm dextrose/100 mL	D_5NS: 10–20 mL/kg
$D_{10}W$ = 10 Gm dextrose/100 mL	$D_{10}W$: 5–10 mL/kg IV slowly
$D_{25}W$ = 25 Gm dextrose/100 mL	$D_{25}W$: 2–4 mL/kg IV slowly
$D_{50}W$ = 50 Gm dextrose/100 mL	$D_{50}W$: 1 mL/kg IV slowly
hydrocortisone *Solucortef* (stress dose; adrenal insufficiency)	2–3 mg/kg IV/IO slowly; max 100 mg

COMMON LOCAL ANESTHETICS (LA)

bupivacaine *Marcaine*	0.25–0.5%
lidocaine	0.5–2%
ropivacaine *Naropin*	0.2–0.5%

LOCAL ANESTHETIC (LA) MAXIMUMS

bupivacaine	*Marcaine*	3 mg/kg	3-5 mg/kg with epinephrine
chloroprocaine	*Nesacaine*	11 mg/kg	-
lidocaine		5 mg/kg	7 mg/kg with epinephrine
ropivacaine	*Naropin*	3 mg/kg	-
tetracaine	*Pontocaine*	2 mg/kg	-

epinephrine with local anesthetics	10 mcg/kg with LA
1:100,000 = 10 mcg/mL (0.01 mg/mL)	
1:200,000 = 5 mcg/mL (0.005 mg/mL)	

Local Anesthetic Toxicity

Signs and symptoms:

CNS excitation: agitation, confusion, twitching, seizure

Then...

CNS depression: drowsiness, obtundation, coma, or apnea

Ventricular ectopy

Progressive hypotension and bradycardia

Treatment of LA toxicity:

Stop local anesthetic, control airway, give 100% FiO_2, and confirm adequate IV access

Avoid calcium-channel blockers, phenytoin, breytelium

Intralipid dosing:

Bolus intralipid 29%: 1.5 mL/kg over 1 min

Start intralipid infusion: 0.25 mL/kg/min

Repeat intralipid bolus q 3-5 min until circulation is restored (max: 3 mL/kg total dose)

Increase infusion rate to 0.5 mL/kg/min if BP remains low

Max total intralipid 20% dose: 8 mL/kg

Rate of LA Absorption (greatest to lowest): intercostal, intratracheal, caudal, epidural, brachial plexus, and subcutaneous

Example: Caudal LA Dose and Level of Analgesia (i.e., bupivacaine 0.25% with epi)

Volume	Level of Sensory Block	Surgical Example
0.5 mL/kg	Sacral roots	Circumcision, lower limbs (max: 25 mL)
1 mL/kg	Sacral up to lower thorax	Inguinal hernia repair, orchiopexy
1.25 mL/kg	Sacral up to mid thorax	Ureteral reimplantation

Toxic dose of bupivacaine in a child is 3.0 mg/kg; for a neonate it is 1.5 mg/kg
Epidural drugs and boluses in a child <2 y old: dosages should be cut in half for a neonate

EPIDURAL AGENTS

bupivacaine *Marcaine*	Bolus: 0.5-1.25 mg/kg Infusion: <6 mo: 0.25 mg/kg/**hr** >6 mo to older: 0.5 mg/kg/**hr**
clonidine *Catapres*	Bolus: 1 mcg/kg Infusion: 0.05-0.2 mcg/kg/**hr**
fentanyl *Sublimaze*	Infusion: 0.5-1 mcg/kg/**hr**
morphine *Duramorph* (preservative free)	Bolus: 0.03-0.05 mg/kg epidurally; Max: 0.1 mg/kg/dose up to 5 mg/24 hr

IO: interosseous; PR: per rectum; SQ: subcutaneous.

◼ Emergency drugs

ANTIHYPERTENSIVES IV PUSH

clonidine *Catapres*	Bolus: 1-5 mcg /kg IV slowly; avg 3 mcg/kg
esmolol *Brevibloc* *See also cardiac infusions*	Bolus: 500 mcg/kg IV over 2 min

hydralazine *Apresoline*	Bolus: 0.1-0.2 mg/kg/dose IV slowly Max: 2 mg/kg q 6 hr
labetalol *Normodyne, Trandate*	Bolus: 0.2-1.0 mg/kg IV slowly q 10 min Start 0.2 mg/kg max 20 mg/dose; 3 mg/kg/hr
nicardipine *Cardene* (off-label)	Bolus: 0.5-3 mcg/kg/min IV slowly

EMERGENCY MEDICATIONS: BOLUS

adenosine *Adenocard* First dose:	100 mcg/kg rapid IV push (0.1 mg/kg) and rapid flush; max: 6 mg
Repeat dose:	200 mcg/kg rapid IV push (0.2 mg/kg) and rapid flush; max: 12 mg
amiodarone *Cordarone SVT, VT, VF* *See also cardiac infusions*	5 mg/kg IV/IO over 20-60 min; max: 300 mg/dose Repeat to daily max of 15 mg/kg
atropine There is some debate regarding minimum dosing of atropine; it is listed here for your information.	0.02 mg/kg slow IV/IO/IM (10-20 mcg/kg) Minimum dose: 0.1 mg; max single dose: 0.5 mg May repeat q 5 min; max: 1.0 child, 2.0 mg adolescent 20-30 mcg/kg IM/PO 0.04-0.06 mg/kg ETT; 2-3 × IV/IO dose Optimal max ETT dose not established
calcium chloride 10% *3 times as potent as calcium gluconate*	20 mg/kg IV/IO slowly of 10% solution; may repeat × 1 Slowly: 100 mg/min
calcium gluconate 10% (100 mg/mL)	60-100 mg/kg/dose IV/IO slowly Can give q 10 min; max: 800 mg/dose; 3 Gm/episode
dantrolene *Dantrium*	2.5 mg/kg IV q 5 min; max: 30 mg/kg
ephedrine (hypotension and bradycardia: range 0.1-0.2 mg/kg)	0.15 mg/kg IV slowly

epinephrine *Adrenalin* 1:1,000 = 1 mg/mL 1:10,000 = 0.1 mg/mL *See also cardiac infusions*	*Pulseless arrest or bradycardia:* 0.01 mg/kg IV/IO (0.1 mL/kg of 1:10,000); same as 10 mcg/kg Can repeat q 3-5 min; max: 1 mg 0.1 mg/kg (0.1 mL/kg) 1:1,000 ETT q 3-5 min ETT dose of epinephrine is 10 × IV/IO dose Max dose ETT epinephrine: 2.5 mg/dose
lidocaine *Xylocaine* *See also cardiac infusions*	1 mg/kg IV/IO slowly; may repeat × 1 in 15 min 2-3 mg/kg ETT
magnesium sulfate	25-50 mg/kg IV/IO infuse over 15 min; max: 2 Gm
phenylephrine *Neosynephrine* *See also cardiac infusions*	5-20 mcg/kg/dose IV bolus q 10-15 min as needed; max: 5 mg
sodium bicarbonate NaHCO$_3$ (BW × BD × 0.3/2)	**1 mEq**/kg IV/IO very slowly; max: 50 mEq Not routinely given; guide by bicarbonate concentration
vasopressin *ADH* *Vasopressin is given after at least two doses of epinephrine have been given.*	*Cardiac arrest:* 0.4 units/kg IV/IO; max: 40 units *Vasopressin can be given via ETT but human studies regarding dosing are limited.*
verapamil *Isoptin SVT*	<1 y: 0.1-0.2 mg/kg/dose IV over 2 min 1-15 y: 0.1-0.3 mg/kg/dose max 5 mg

EMERGENCY MEDICATIONS: INFUSIONS

amiodarone *Cordarone*	Load: 5 mg/kg IV over 50-60 min Infusion: 5-15 mcg/kg/min IV
dobutamine *Dobutrex*	2-20 mcg/kg/min IV infusion; start at 0.5-1 mcg/kg/min
dopamine *Intropin*	2-20 mcg/kg/min IV infusion
epinephrine *Adrenalin*	Hypotensive shock: 0.1-1 mcg/kg/min IV/IO infusion

6   Pediatric Pharmacology: Perioperative and Emergency Drugs

esmolol *Brevibloc*	Infusion: 50-150 mcg/kg/min IV infusion; max: 300 mcg/kg/min
isoproterenol *Isuprel* (off-label)	0.05 mcg/kg/min IV, increase by 0.1 mcg/kg/min q 5-10 min; max: 2 mcg/kg/min
lidocaine *Xylocaine*	20-50 mcg/kg/min IV/IO infusion
milrinone *Primacor*	Load: 50-75 mcg/kg slow IV/IO over ≥ 15 min Infusion: 0.5-0.75 mcg/kg/min IV/IO infusion
nitroglycerin	0.5-2.0 mcg/kg/min IV/IO infusion; max: 6 mcg/kg/min
nitroprusside	0.5-10 mcg/kg/min IV infusion
norepinephrine *Levophed*	0.1-2.0 mcg/kg/min IV/IO infusion; max: 2 mcg/kg/min
phenylephrine *Neosynephrine*	0.1-0.5 mcg/kg/min IV infusion
procainamide *Pronestyl*	Load: 15 mg/kg IV/IO over 30-60 min; max: 500 mg in 30 min Infusion: 20-80 mcg/kg min infusion; max: 2 Gm/day
prostaglandin E₁ *PGE-1*	0.05-0.1 mcg/kg/min infusion
vasopressin *ADH*	Hypotensive shock: 0.0003-0.002 units/kg/min infusion Same as 0.3-2 milliunits/kg/min infusion

IM: intramuscular; IN: intranasal; IO: interosseous; IV: intravenous; PR: per rectum; RSI: rapid sequence induction; SQ: subcutaneous.

CARDIOVERSION/DEFIBRILLATION

cardioversion	0.5 J/kg; repeat 1-2 J/kg
defibrillation	2 J/kg; repeat 4 J/kg

450 GMS (0.45 KG) MAINTENANCE IV FLUIDS: 1.8 ML/HR

drug	route	dose	mg to pt	supplied	mL to give
VAGOLYTIC/ANTISIALAGOGUE					
ATROPINE	IV	0.02 mg/kg	0.009 mg	0.4 mg/mL	0.0225 mL
GLYCOPYRROLATE	IV	0.004 mg/kg	0.0018 mg	0.2 mg/mL	0.009 mL
PROPOFOL	IV	3 mg/kg	1.35 mg	10 mg/mL	0.135 mL
KETAMINE	IV	2 mg/kg	0.9 mg	10 mg/mL	0.09 mL
KETAMINE	IM/PR	5 mg/kg	2.25 mg	10 mg/mL	0.225 mL
FENTANYL	IV	1 mcg/kg	0.45 mcg	50 mcg/mL	0.009 mL
FENTANYL	IN	2 mcg/kg	0.9 mcg	50 mcg/mL	0.018 mL
FENTANYL	IV	high dose	4 mcg/kg	1.8 mcg	50 mcg/mL	0.036 mL
FENTANYL	IV	cardiac	10 mcg/kg	4.5 mcg	50 mcg/mL	0.09 mL
ACETAMINOPHEN	PR	20 mg/kg	9 mg		
SUCCINYLCHOLINE	IV	2 mg/kg	0.9 mg	20 mg/mL	0.045 mL
SUCCINYLCHOLINE	IM	4 mg/kg	1.8 mg	20 mg/mL	0.09 mL
CISATRACURIUM	IV	0.1 mg/kg	0.045 mg	2 mg/mL	0.0225 mL
PANCURONIUM	IV	> 1 mo	0.02 mg/kg	0.009 mg	1 mg/mL	0.009 mL
PANCURONIUM	IV	< 1 mo	0.1 mg/kg	0.045 mg	1 mg/mL	0.045 mL
ROCURONIUM	IV	0.6 mg/kg	0.27 mg	10 mg/mL	0.027 mL
VECURONIUM	IV	0.1 mg/kg	0.045 mg	1 mg/mL	0.045 mL
AMPICILLIN	IV	50 mg/kg	22.5 mg		
CEFAZOLIN	IV	25 mg/kg	11.25 mg		
CLINDAMYCIN	IV	10 mg/kg	4.5 mg		
GENTAMICIN	IV	2 mg/kg	0.9 mg		
METRONIDAZOLE	IV	10 mg/kg	4.5 mg		
VANCOMYCIN	IV	15 mg/kg	6.75 mg		
ATROPINE	IV	0.02 mg/kg	0.009 mg	0.4 mg/mL	0.0225 mL
GLYCOPYRROLATE	IV	0.007 mg/kg	0.00315 mg	0.2 mg/mL	0.01575 mL
NEOSTIGMINE	IV	0.07 mg/kg	0.0315 mg	1 mg/mL	0.0315 mL
EDROPHONIUM	IV	< 2 mo	0.1 mg		single dose	
PRIMARY ANESTHESIA FOR NEONATES: HIGH DOSE FENTANYL AND PANCURONIUM					

450 GMS (0.45 KG)

Ventilation: trained rescuer	1 breath q 6-8 sec (8-10 breaths/minute) about 1 second/ breath-visible chest rise; if intubated, continuous compressions without pause for ventilations
Pulse check	brachial/femoral
Compression	2-3 fingers–1 finger width below nipples *Wrap hands around chest if possible, compress with thumbs*
Depth	1.5 inch (4 cm) or at least 1/3 chest depth
Rate	at least 100 compressions per minute
Compress/vent ratio	30:2 with 1 or 2 rescuers
Foreign body obstruction	5 back blows at level of scapula, support head; alternate with 5 chest compressions
	Never perform a blind finger-sweep. Open the mouth and look for object; if you see it, remove it.

sync cardioversion		0.5 J/kg	0.225 J
	repeat	1 J/kg	0.45 J
defibrillation		2 J/kg	0.9 J
	repeat	4 J/kg	1.8 J

IV Bolus Drugs		dose	mg to pt	supplied	mL to give
ADENOSINE	IV	0.1 mg/kg	0.045 mg	3 mg/mL	0.02 mL
ADENOSINE repeat dose	IV	0.2 mg/kg	0.09 mg	3 mg/mL	0.03 mL
AMIODARONE	IV/IO	5 mg/kg	2.25 mg	50 mg/mL	0.05 mL
ATROPINE	IV/IM	0.02 mg/kg	0.009 mg	0.4 mg/mL	0.02 mL
ATROPINE	ETT	0.04 mg/kg	0.018 mg	0.4 mg/mL	0.05 mL
CALCIUM CHLORIDE	IV	20 mg/kg	9 mg	100 mg/mL	0.09 mL
CALCIUM GLUCONATE	IV/IO	60 mg/kg	27 mg	100 mg/mL	0.27 mL
DANTROLENE	IV	2.5 mg/kg	1.125 mg		
EPHEDRINE	IV	0.15 mg/kg	0.0675 mg	10 mg/mL	0.01 mL
EPINEPHRINE (1:10,000)	IV/IO	0.01 mg/kg	0.0045 mg	0.1 mg/mL	0.05 mL
EPINEPHRINE (1:1,000)	ETT	0.1 mg/kg	0.045 mg	1 mg/mL	0.05 mL
ESMOLOL	IV	0.5 mg/kg	0.225 mg	10 mg/mL	0.02 mL
LABETALOL	IV	0.2 mg/kg	0.09 mg	5 mg/mL	0.02 mL
LIDOCAINE	IV/IO	1 mg/kg	0.45 mg	20 mg/mL	0.02 mL
NEOSYNEPHRINE	IV	5 mcg/kg	2.25 mcg	100 mcg/mL	0.02 mL
ROMAZICON	IV	0.01 mg/kg	0.0045 mg	0.1 mg/mL	0.05 mL
VASOPRESSIN	IV/IO	0.4 unit/kg	0.18 units	20 u/mL	0.01 mL

500 GMS (0.5 KG) MAINTENANCE IV FLUIDS: 2 ML/HR

drug	route	dose	mg to pt	supplied	mL to give
VAGOLYTIC/ANTISIALAGOGUE					
ATROPINE	IV	0.02 mg/kg	0.01 mg	0.4 mg/mL	0.025 mL
GLYCOPYRROLATE	IV	0.004 mg/kg	0.002 mg	0.2 mg/mL	0.01 mL
PROPOFOL	IV	3 mg/kg	1.5 mg	10 mg/mL	0.15 mL
KETAMINE	IV	2 mg/kg	1 mg	10 mg/mL	0.1 mL
KETAMINE	IM/PR	5 mg/kg	2.5 mg	10 mg/mL	0.25 mL
FENTANYL	IV	1 mcg/kg	0.5 mcg	50 mcg/mL	0.01 mL
FENTANYL	IN	2 mcg/kg	1 mcg	50 mcg/mL	0.02 mL
FENTANYL	IV high dose	4 mcg/kg	2 mcg	50 mcg/mL	0.04 mL
FENTANYL	IV cardiac	10 mcg/kg	5 mcg	50 mcg/mL	0.1 mL
ACETAMINOPHEN	PR	20 mg/kg	10 mg		
SUCCINYLCHOLINE	IV	2 mg/kg	1 mg	20 mg/mL	0.05 mL
SUCCINYLCHOLINE	IM	4 mg/kg	2 mg	20 mg/mL	0.1 mL
CISATRACURIUM	IV	0.1 mg/kg	0.05 mg	2 mg/mL	0.025 mL
PANCURONIUM	IV < 1 mo	0.02 mg/kg	0.01 mg	1 mg/mL	0.01 mL
PANCURONIUM	IV > 1 mo	0.1 mg/kg	0.05 mg	1 mg/mL	0.05 mL
ROCURONIUM	IV	0.6 mg/kg	0.3 mg	10 mg/mL	0.03 mL
VECURONIUM	IV	0.1 mg/kg	0.05 mg	1 mg/mL	0.05 mL
AMPICILLIN	IV	50 mg/kg	25 mg		
CEFAZOLIN	IV	25 mg/kg	12.5 mg		
CLINDAMYCIN	IV	10 mg/kg	5 mg		
GENTAMICIN	IV	2 mg/kg	1 mg		
METRONIDAZOLE	IV	10 mg/kg	5 mg		
VANCOMYCIN	IV	15 mg/kg	7.5 mg		
ATROPINE	IV	0.02 mg/kg	0.01 mg	0.4 mg/mL	0.025 mL
GLYCOPYRROLATE	IV	0.007 mg/kg	0.005 mg	0.2 mg/mL	0.0175 mL
NEOSTIGMINE	IV	0.07 mg/kg	0.035 mg	1 mg/mL	0.035 mL
EDROPHONIUM	IV < 2 mo		0.1 mg	single dose	

PRIMARY ANESTHESIA FOR NEONATES: HIGH DOSE FENTANYL AND PANCURONIUM

500 GMS (0.5 KG)

Ventilation: trained rescuer	1 breath q 6-8 sec (8-10 breaths/minute) about 1 second/ breath-visible chest rise; if intubated, continuous compressions without pause for ventilations
Pulse check	brachial/femoral
Compression	2-3 fingers-1 finger width below nipples; *Wrap hands around chest if possible, compress with thumbs*
Depth	1.5 inch (4 cm) or at least 1/3 chest depth
Rate	at least 100 compressions per minute
Compress/vent ratio	30:2 with 1 or 2 rescuers
Foreign body obstruction	5 back blows at level of scapula, support head; alternate with 5 chest compressions *Never perform a blind finger-sweep. Open the mouth and look for object; if you see it, remove it.*

sync cardioversion	0.5 J/kg	0.25 J
repeat	1 J/kg	0.5 J
defibrillation	2 J/kg	1 J
repeat	4 J/kg	2 J

IV Bolus Drugs		dose	mg to pt	supplied	mL to give
ADENOSINE	IV	0.1 mg/kg	0.05 mg	3 mg/mL	0.02 mL
ADENOSINE repeat dose	IV	0.2 mg/kg	0.1 mg	3 mg/mL	0.03 mL
AMIODARONE	IV/IO	5 mg/kg	2.5 mg	50 mg/mL	0.05 mL
ATROPINE	IV/IM	0.02 mg/kg	0.01 mg	0.4 mg/mL	0.05 mL
ATROPINE	ETT	0.04 mg/kg	0.02 mg	0.4 mg/mL	0.05 mL
CALCIUM CHLORIDE	IV	20 mg/kg	10 mg	100 mg/mL	0.10 mL
CALCIUM GLUCONATE	IV/IO	60 mg/kg	30 mg	100 mg/mL	0.30 mL
DANTROLENE	IV	2.5 mg/kg	1.25 mg		
EPHEDRINE	IV	0.15 mg/kg	0.075 mg	10 mg/mL	0.01 mL
EPINEPHRINE (1:10,000)	IV/IO	0.01 mg/kg	0.005 mg	0.1 mg/mL	0.05 mL
EPINEPHRINE (1:1,000)	ETT	0.1 mg/kg	0.05 mg	1 mg/mL	0.05 mL
ESMOLOL	IV	0.5 mg/kg	0.25 mg	10 mg/mL	0.03 mL
LABETALOL	IV	0.2 mg/kg	0.1 mg	5 mg/mL	0.02 mL
LIDOCAINE	IV/IO	1 mg/kg	0.5 mg	20 mg/mL	0.03 mL
NEOSYNEPHRINE	IV	5 mcg/kg	2.5 mcg	100 mcg/mL	0.03 mL
ROMAZICON	IV	0.01 mg/kg	0.005 mg	0.1 mg/mL	0.05 mL
VASOPRESSIN	IV/IO	0.4 unit/kg	0.2 units	20 u/mL	0.01 mL

550 GMS (0.55 KG) MAINTENANCE IV FLUIDS: 2.2 ML/HR

drug		route	dose	mg to pt	supplied	mL to give
VAGOLYTIC/ANTISIALAGOGUE						
ATROPINE		IV	0.02 mg/kg	0.011 mg	0.4 mg/mL	0.0275 mL
GLYCOPYRROLATE		IV	0.004 mg/kg	0.0022 mg	0.2 mg/mL	0.011 mL
PROPOFOL		IV	3 mg/kg	1.65 mg	10 mg/mL	0.165 mL
KETAMINE		IV	2 mg/kg	1.1 mg	10 mg/mL	0.11 mL
KETAMINE		IM/PR	5 mg/kg	2.75 mg	10 mg/mL	0.275 mL
FENTANYL		IV	1 mcg/kg	0.55 mcg	50 mcg/mL	0.011 mL
FENTANYL		IN	2 mcg/kg	1.1 mcg	50 mcg/mL	0.022 mL
FENTANYL	high dose	IV	4 mcg/kg	2.2 mcg	50 mcg/mL	0.044 mL
FENTANYL	cardiac	IV	10 mcg/kg	5.5 mcg	50 mcg/mL	0.11 mL
ACETAMINOPHEN		PR	20 mg/kg	11 mg		
SUCCINYLCHOLINE		IV	2 mg/kg	1.1 mg	20 mg/mL	0.055 mL
SUCCINYLCHOLINE		IM	4 mg/kg	2.2 mg	20 mg/mL	0.11 mL
CISATRACURIUM		IV	0.1 mg/kg	0.055 mg	2 mg/mL	0.0275 mL
PANCURONIUM	<1 mo	IV	0.02 mg/kg	0.011 mg	1 mg/mL	0.011 mL
PANCURONIUM	>1 mo	IV	0.1 mg/kg	0.055 mg	1 mg/mL	0.055 mL
ROCURONIUM		IV	0.6 mg/kg	0.33 mg	10 mg/mL	0.033 mL
VECURONIUM		IV	0.1 mg/kg	0.055 mg	1 mg/mL	0.055 mL
AMPICILLIN		IV	50 mg/kg	27.5 mg		
CEFAZOLIN		IV	25 mg/kg	13.75 mg		
CLINDAMYCIN		IV	10 mg/kg	5.5 mg		
GENTAMICIN		IV	2 mg/kg	1.1 mg		
METRONIDAZOLE		IV	10 mg/kg	5.5 mg		
VANCOMYCIN		IV	15 mg/kg	8.25 mg		
ATROPINE		IV	0.02 mg/kg	0.011 mg	0.4 mg/mL	0.0275 mL
GLYCOPYRROLATE		IV	0.007 mg/kg	0.00385 mg	0.2 mg/mL	0.01925 mL
NEOSTIGMINE		IV	0.07 mg/kg	0.0385 mg	1 mg/mL	0.0385 mL
EDROPHONIUM	<2 mo	IV	0.1 mg	single dose		

PRIMARY ANESTHESIA FOR NEONATES: HIGH DOSE FENTANYL AND PANCURONIUM

6 Pediatric Pharmacology: Perioperative and Emergency Drugs 63

550 GMS (0.55 KG)

Ventilation: trained rescuer	1 breath q 6-8 sec (8-10 breaths/minute) about 1 second/ breath-visible chest rise; if intubated, continuous compressions without pause for ventilations
Pulse check	brachial/femoral
Compression	2-3 fingers–1 finger width below nipples / *Wrap hands around chest if possible, compress with thumbs*
Depth	1.5 inch (4 cm) or at least 1/3 chest depth
Rate	at least 100 compressions per minute
Compress/vent ratio	30:2 with 1 or 2 rescuers
Foreign body obstruction	5 back blows at level of scapula, support head; alternate with 5 chest compressions / Never perform a blind finger-sweep. Open the mouth and look for object; if you see it, remove it.

sync cardioversion	0.5 J/kg	0.275 J
defibrillation	1 J/kg	0.55 J
repeat	2 J/kg	1.1 J
repeat	4 J/kg	2.2 J

IV Bolus Drugs		dose	mg to pt	supplied	mL to give
ADENOSINE	IV	0.1 mg/kg	0.055 mg	3 mg/mL	0.02 mL
ADENOSINE repeat dose	IV	0.2 mg/kg	0.11 mg	3 mg/mL	0.04 mL
AMIODARONE	IV/IO	5 mg/kg	2.75 mg	50 mg/mL	0.06 mL
ATROPINE	IV/IM	0.02 mg/kg	0.011 mg	0.4 mg/mL	0.03 mL
ATROPINE	ETT	0.04 mg/kg	0.022 mg	0.4 mg/mL	0.06 mL
CALCIUM CHLORIDE	IV	20 mg/kg	11 mg	100 mg/mL	0.11 mL
CALCIUM GLUCONATE	IV/IO	60 mg/kg	33 mg	100 mg/mL	0.33 mL
DANTROLENE	IV	2.5 mg/kg	1.375 mg		
EPHEDRINE	IV	0.15 mg/kg	0.0825 mg	10 mg/mL	0.01 mL
EPINEPHRINE (1:10,000)	IV/IO	0.01 mg/kg	0.0055 mg	0.1 mg/mL	0.06 mL
EPINEPHRINE (1:1,000)	ETT	0.1 mg/kg	0.055 mg	1 mg/mL	0.06 mL
ESMOLOL	IV	0.5 mg/kg	0.275 mg	10 mg/mL	0.03 mL
LABETALOL	IV	0.2 mg/kg	0.11 mg	5 mg/mL	0.03 mL
LIDOCAINE	IV/IO	1 mg/kg	0.55 mg	20 mg/mL	0.03 mL
NEOSYNEPHRINE	IV	5 mcg/kg	2.75 mcg	100 mcg/mL	0.03 mL
ROMAZICON	IV	0.01 mg/kg	0.0055 mg	0.1 mg/mL	0.06 mL
VASOPRESSIN	IV/IO	0.4 unit/kg	0.22 units	20 u/mL	0.01 mL

600 GMS (0.6 KG) MAINTENANCE IV FLUIDS: 2.4 ML/HR

drug		route	dose	mg to pt	supplied	mL to give
VAGOLYTIC/ANTISIALAGOGUE						
ATROPINE		IV	0.02 mg/kg	0.012 mg	0.4 mg/mL	0.03 mL
GLYCOPYRROLATE		IV	0.004 mg/kg	0.0024 mg	0.2 mg/mL	0.012 mL
PROPOFOL		IV	3 mg/kg	1.8 mg	10 mg/mL	0.18 mL
KETAMINE		IV	2 mg/kg	1.2 mg	10 mg/mL	0.12 mL
KETAMINE		IM/PR	5 mg/kg	3 mg	10 mg/mL	0.3 mL
FENTANYL		IV	1 mcg/kg	0.6 mcg	50 mcg/mL	0.012 mL
FENTANYL		IN	2 mcg/kg	1.2 mcg	50 mcg/mL	0.024 mL
FENTANYL	high dose	IV	4 mcg/kg	2.4 mcg	50 mcg/mL	0.048 mL
FENTANYL	cardiac	IV	10 mcg/kg	6 mcg	50 mcg/mL	0.12 mL
ACETAMINOPHEN		PR	20 mg/kg	12 mg		
SUCCINYLCHOLINE		IV	2 mg/kg	1.2 mg	20 mg/mL	0.06 mL
SUCCINYLCHOLINE		IM	4 mg/kg	2.4 mg	20 mg/mL	0.12 mL
CISATRACURIUM		IV	0.1 mg/kg	0.06 mg	2 mg/mL	0.03 mL
PANCURONIUM	<1 mo	IV	0.02 mg/kg	0.012 mg	1 mg/mL	0.012 mL
PANCURONIUM	>1 mo	IV	0.1 mg/kg	0.06 mg	1 mg/mL	0.06 mL
ROCURONIUM		IV	0.6 mg/kg	0.36 mg	10 mg/mL	0.036 mL
VECURONIUM		IV	0.1 mg/kg	0.06 mg	1 mg/mL	0.06 mL
AMPICILLIN		IV	50 mg/kg	30 mg		
CEFAZOLIN		IV	25 mg/kg	15 mg		
CLINDAMYCIN		IV	10 mg/kg	6 mg		
GENTAMICIN		IV	2 mg/kg	1.2 mg		
METRONIDAZOLE		IV	10 mg/kg	6 mg		
VANCOMYCIN		IV	15 mg/kg	9 mg		
ATROPINE		IV	0.02 mg/kg	0.012 mg	0.4 mg/mL	0.03 mL
GLYCOPYRROLATE		IV	0.007 mg/kg	0.0042 mg	0.2 mg/mL	0.021 mL
NEOSTIGMINE		IV	0.07 mg/kg	0.042 mg	1 mg/mL	0.042 mL
EDROPHONIUM	<2 mo	IV	0.1 mg	single dose		

PRIMARY ANESTHESIA FOR NEONATES: HIGH DOSE FENTANYL AND PANCURONIUM

600 GMS (0.6 KG)

Ventilation: trained rescuer	1 breath q 6-8 sec (8-10 breaths/minute) about 1 second/ breath-visible chest rise; if intubated, continuous compressions without pause for ventilations
Pulse check	brachial/femoral
Compression	2-3 fingers–1 finger width below nipples *Wrap hands around chest if possible, compress with thumbs*
Depth	1.5 inch (4 cm) or at least 1/3 chest depth
Rate	at least 100 compressions per minute
Compress/vent ratio	30:2 with 1 or 2 rescuers
Foreign body obstruction	5 back blows at level of scapula, support head; alternate with 5 chest compressions *Never perform a blind finger-sweep. Open the mouth and look for object; if you see it, remove it.*

sync cardioversion	0.5 J/kg	0.3 J
defibrillation	1 J/kg	0.6 J
repeat	2 J/kg	1.2 J
repeat	4 J/kg	2.4 J

IV Bolus Drugs		dose	mg to pt	supplied	mL to give
ADENOSINE	IV	0.1 mg/kg	0.06 mg	3 mg/mL	0.02 mL
ADENOSINE repeat dose	IV	0.2 mg/kg	0.12 mg	3 mg/mL	0.04 mL
AMIODARONE	IV/IO	5 mg/kg	3 mg	50 mg/mL	0.06 mL
ATROPINE	IM	0.02 mg/kg	0.012 mg	0.4 mg/mL	0.03 mL
ATROPINE	ETT	0.04 mg/kg	0.024 mg	0.4 mg/mL	0.06 mL
CALCIUM CHLORIDE	IV	20 mg/kg	12 mg	100 mg/mL	0.12 mL
CALCIUM GLUCONATE	IV/IO	60 mg/kg	36 mg	100 mg/mL	0.36 mL
DANTROLENE	IV	2.5 mg/kg	1.5 mg		
EPHEDRINE	IV	0.15 mg/kg	0.09 mg	10 mg/mL	0.01 mL
EPINEPHRINE (1:10,000)	IV/IO	0.01 mg/kg	0.006 mg	0.1 mg/mL	0.06 mL
EPINEPHRINE (1:1,000)	ETT	0.1 mg/kg	0.06 mg	1 mg/mL	0.06 mL
ESMOLOL	IV	0.5 mg/kg	0.3 mg	10 mg/mL	0.03 mL
LABETALOL	IV	0.2 mg/kg	0.12 mg	5 mg/mL	0.02 mL
LIDOCAINE	IV/IO	1 mg/kg	0.6 mg	20 mcg/mL	0.03 mL
NEOSYNEPHRINE	IV	5 mcg/kg	3 mcg	100 mg/mL	0.03 mL
ROMAZICON	IV	0.01 mg/kg	0.006 mg	0.1 mg/mL	0.06 mL
VASOPRESSIN	IV/IO	0.4 unit/kg	0.24 units	20 u/mL	0.01 mL

650 GMS (0.65 KG) MAINTENANCE IV FLUIDS: 2.6 ML/HR

drug		route	dose	mg to pt	supplied	mL to give
VAGOLYTIC/ANTISIALAGOGUE						
ATROPINE		IV	0.02 mg/kg	0.013 mg	0.4 mg/mL	0.0325 mL
GLYCOPYRROLATE		IV	0.004 mg/kg	0.0026 mg	0.2 mg/mL	0.013 mL
PROPOFOL		IV	3 mg/kg	1.95 mg	10 mg/mL	0.195 mL
KETAMINE		IV	2 mg/kg	1.3 mg	10 mg/mL	0.13 mL
KETAMINE		IM/PR	5 mg/kg	3.25 mg	10 mg/mL	0.325 mL
FENTANYL		IV	1 mcg/kg	0.65 mcg	50 mcg/mL	0.013 mL
FENTANYL		IN	2 mcg/kg	1.3 mcg	50 mcg/mL	0.026 mL
FENTANYL	high dose	IV	4 mcg/kg	2.6 mcg	50 mcg/mL	0.052 mL
FENTANYL	cardiac	IV	10 mcg/kg	6.5 mcg	50 mcg/mL	0.13 mL
ACETAMINOPHEN		PR	20 mg/kg	13 mg		
SUCCINYLCHOLINE		IV	2 mg/kg	1.3 mg	20 mg/mL	0.065 mL
SUCCINYLCHOLINE		IM	4 mg/kg	2.6 mg	20 mg/mL	0.13 mL
CISATRACURIUM		IV	0.1 mg/kg	0.065 mg	2 mg/mL	0.0325 mL
PANCURONIUM	<1 mo	IV	0.02 mg/kg	0.013 mg	1 mg/mL	0.013 mL
PANCURONIUM	>1 mo	IV	0.1 mg/kg	0.065 mg	1 mg/mL	0.065 mL
ROCURONIUM		IV	0.6 mg/kg	0.39 mg	10 mg/mL	0.039 mL
VECURONIUM		IV	0.1 mg/kg	0.065 mg	1 mg/mL	0.065 mL
AMPICILLIN		IV	50 mg/kg	32.5 mg		
CEFAZOLIN		IV	25 mg/kg	16.25 mg		
CLINDAMYCIN		IV	10 mg/kg	6.5 mg		
GENTAMICIN		IV	2 mg/kg	1.3 mg		
METRONIDAZOLE		IV	10 mg/kg	6.5 mg		
VANCOMYCIN		IV	15 mg/kg	9.75 mg		
ATROPINE		IV	0.02 mg/kg	0.013 mg	0.4 mg/mL	0.0325 mL
GLYCOPYRROLATE		IV	0.007 mg/kg	0.00455 mg	0.2 mg/mL	0.02275 mL
NEOSTIGMINE		IV	0.07 mg/kg	0.0455 mg	1 mg/mL	0.0455 mL
EDROPHONIUM	<2 mo	IV	0.1 mg	single dose		
PRIMARY ANESTHESIA FOR NEONATES: HIGH DOSE FENTANYL AND PANCURONIUM						

650 GMS (0.65 KG)

Ventilation: trained rescuer	1 breath q 6-8 sec (8-10 breaths/minute) about 1 second/breath-visible chest rise; if intubated, continuous compressions without pause for ventilations
Pulse check	brachial/femoral
Compression	2-3 fingers—1 finger width below nipples Wrap hands around chest if possible, compress with thumbs
Depth	1.5 inch (4 cm) or at least 1/3 chest depth
Rate	at least 100 compressions per minute
Compress/vent ratio	30:2 with 1 or 2 rescuers
Foreign body obstruction	5 back blows at level of scapula, support head; alternate with 5 chest compressions Never perform a blind finger-sweep. Open the mouth and look for object; if you see it, remove it.

sync cardioversion	0.5 J/kg	0.325 J	
	repeat	1 J/kg	0.65 J
defibrillation	2 J/kg	1.3 J	
	repeat	4 J/kg	2.6 J

IV Bolus Drugs		dose	mg to pt	supplied	mL to give
ADENOSINE	IV	0.1 mg/kg	0.065 mg	3 mg/mL	0.02 mL
ADENOSINE repeat dose	IV	0.2 mg/kg	0.13 mg	3 mg/mL	0.04 mL
AMIODARONE	IV/IO	5 mg/kg	3.25 mg	50 mg/mL	0.07 mL
ATROPINE	IV/IM	0.02 mg/kg	0.013 mg	0.4 mg/mL	0.03 mL
ATROPINE	ETT	0.04 mg/kg	0.026 mg	0.4 mg/mL	0.07 mL
CALCIUM CHLORIDE	IV	20 mg/kg	13 mg	100 mg/mL	0.13 mL
CALCIUM GLUCONATE	IV/IO	60 mg/kg	39 mg	100 mg/mL	0.39 mL
DANTROLENE	IV	2.5 mg/kg	1.625 mg		
EPHEDRINE	IV	0.15 mg/kg	0.0975 mg	10 mg/mL	0.01 mL
EPINEPHRINE (1:10,000)	IV/IO	0.01 mg/kg	0.0065 mg	0.1 mg/mL	0.07 mL
EPINEPHRINE (1:1,000)	ETT	0.1 mg/kg	0.065 mg	1 mg/mL	0.07 mL
ESMOLOL	IV	0.5 mg/kg	0.325 mg	10 mg/mL	0.03 mL
LABETALOL	IV	0.2 mg/kg	0.13 mg	5 mg/mL	0.03 mL
LIDOCAINE	IV/IO	1 mg/kg	0.65 mg	20 mg/mL	0.03 mL
NEOSYNEPHRINE	IV	5 mcg/kg	3.25 mcg	100 mcg/mL	0.03 mL
ROMAZICON	IV	0.01 mg/kg	0.0065 mg	0.1 mg/mL	0.07 mL
VASOPRESSIN	IV/IO	0.4 unit/kg	0.26 units	20 u/mL	0.01 mL

700 GMS (0.7 KG) MAINTENANCE IV FLUIDS: 2.8 ML/HR

drug		route	dose	mg to pt	supplied	mL to give
VAGOLYTIC/ANTISIALAGOGUE						
ATROPINE		IV	0.02 mg/kg	0.014 mg	0.4 mg/mL	0.035 mL
GLYCOPYRROLATE		IV	0.004 mg/kg	0.0028 mg	0.2 mg/mL	0.014 mL
PROPOFOL		IV	3 mg/kg	2.1 mg	10 mg/mL	0.21 mL
KETAMINE		IV	2 mg/kg	1.4 mg	10 mg/mL	0.14 mL
KETAMINE		IM/PR	5 mg/kg	3.5 mg	10 mg/mL	0.35 mL
FENTANYL		IV	1 mcg/kg	0.7 mcg	50 mcg/mL	0.014 mL
FENTANYL		IN	2 mcg/kg	1.4 mcg	50 mcg/mL	0.028 mL
FENTANYL	high dose	IV	4 mcg/kg	2.8 mcg	50 mcg/mL	0.056 mL
FENTANYL	cardiac	IV	10 mcg/kg	7 mcg	50 mcg/mL	0.14 mL
ACETAMINOPHEN		PR	20 mg/kg	14 mg		
SUCCINYLCHOLINE		IV	2 mg/kg	1.4 mg	20 mg/mL	0.07 mL
SUCCINYLCHOLINE		IM	4 mg/kg	2.8 mg	20 mg/mL	0.14 mL
CISATRACURIUM		IV	0.1 mg/kg	0.07 mg	2 mg/mL	0.035 mL
PANCURONIUM	<1 mo	IV	0.02 mg/kg	0.014 mg	1 mg/mL	0.014 mL
PANCURONIUM	>1 mo	IV	0.1 mg/kg	0.07 mg	1 mg/mL	0.07 mL
ROCURONIUM		IV	0.6 mg/kg	0.42 mg	10 mg/mL	0.042 mL
VECURONIUM		IV	0.1 mg/kg	0.07 mg	1 mg/mL	0.07 mL
AMPICILLIN		IV	50 mg/kg	35 mg		
CEFAZOLIN		IV	25 mg/kg	17.5 mg		
CLINDAMYCIN		IV	10 mg/kg	7 mg		
GENTAMICIN		IV	2 mg/kg	1.4 mg		
METRONIDAZOLE		IV	10 mg/kg	7 mg		
VANCOMYCIN		IV	15 mg/kg	10.5 mg		
ATROPINE		IV	0.02 mg/kg	0.014 mg	0.4 mg/mL	0.035 mL
GLYCOPYRROLATE		IV	0.007 mg/kg	0.0049 mg	0.2 mg/mL	0.0225 mL
NEOSTIGMINE		IV	0.07 mg/kg	0.049 mg	1 mg/mL	0.049 mL
EDROPHONIUM	<2 mo	IV	0.1 mg	single dose		

PRIMARY ANESTHESIA FOR NEONATES: HIGH DOSE FENTANYL AND PANCURONIUM

6 Pediatric Pharmacology: Perioperative and Emergency Drugs

700 GMS (0.7 KG)

Ventilation: trained rescuer	1 breath q 6-8 sec (8-10 breaths/minute) about 1 second/ breath-visible chest rise; if intubated, continuous compressions without pause for ventilations
Pulse check	brachial/femoral
Compression	2-3 fingers−1 finger width below nipples Wrap hands around chest if possible, compress with thumbs
Depth	1.5 inch (4 cm) or at least 1/3 chest depth
Rate	at least 100 compressions per minute
Compress/vent ratio	30:2 with 1 or 2 rescuers
Foreign body obstruction	5 back blows at level of scapula, support head; alternate with 5 chest compressions Never perform a blind finger-sweep. Open the mouth and look for object; if you see it, remove it.

sync cardioversion	0.5 J/kg	0.35 J
defibrillation	1 J/kg	0.7 J
repeat	2 J/kg	1.4 J
repeat	4 J/kg	2.8 J

IV Bolus Drugs		dose	mg to pt	supplied	mL to give
ADENOSINE	IV	0.1 mg/kg	0.07 mg	3 mg/mL	0.02 mL
ADENOSINE repeat dose	IV	0.2 mg/kg	0.14 mg	3 mg/mL	0.05 mL
AMIODARONE	IV/IO	5 mg/kg	3.5 mg	50 mg/mL	0.07 mL
ATROPINE	IV/IM	0.02 mg/kg	0.014 mg	0.4 mg/mL	0.04 mL
ATROPINE	ETT	0.04 mg/kg	0.028 mg	0.4 mg/mL	0.07 mL
CALCIUM CHLORIDE	IV	20 mg/kg	14 mg	100 mg/mL	0.14 mL
CALCIUM GLUCONATE	IV/IO	60 mg/kg	42 mg	100 mg/mL	0.42 mL
DANTROLENE	IV	2.5 mg/kg	1.75 mg		
EPHEDRINE	IV	0.15 mg/kg	0.105 mg	10 mg/mL	0.01 mL
EPINEPHRINE (1:10,000)	IV/IO	0.01 mg/kg	0.007 mg	0.1 mg/mL	0.07 mL
EPINEPHRINE (1:1,000)	ETT	0.1 mg/kg	0.07 mg	1 mg/mL	0.07 mL
ESMOLOL	IV	0.5 mg/kg	0.35 mg	10 mg/mL	0.03 mL
LABETALOL	IV	0.2 mg/kg	0.14 mg	5 mg/mL	0.03 mL
LIDOCAINE	IV/IO	1 mg/kg	0.7 mg	20 mg/mL	0.04 mL
NEOSYNEPHRINE	IV	5 mcg/kg	3.5 mcg	100 mcg/mL	0.04 mL
ROMAZICON	IV	0.01 mg/kg	0.007 mg	0.1 mg/mL	0.07 mL
VASOPRESSIN	IV/IO	0.4 unit/kg	0.28 units	20 u/mL	0.01 mL

750 GMS (0.75 KG) MAINTENANCE IV FLUIDS: 3 ML/HR

drug		route	dose	mg to pt	supplied	mL to give
VAGOLYTIC/ANTISIALAGOGUE						
ATROPINE		IV	0.02 mg/kg	0.015 mg	0.4 mg/mL	0.0375 mL
GLYCOPYRROLATE		IV	0.004 mg/kg	0.003 mg	0.2 mg/mL	0.015 mL
PROPOFOL		IV	3 mg/kg	2.25 mg	10 mg/mL	0.225 mL
KETAMINE		IV	2 mg/kg	1.5 mg	10 mg/mL	0.15 mL
KETAMINE		IM/PR	5 mg/kg	3.75 mg	10 mg/mL	0.375 mL
FENTANYL		IV	1 mcg/kg	0.75 mcg	50 mcg/mL	0.015 mL
FENTANYL		IN	2 mcg/kg	1.5 mcg	50 mcg/mL	0.03 mL
FENTANYL	high dose	IV	4 mcg/kg	3 mcg	50 mcg/mL	0.06 mL
FENTANYL	cardiac	IV	10 mcg/kg	7.5 mcg	50 mcg/mL	0.15 mL
ACETAMINOPHEN		PR	20 mg/kg	15 mg		
SUCCINYLCHOLINE		IV	2 mg/kg	1.5 mg	20 mg/mL	0.075 mL
SUCCINYLCHOLINE		IM	4 mg/kg	3 mg	20 mg/mL	0.15 mL
CISATRACURIUM		IV	0.1 mg/kg	0.075 mg	2 mg/mL	0.0375 mL
PANCURONIUM	<1 mo	IV	0.02 mg/kg	0.015 mg	1 mg/mL	0.015 mL
PANCURONIUM	>1 mo	IV	0.1 mg/kg	0.075 mg	1 mg/mL	0.075 mL
ROCURONIUM		IV	0.6 mg/kg	0.45 mg	10 mg/mL	0.045 mL
VECURONIUM		IV	0.1 mg/kg	0.075 mg	1 mg/mL	0.075 mL
AMPICILLIN		IV	50 mg/kg	37.5 mg		
CEFAZOLIN		IV	25 mg/kg	18.75 mg		
CLINDAMYCIN		IV	10 mg/kg	7.5 mg		
GENTAMICIN		IV	2 mg/kg	1.5 mg		
METRONIDAZOLE		IV	10 mg/kg	7.5 mg		
VANCOMYCIN		IV	15 mg/kg	11.25 mg		
ATROPINE		IV	0.02 mg/kg	0.015 mg	0.4 mg/mL	0.0375 mL
GLYCOPYRROLATE		IV	0.007 mg/kg	0.00525 mg	0.2 mg/mL	0.02625 mL
NEOSTIGMINE		IV	0.07 mg/kg	0.0525 mg	1 mg/mL	0.0525 mL
EDROPHONIUM	<2 mo	IV	0.1 mg	single dose		

PRIMARY ANESTHESIA FOR NEONATES: HIGH DOSE FENTANYL AND PANCURONIUM

750 GMS (0.75 KG)

Ventilation: trained rescuer:	1 breath q 6-8 sec (8-10 breaths/minute) about 1 second/breath-visible chest rise; if intubated, continuous compressions without pause for ventilations
Pulse check	brachial/femoral
Compression	2-3 fingers–1 finger width below nipples *Wrap hands around chest if possible, compress with thumbs*
Depth	1.5 inch (4 cm) or at least 1/3 chest depth
Rate	at least 100 compressions per minute
Compress/vent ratio	30:2 with 1 or 2 rescuers
Foreign body obstruction	5 back blows at level of scapula, support head; alternate with 5 chest compressions. Never perform a blind finger-sweep. Open the mouth and look for object; if you see it, remove it.

sync cardioversion	0.5 J/kg	0.375 J
	repeat 1 J/kg	0.75 J
defibrillation	2 J/kg	1.5 J
	repeat 4 J/kg	3 J

IV Bolus Drugs		dose	mg to pt	supplied	mL to give
ADENOSINE	IV	0.1 mg/kg	0.075 mg	3 mg/mL	0.03 mL
ADENOSINE repeat dose	IV	0.2 mg/kg	0.15 mg	3 mg/mL	0.05 mL
AMIODARONE	IV/IO	5 mg/kg	3.75 mg	50 mg/mL	0.08 mL
ATROPINE	IV/IM	0.02 mg/kg	0.015 mg	0.4 mg/mL	0.04 mL
ATROPINE	ETT	0.04 mg/kg	0.03 mg	0.4 mg/mL	0.08 mL
CALCIUM CHLORIDE	IV	20 mg/kg	15 mg	100 mg/mL	0.15 mL
CALCIUM GLUCONATE	IV/IO	60 mg/kg	45 mg	100 mg/mL	0.45 mL
DANTROLENE	IV	2.5 mg/kg	1.875 mg		
EPHEDRINE	IV	0.15 mg/kg	0.1125 mg	10 mg/mL	0.01 mL
EPINEPHRINE (1:10,000)	IV/IO	0.01 mg/kg	0.0075 mg	0.1 mg/mL	0.08 mL
EPINEPHRINE (1:1,000)	ETT	0.1 mg/kg	0.075 mg	1 mg/mL	0.08 mL
ESMOLOL	IV	0.5 mg/kg	0.375 mg	10 mg/mL	0.04 mL
LABETALOL	IV	0.2 mg/kg	0.15 mg	5 mg/mL	0.03 mL
LIDOCAINE	IV/IO	1 mg/kg	0.75 mg	20 mg/mL	0.04 mL
NEOSYNEPHRINE	IV	5 mcg/kg	3.75 mcg	100 mcg/mL	0.04 mL
ROMAZICON	IV	0.01 mg/kg	0.0075 mg	0.1 mg/mL	0.08 mL
VASOPRESSIN	IV/IO	0.4 unit/kg	0.3 units	20 u/mL	0.02 mL

800 GMS (0.8 KG) MAINTENANCE IV FLUIDS: 3.2 ML/HR

drug		route	dose	mg to pt	supplied	mL to give
VAGOLYTIC/ANTISIALAGOGUE						
ATROPINE		IV	0.02 mg/kg	0.016 mg	0.4 mg/mL	0.04 mL
GLYCOPYRROLATE		IV	0.004 mg/kg	0.0032 mg	0.2 mg/mL	0.016 mL
PROPOFOL		IV	3 mg/kg	2.4 mg	10 mg/mL	0.24 mL
KETAMINE		IV	2 mg/kg	1.6 mg	10 mg/mL	0.16 mL
KETAMINE		IM/PR	5 mg/kg	4 mg	10 mg/mL	0.4 mL
FENTANYL		IV	1 mcg/kg	0.8 mcg	50 mcg/mL	0.016 mL
FENTANYL		IN	2 mcg/kg	1.6 mcg	50 mcg/mL	0.032 mL
FENTANYL	high dose	IV	4 mcg/kg	3.2 mcg	50 mcg/mL	0.064 mL
FENTANYL	cardiac	IV	10 mcg/kg	8 mcg	50 mcg/mL	0.16 mL
ACETAMINOPHEN		PR	20 mg/kg	16 mg		
SUCCINYLCHOLINE		IV	2 mg/kg	1.6 mg	20 mg/mL	0.08 mL
SUCCINYLCHOLINE		IM	4 mg/kg	3.2 mg	20 mg/mL	0.16 mL
CISATRACURIUM		IV	0.1 mg/kg	0.08 mg	2 mg/mL	0.04 mL
PANCURONIUM	<1 mo	IV	0.02 mg/kg	0.016 mg	1 mg/mL	0.016 mL
PANCURONIUM	>1 mo	IV	0.1 mg/kg	0.08 mg	1 mg/mL	0.08 mL
ROCURONIUM		IV	0.6 mg/kg	0.48 mg	10 mg/mL	0.048 mL
VECURONIUM		IV	0.1 mg/kg	0.08 mg	1 mg/mL	0.08 mL
AMPICILLIN		IV	50 mg/kg	40 mg		
CEFAZOLIN		IV	25 mg/kg	20 mg		
CLINDAMYCIN		IV	10 mg/kg	8 mg		
GENTAMICIN		IV	2 mg/kg	1.6 mg		
METRONIDAZOLE		IV	10 mg/kg	8 mg		
VANCOMYCIN		IV	15 mg/kg	12 mg		
ATROPINE		IV	0.02 mg/kg	0.016 mg	0.4 mg/mL	0.04 mL
GLYCOPYRROLATE		IV	0.007 mg/kg	0.0056 mg	0.2 mg/mL	0.028 mL
NEOSTIGMINE		IV	0.07 mg/kg	0.056 mg	1 mg/mL	0.056 mL
EDROPHONIUM	<2 mo	IV	0.1 mg	single dose		

PRIMARY ANESTHESIA FOR NEONATES: HIGH DOSE FENTANYL AND PANCURONIUM

 6 Pediatric Pharmacology: Perioperative and Emergency Drugs

800 GMS (0.8 KG)

Ventilation: trained rescuer:	1 breath q 6-8 sec (8-10 breaths/minute) about 1 second/breath-visible chest rise; if intubated, continuous compressions without pause for ventilations
Pulse check	brachial/femoral
Compression	2-3 fingers–1 finger width below nipples; *Wrap hands around chest if possible, compress with thumbs*
Depth	1.5 inch (4 cm) or at least 1/3 chest depth
Rate	at least 100 compressions per minute
Compress/vent ratio	30:2 with 1 or 2 rescuers
Foreign body obstruction	5 back blows at level of scapula, support head; alternate with 5 chest compressions. Never perform a blind finger-sweep. Open the mouth and look for object; if you see it, remove it.

sync cardioversion	0.5 J/kg		0.4 J
defibrillation	1 J/kg		0.8 J
	repeat	2 J/kg	1.6 J
	repeat	4 J/kg	3.2 J

IV Bolus Drugs		dose	mg to pt	supplied	mL to give
ADENOSINE	IV	0.1 mg/kg	0.08 mg	3 mg/mL	0.03 mL
ADENOSINE repeat dose	IV	0.2 mg/kg	0.16 mg	3 mg/mL	0.05 mL
AMIODARONE	IV/IO	5 mg/kg	4 mg	50 mg/mL	0.08 mL
ATROPINE	IV/IM	0.02 mg/kg	0.016 mg	0.4 mg/mL	0.04 mL
ATROPINE	ETT	0.04 mg/kg	0.032 mg	0.4 mg/mL	0.08 mL
CALCIUM CHLORIDE	IV	20 mg/kg	16 mg	100 mg/mL	0.16
CALCIUM GLUCONATE	IV/IO	60 mg/kg	48 mg	100 mg/mL	0.48 mL
DANTROLENE	IV	2.5 mg/kg	2 mg		
EPHEDRINE	IV	0.15 mg/kg	0.12 mg	10 mg/mL	0.01 mL
EPINEPHRINE (1:10,000)	IV/IO	0.01 mg/kg	0.008 mg	0.1 mg/mL	0.08 mL
EPINEPHRINE (1:1,000)	ETT	0.1 mg/kg	0.08 mg	1 mg/mL	0.08 mL
ESMOLOL	IV	0.5 mg/kg	0.4 mg	10 mg/mL	0.03 mL
LABETALOL	IV	0.2 mg/kg	0.16 mg	5 mg/mL	0.03 mL
LIDOCAINE	IV/IO	1 mg/kg	0.8 mg	20 mg/mL	0.04 mL
NEOSYNEPHRINE	IV	5 mcg/kg	4 mcg	100 mcg/mL	0.04 mL
ROMAZICON	IV	0.01 mg/kg	0.008 mg	0.1 mg/mL	0.08 mL
VASOPRESSIN	IV/IO	0.4 unit/kg	0.32 units	20 u/mL	0.02 mL

850 GMS (0.85 KG) MAINTENANCE IV FLUIDS: 3.4 ML/HR

drug		route	dose	mg to pt	supplied	mL to give
VAGOLYTIC/ANTISIALAGOGUE						
ATROPINE		IV	0.02 mg/kg	0.017 mg	0.4 mg/mL	0.0425 mL
GLYCOPYRROLATE		IV	0.004 mg/kg	0.0034 mg	0.2 mg/mL	0.017 mL
PROPOFOL		IV	3 mg/kg	2.55 mg	10 mg/mL	0.255 mL
KETAMINE		IV	2 mg/kg	1.7 mg	10 mg/mL	0.17 mL
KETAMINE		IM/PR	5 mg/kg	4.25 mg	10 mg/mL	0.425 mL
FENTANYL		IV	1 mcg/kg	0.85 mcg	50 mcg/mL	0.017 mL
FENTANYL		IN	2 mcg/kg	1.7 mcg	50 mcg/mL	0.034 mL
FENTANYL	high dose	IV	4 mcg/kg	3.4 mcg	50 mcg/mL	0.068 mL
FENTANYL	cardiac	IV	10 mcg/kg	8.5 mcg	50 mcg/mL	0.17 mL
ACETAMINOPHEN		PR	20 mg/kg	17 mg		
SUCCINYLCHOLINE		IV	2 mg/kg	1.7 mg	20 mg/mL	0.085 mL
SUCCINYLCHOLINE		IM	4 mg/kg	3.4 mg	20 mg/mL	0.17 mL
CISATRACURIUM		IV	0.1 mg/kg	0.085 mg	2 mg/mL	0.0425 mL
PANCURONIUM	<1 mo	IV	0.02 mg/kg	0.017 mg	1 mg/mL	0.017 mL
PANCURONIUM	>1 mo	IV	0.1 mg/kg	0.085 mg	1 mg/mL	0.085 mL
ROCURONIUM		IV	0.6 mg/kg	0.51 mg	10 mg/mL	0.051 mL
VECURONIUM		IV	0.1 mg/kg	0.085 mg	1 mg/mL	0.085 mL
AMPICILLIN		IV	50 mg/kg	42.5 mg		
CEFAZOLIN		IV	25 mg/kg	21.25 mg		
CLINDAMYCIN		IV	10 mg/kg	8.5 mg		
GENTAMICIN		IV	2 mg/kg	1.7 mg		
METRONIDAZOLE		IV	10 mg/kg	8.5 mg		
VANCOMYCIN		IV	15 mg/kg	12.75 mg		
ATROPINE		IV	0.02 mg/kg	0.017 mg	0.4 mg/mL	0.0425 mL
GLYCOPYRROLATE		IV	0.007 mg/kg	0.00595 mg	0.2 mg/mL	0.02975 mL
NEOSTIGMINE		IV	0.07 mg/kg	0.0595 mg	1 mg/mL	0.0595 mL
EDROPHONIUM	<2 mo	IV	0.1 mg	single dose		

PRIMARY ANESTHESIA FOR NEONATES: HIGH DOSE FENTANYL AND PANCURONIUM

 6 Pediatric Pharmacology: Perioperative and Emergency Drugs

850 GMS (0.85 KG)

Ventilation: trained rescuer	1 breath q 6-8 sec (8-10 breaths/minute) about 1 second/ breath-visible chest rise; if intubated, continuous compressions without pause for ventilations
Pulse check	brachial/femoral
Compression	2-3 fingers-1 finger width below nipples *Wrap hands around chest if possible, compress with thumbs*
Depth	1.5 inch (4 cm) or at least 1/3 chest depth
Rate	at least 100 compressions per minute
Compress/vent ratio	30:2 with 1 or 2 rescuers
Foreign body obstruction	5 back blows at level of scapula, support head; alternate with 5 chest compressions Never perform a blind finger-sweep. Open the mouth and look for object; if you see it, remove it.

sync cardioversion	0.5 J/kg	0.425 J
defibrillation	1 J/kg	0.85 J
repeat	2 J/kg	1.7 J
repeat	4 J/kg	3.4 J

IV Bolus Drugs		dose	mg to pt	supplied	mL to give
ADENOSINE	IV	0.1 mg/kg	0.085 mg	3 mg/mL	0.03 mL
ADENOSINE repeat dose	IV	0.2 mg/kg	0.17 mg	3 mg/mL	0.06 mL
AMIODARONE	IV/IO	5 mg/kg	4.25 mg	50 mg/mL	0.09 mL
ATROPINE	IV/IM	0.02 mg/kg	0.017 mg	0.4 mg/mL	0.04 mL
ATROPINE	ETT	0.04 mg/kg	0.034 mg	0.4 mg/mL	0.09 mL
CALCIUM CHLORIDE	IV	20 mg/kg	17 mg	100 mg/mL	0.17 mL
CALCIUM GLUCONATE	IV/IO	60 mg/kg	51 mg	100 mg/mL	0.51 mL
DANTROLENE	IV	2.5 mg/kg	2.125 mg		
EPHEDRINE	IV	0.15 mg/kg	0.1275 mg	10 mg/mL	0.01 mL
EPINEPHRINE (1:10,000)	IV/IO	0.01 mg/kg	0.0085 mg	0.1 mg/mL	0.09 mL
EPINEPHRINE (1:1,000)	ETT	0.1 mg/kg	0.085 mg	1 mg/mL	0.09 mL
ESMOLOL	IV	0.5 mg/kg	0.425 mg	10 mg/mL	0.03 mL
LABETALOL	IV	0.2 mg/kg	0.17 mg	5 mg/mL	0.03 mL
LIDOCAINE	IV/IO	1 mg/kg	0.85 mg	20 mg/mL	0.04 mL
NEOSYNEPHRINE	IV	5 mcg/kg	4.25 mcg	100 mcg/mL	0.04 mL
ROMAZICON	IV	0.01 mg/kg	0.0085 mg	0.1 mg/mL	0.09 mL
VASOPRESSIN	IV/IO	0.4 unit/kg	0.34 units	20 u/mL	0.02 mL

900 GMS (0.9 KG) MAINTENANCE IV FLUIDS: 3.6 ML/HR

drug		route	dose	mg to pt	supplied	mL to give
VAGOLYTIC/ANTISIALAGOGUE						
ATROPINE		IV	0.02 mg/kg	0.018 mg	0.4 mg/mL	0.045 mL
GLYCOPYRROLATE		IV	0.004 mg/kg	0.0036 mg	0.2 mg/mL	0.018 mL
PROPOFOL		IV	3 mg/kg	2.7 mg	10 mg/mL	0.27 mL
KETAMINE		IV	2 mg/kg	1.8 mg	10 mg/mL	0.18 mL
KETAMINE		IM/PR	5 mg/kg	4.5 mg	10 mg/mL	0.45 mL
FENTANYL		IV	1 mcg/kg	0.9 mcg	50 mcg/mL	0.018 mL
FENTANYL		IN	2 mcg/kg	1.8 mcg	50 mcg/mL	0.036 mL
FENTANYL	high dose	IV	4 mcg/kg	3.6 mcg	50 mcg/mL	0.072 mL
FENTANYL	cardiac	IV	10 mcg/kg	9 mcg	50 mcg/mL	0.18 mL
ACETAMINOPHEN		PR	20 mg/kg	18 mg		
SUCCINYLCHOLINE		IV	2 mg/kg	1.8 mg	20 mg/mL	0.09 mL
SUCCINYLCHOLINE		IM	4 mg/kg	3.6 mg	20 mg/mL	0.18 mL
CISATRACURIUM		IV	0.1 mg/kg	0.09 mg	2 mg/mL	0.045 mL
PANCURONIUM	<1 mo	IV	0.02 mg/kg	0.018 mg	1 mg/mL	0.018 mL
PANCURONIUM	>1 mo	IV	0.1 mg/kg	0.09 mg	1 mg/mL	0.09 mL
ROCURONIUM		IV	0.6 mg/kg	0.54 mg	10 mg/mL	0.054 mL
VECURONIUM		IV	0.1 mg/kg	0.09 mg	1 mg/mL	0.09 mL
AMPICILLIN		IV	50 mg/kg	45 mg		
CEFAZOLIN		IV	25 mg/kg	22.5 mg		
CLINDAMYCIN		IV	10 mg/kg	9 mg		
GENTAMICIN		IV	2 mg/kg	1.8 mg		
METRONIDAZOLE		IV	10 mg/kg	9 mg		
VANCOMYCIN		IV	15 mg/kg	13.5 mg		
ATROPINE		IV	0.02 mg/kg	0.018 mg	0.4 mg/mL	0.045 mL
GLYCOPYRROLATE		IV	0.007 mg/kg	0.0063 mg	0.2 mg/mL	0.0315 mL
NEOSTIGMINE		IV	0.07 mg/kg	0.063 mg	1 mg/mL	0.063 mL
EDROPHONIUM	<2 mo	IV	0.1 mg	single dose		

PRIMARY ANESTHESIA FOR NEONATES: HIGH DOSE FENTANYL AND PANCURONIUM

6 Pediatric Pharmacology: Perioperative and Emergency Drugs 77

900 GMS (0.9 KG)

Ventilation: trained rescuer	1 breath q 6-8 sec (8-10 breaths/minute) about 1 second/ breath-visible chest rise; if intubated, continuous compressions without pause for ventilations
Pulse check	brachial/femoral
Compression	2-3 fingers–1 finger width below nipples *Wrap hands around chest if possible, compress with thumbs*
Depth	1.5 inch (4 cm) or at least 1/3 chest depth
Rate	at least 100 compressions per minute
Compress/vent ratio	30:2 with 1 or 2 rescuers
Foreign body obstruction	5 back blows at level of scapula, support head; alternate with 5 chest compressions Never perform a blind finger-sweep. Open the mouth and look for object; if you see it, remove it.

sync cardioversion	0.5 J/kg	0.45 J
defibrillation	1 J/kg	0.9 J
repeat	2 J/kg	1.8 J
repeat	4 J/kg	3.6 J

IV Bolus Drugs		dose	mg to pt	supplied	mL to give
ADENOSINE	IV	0.1 mg/kg	0.09 mg	3 mg/mL	0.03 mL
ADENOSINE repeat dose	IV	0.2 mg/kg	0.18 mg	3 mg/mL	0.06 mL
AMIODARONE	IV/IO	5 mg/kg	4.5 mg	50 mg/mL	0.09 mL
ATROPINE	IV/IM	0.02 mg/kg	0.018 mg	0.4 mg/mL	0.04 mL
ATROPINE	ETT	0.04 mg/kg	0.036 mg	0.4 mg/mL	0.09 mL
CALCIUM CHLORIDE	IV	20 mg/kg	18 mg	100 mg/mL	0.18 mL
CALCIUM GLUCONATE	IV/IO	60 mg/kg	54 mg	100 mg/mL	0.54 mL
DANTROLENE	IV	2.5 mg/kg	2.25 mg		
EPHEDRINE	IV	0.15 mg/kg	0.135 mg	10 mg/mL	0.01 mL
EPINEPHRINE (1:10,000)	IV/IO	0.01 mg/kg	0.009 mg	0.1 mg/mL	0.09 mL
EPINEPHRINE (1:1,000)	ETT	0.1 mg/kg	0.09 mg	1 mg/mL	0.09 mL
ESMOLOL	IV	0.5 mg/kg	0.45 mg	10 mg/mL	0.05 mL
LABETALOL	IV	0.2 mg/kg	0.18 mg	5 mg/mL	0.04 mL
LIDOCAINE	IV/IO	1 mg/kg	0.9 mg	20 mg/mL	0.05 mL
NEOSYNEPHRINE	IV	5 mcg/kg	4.5 mcg	100 mcg/mL	0.05 mL
ROMAZICON	IV	0.01 mg/kg	0.009 mg	0.1 mg/mL	0.09 mL
VASOPRESSIN	IV/IO	0.4 unit/kg	0.36 units	20 u/mL	0.02 mL

950 GMS (0.95 KG) MAINTENANCE IV FLUIDS: 3.8 ML/HR

drug	route	dose	mg to pt	supplied	mL to give
VAGOLYTIC/ANTISIALAGOGUE					
ATROPINE	IV	0.02 mg/kg	0.019 mg	0.4 mg/mL	0.0475 mL
GLYCOPYRROLATE	IV	0.004 mg/kg	0.0038 mg	0.2 mg/mL	0.019 mL
PROPOFOL	IV	3 mg/kg	2.85 mg	10 mg/mL	0.285 mL
KETAMINE	IV	2 mg/kg	1.9 mg	10 mg/mL	0.19 mL
KETAMINE	IM/PR	5 mg/kg	4.75 mg	10 mg/mL	0.475 mL
FENTANYL	IV	1 mcg/kg	0.95 mcg	50 mcg/mL	0.019 mL
FENTANYL	IN	2 mcg/kg	1.9 mcg	50 mcg/mL	0.038 mL
FENTANYL high dose	IV	4 mcg/kg	3.8 mcg	50 mcg/mL	0.076 mL
FENTANYL cardiac	IV	10 mcg/kg	9.5 mcg	50 mcg/mL	0.19 mL
ACETAMINOPHEN	PR	20 mg/kg	19 mg		
SUCCINYLCHOLINE	IV	2 mg/kg	1.9 mg	20 mg/mL	0.095 mL
SUCCINYLCHOLINE	IM	4 mg/kg	3.8 mg	20 mg/mL	0.19 mL
CISATRACURIUM	IV	0.1 mg/kg	0.095 mg	2 mg/mL	0.0475 mL
PANCURONIUM <1 mo	IV	0.02 mg/kg	0.019 mg	1 mg/mL	0.019 mL
PANCURONIUM >1 mo	IV	0.1 mg/kg	0.095 mg	1 mg/mL	0.095 mL
ROCURONIUM	IV	0.6 mg/kg	0.57 mg	10 mg/mL	0.057 mL
VECURONIUM	IV	0.1 mg/kg	0.095 mg	1 mg/mL	0.095 mL
AMPICILLIN	IV	50 mg/kg	47.5 mg		
CEFAZOLIN	IV	25 mg/kg	23.75 mg		
CLINDAMYCIN	IV	10 mg/kg	9.5 mg		
GENTAMICIN	IV	2 mg/kg	1.9 mg		
METRONIDAZOLE	IV	10 mg/kg	9.5 mg		
VANCOMYCIN	IV	15 mg/kg	14.25 mg		
ATROPINE	IV	0.02 mg/kg	0.019 mg	0.4 mg/mL	0.0475 mL
GLYCOPYRROLATE	IV	0.007 mg/kg	0.00665 mg	0.2 mg/mL	0.03325 mL
NEOSTIGMINE	IV	0.07 mg/kg	0.0665 mg	1 mg/mL	0.0665 mL
EDROPHONIUM <2 mo	IV	0.1 mg	single dose		

PRIMARY ANESTHESIA FOR NEONATES: HIGH DOSE FENTANYL AND PANCURONIUM

6 Pediatric Pharmacology: Perioperative and Emergency Drugs

950 GMS (0.95 KG)

Ventilation:	1 breath q 6-8 sec (8-10 breaths/minute) about 1 second/ breath-visible chest rise; if intubated, continuous compressions without pause for ventilations
Pulse check	brachial/femoral
Compression	2-3 fingers-1 finger width below nipples
Depth	1.5 inch (4 cm) or at least 1/3 chest depth
Rate	at least 100 compressions per minute
Compress/vent ratio	30:2 with 1 or 2 rescuers
Foreign body obstruction	5 back blows at level of scapula, support head; alternate with 5 chest compressions
	Never perform a blind finger-sweep. Open the mouth and look for object; if you see it, remove it.

sync cardioversion	0.5 J/kg	0.475 J	
	repeat	1 J/kg	0.95 J
defibrillation	2 J/kg	1.9 J	
	repeat	4 J/kg	3.8 J

IV Bolus Drugs		dose	mg to pt	supplied	mL to give
ADENOSINE	IV	0.1 mg/kg	0.095 mg	3 mg/mL	0.03 mL
ADENOSINE	repeat dose	0.2 mg/kg	0.19 mg	3 mg/mL	0.06 mL
AMIODARONE	IV/IO	5 mg/kg	4.75 mg	50 mg/mL	0.10 mL
ATROPINE	IV/IM	0.02 mg/kg	0.019 mg	0.4 mg/mL	0.05 mL
ATROPINE	ETT	0.04 mg/kg	0.038 mg	0.4 mg/mL	0.10 mL
CALCIUM CHLORIDE	IV	20 mg/kg	19 mg	100 mg/mL	0.19 mL
CALCIUM GLUCONATE	IV/IO	60 mg/kg	57 mg	100 mg/mL	0.57 mL
DANTROLENE	IV	2.5 mg/kg	2.375 mg		
EPHEDRINE	IV	0.15 mg/kg	0.1425 mg	10 mg/mL	0.01 mL
EPINEPHRINE (1:10,000)	IV/IO	0.01 mg/kg	0.0095 mg	0.1 mg/mL	0.10 mL
EPINEPHRINE (1:1,000)	ETT	0.1 mg/kg	0.095 mg	1 mg/mL	0.10 mL
ESMOLOL	IV	0.5 mg/kg	0.475 mg	10 mg/mL	0.04 mL
LABETALOL	IV	0.2 mg/kg	0.19 mg	5 mg/mL	0.04 mL
LIDOCAINE	IV/IO	1 mg/kg	0.95 mg	20 mg/mL	0.05 mL
NEOSYNEPHRINE	IV	5 mcg/kg	4.75 mcg	100 mcg/mL	0.05 mL
ROMAZICON	IV	0.1 mg/kg	0.095 mg	0.1 mg/mL	0.10 mL
VASOPRESSIN	IV/IO	0.4 unit/kg	0.38 units	20 u/mL	0.02 mL

1 KG MAINTENANCE IV FLUIDS: 4 ML/HR

common pediatric drugs		route	dose	mg to pt	supplied	mL to give
ATROPINE	vagolytic	IV	0.02 mg/kg	0.02 mg	0.4 mg/mL	0.05 mL
GLYCOPYRROLATE	vagolytic	IV	0.004 mg/kg	0.004 mg	0.2 mg/mL	0.02 mL
MIDAZOLAM		IV	0.05 mg/kg	0.05 mg	1 mg/mL	0.05 mL
MIDAZOLAM		PO	0.5 mg/kg	0.5 mg	1 mg/mL	0.5 mL
MIDAZOLAM		IN	0.2 mg/kg	0.2 mg	1 mg/mL	0.2 mL
SUCCINYLCHOLINE		IV	2 mg/kg	2 mg	20 mg/mL	0.1 mL
SUCCINYLCHOLINE		IM	4 mg/kg	4 mg	20 mg/mL	0.2 mL
PROPOFOL		IV	3 mg/kg	3 mg	10 mg/mL	0.3 mL
ETOMIDATE	>10 y	IV	0.3 mg/kg	0.3 mg	2 mg/mL	0.15 mL
FENTANYL		IV	1 mcg/kg	1 mcg	50 mcg/mL	0.02 mL
FENTANYL		IN	2 mcg/kg	2 mcg	50 mcg/mL	0.04 mL
MORPHINE	<6 mo	IV/IM	0.05 mg/kg	0.05 mg	10 mg/mL	0.005 mL
MORPHINE	>6 mo	IV/IM	0.1 mg/kg	0.1 mg	10 mg/mL	0.01 mL
TORADOL	>2-16 y	IV	0.5 mg/kg	0.5 mg	30 mg/mL	0.0167 mL
TORADOL	>2-16 y	IM	1 mg/kg	1 mg	30 mg/mL	0.0333 mL
ACETAMINOPHEN		PR	20 mg/kg	20 mg		
ACETAMINOPHEN	2-12 y	IV	15 mg/kg	15 mg	10 mg/mL	1.5 mL
CISATRACURIUM		IV	0.1 mg/kg	0.1 mg	2 mg/mL	0.05 mL
PANCURONIUM	<1 mo	IV	0.02 mg/kg	0.02 mg	1 mg/mL	0.02 mL
PANCURONIUM	>1 mo	IV	0.1 mg/kg	0.1 mg	1 mg/mL	0.1 mL
ROCURONIUM		IV	0.6 mg/kg	0.6 mg	10 mg/mL	0.06 mL
ROCURONIUM	RSI	IV	1.2 mg/kg	1.2 mg	10 mg/mL	0.12 mL
VECURONIUM		IV	0.1 mg/kg	0.1 mg	1 mg/mL	0.1 mL
GLYCOPYRROLATE	reversal	IV	0.007 mg/kg	0.007 mg	0.2 mg/mL	0.035 mL
NEOSTIGMINE		IV	0.07 mg/kg	0.07 mg	1 mg/mL	0.07 mL
DEXAMETHASONE		IV	0.25 mg/kg	0.25 mg	10 mg/mL	0.025 mL
ONDANSETRON		IV	0.15 mg/kg	0.15 mg	2 mg/mL	0.075 mL

additional pediatric drugs	route	dose	mg to pt	supplied	mL to give
PREMED/SEDATION; VAGOLYTIC/ANTISIALAGOGUE; GIVE IM 30-60 MIN PREOP					
ATROPINE	IM	0.02 mg/kg	0.02 mg	0.4 mg/mL	0.05 mL
GLYCOPYRROLATE	IM	0.004 mg/kg	0.004 mg	0.2 mg/mL	0.02 mL
MIDAZOLAM	IM	0.1 mg/kg	0.1 mg	1 mg/mL	0.1 mL
DEXMEDETOMIDINE load dose	IV	0.5 mcg/kg	0.5 mcg	4 mcg/mL	0.125 mL
INDUCTION					
KETAMINE	IV	2 mg/kg	2 mg	10 mg/mL	0.2 mL
KETAMINE	IM/PR	5 mg/kg	5 mg	10 mg/mL	0.5 mL
OPIOIDS/NONOPIOIDS					
FENTANYL	high dose	IV	4 mcg/kg	4 mcg	50 mcg/mL	0.08 mL
FENTANYL	cardiac	IV	10 mcg/kg	10 mcg	50 mcg/mL	0.2 mL
HYDROMORPHONE	< 6 mo	SQ/IV	0.005 mg/kg	0.005 mg	10 mg/mL	0.0005 mL
HYDROMORPHONE	> 6 mo	SQ/IV	0.015 mg/kg	0.015 mg	10 mg/mL	0.0015 mL
REMIFENTANIL	IV	0.5 mcg/kg	0.5 mcg	50 mcg/mL	0.01 mL
SUFENTANIL	IV	0.5 mcg/kg	0.5 mcg	50 mcg/mL	0.01 mL
REVERSALS					
ATROPINE	IV	0.02 mg/kg	0.02	0.4 mg/mL	0.05 mL
EDROPHONIUM	neonate	IV	0.1 mg single dose		10 mg/mL	0.01 mL
EDROPHONIUM	> 2 mo	IV	0.04 mg/kg	0.04 mg	10 mg/mL	0.004 mL
FLUMAZENIL	< 1 y	IV	0.01 mg/kg	0.01 mg	0.1 mg/mL	0.1 mL
NALOXONE	< 5 y; > 20 kg	IM/IV	0.1 mg/kg	0.1 mg	0.4 mg/mL	0.25 mL
NALOXONE	< 5 y; > 20 kg	IM	2 mg per dose		0.4 mg/mL	5 mL
NALOXONE	ETT	0.3 mg/kg	0.3 mg	0.4 mg/mL	0.75 mL

additional pediatric drugs		route	dose	mg to pt	supplied	mL to give
ANTIBIOTICS						
AMPICILLIN	<6 y	IV	50 mg/kg	50 mg		
AMPICILLIN	>6 y	IV	50 mg/kg	50 mg		
AMPICILLIN & SULBACTUM	>1 mo	IV	50 mg/kg	50 mg		
CEFAZOLIN		IV	25 mg/kg	25 mg		
CLINDAMYCIN		IV	10 mg/kg	10 mg		
ERTAPENEM	3 mo-12 y	IV	15 mg/kg	15 mg		
ERTAPENEM	>12 y	IV	1 Gm	per dose		
GENTAMICIN		IV	2 mg/kg	2 mg		
LEVOFLOXACIN		IV	10 mg/kg	10 mg		
METRONIDAZOLE		IV	10 mg/kg	10 mg		
PIPERACILLIN & TAZOBACTAM	<40 kg & 2-9 mo	IV	80 mg/kg	80 mg		
PIPERACILLIN & TAZOBACTAM	<40 kg & >9 mo	IV	100 mg/kg	100 mg		
PIPERACILLIN & TAZOBACTAM	>40 kg	IV	3.375 Gm per dose			
VANCOMYCIN		IV	15 mg/kg	15 mg		
ANTINAUSEA						
METOCLOPROMIDE		IV	0.2 mg/kg	0.2 mg	5 mg/mL	0.04 mL
DIPHENHYDRAMINE		IV/IM	1.25 mg/kg	1.25 mg	50 mg/mL	0.025 mL
SCOPOLAMINE		IV/IM	6 mcg/kg	6 mcg	400 mcg/mL	0.015 mL
MISCELLANEOUS MEDS						
AMINOCAPROIC ACID		IV	100 mg/kg	100 mg	250 mg/mL	0.4 mL
DESMOPRESSIN		IV/SQ	0.3 mcg/kg	0.3 mcg	4 mcg/mL	0.075 mL
DEXAMETHASONE	croup	IV	0.6 mg/kg	0.6 mg	4 mg/mL	0.15 mL
HYDROCORTISONE		IV/IO	3 mg/kg	3 mg	100 mg/mL	0.03 mL

1 KG

Ventilation: trained rescuer	1 breath q 6-8 sec (8-10 breaths/minute) about 1 second/breath-visible chest rise; if intubated, continuous compressions without pause for ventilations
Pulse check	brachial/femoral
Compression	2-3 fingers–1 finger width below nipples *Wrap hands around chest if possible, compress with thumbs*
Depth	1.5 inch (4 cm) or at least 1/3 chest depth
Rate	at least 100 compressions per minute
Compress/vent ratio	30:2 with 1 or 2 rescuers
Foreign body obstruction	5 back blows at level of scapula, support head; alternate with 5 chest compressions Never perform a blind finger-sweep. Open the mouth and look for object; if you see it, remove it.

sync cardioversion	0.5 J/kg	0.5 J
repeat	1 J/kg	1 J
defibrillation	2 J/kg	2 J
repeat	4 J/kg	4 J

IV Bolus Drugs

		dose	mg to pt	supplied	mL to give
ADENOSINE	IV	0.1 mg/kg	0.1 mg	3 mg/mL	0.03 mL
ADENOSINE repeat dose	IV	0.2 mg/kg	0.2 mg	3 mg/mL	0.07 mL
AMIODARONE	IV/IO	5 mg/kg	5 mg	50 mg/mL	0.10 mL
ATROPINE	IM/IV	0.02 mg/kg	0.02 mg	0.4 mg/mL	0.05 mL
ATROPINE	ETT	0.04 mg/kg	0.04 mg	0.4 mg/mL	0.10 mL
CALCIUM CHLORIDE	IV	20 mg/kg	20 mg	100 mg/mL	0.20 mL
CALCIUM GLUCONATE	IV/IO	60 mg/kg	60 mg	100 mg/mL	0.60 mL
DANTROLENE	IV	2.5 mg/kg	2.5 mg		
EPHEDRINE	IV	0.15 mg/kg	0.15 mg	10 mg/mL	0.02 mL
EPINEPHRINE (1:10,000)	IV/IO	0.01 mg/kg	0.01 mg	0.1 mg/mL	0.10 mL
EPINEPHRINE (1:1,000)	ETT	0.1 mg/kg	0.1 mg	1 mg/mL	0.10 mL
ESMOLOL	IV	0.5 mg/kg	0.5 mg	10 mg/mL	0.05 mL
LABETALOL	IV	0.2 mg/kg	0.2 mg	5 mg/mL	0.04 mL
LIDOCAINE	IV/IO	1 mg/kg	1 mg	20 mg/mL	0.05 mL
NEOSYNEPHRINE	IV	5 mcg/kg	5 mcg	100 mcg/mL	0.05 mL
ROMAZICON	IV	0.01 mg/kg	0.01 mg	0.1 mg/mL	0.10 mL
VASOPRESSIN	IV/IO	0.4 unit/kg	0.4 units	20 u/mL	0.02 mL

1.5 KG MAINTENANCE IV FLUIDS: 6 ML/HR

common pediatric drugs		route	dose	mg to pt	supplied	mL to give
ATROPINE	vagolytic	IV	0.02 mg/kg	0.03 mg	0.4 mg/mL	0.075 mL
GLYCOPYRROLATE	vagolytic	IV	0.004 mg/kg	0.006 mg	0.2 mg/mL	0.03 mL
MIDAZOLAM		IV	0.05 mg/kg	0.075 mg	1 mg/mL	0.075 mL
MIDAZOLAM		PO	0.5 mg/kg	0.75 mg	1 mg/mL	0.75 mL
MIDAZOLAM		IN	0.2 mg/kg	0.3 mg	1 mg/mL	0.3 mL
SUCCINYLCHOLINE		IV	2 mg/kg	3 mg	20 mg/mL	0.15 mL
SUCCINYLCHOLINE		IM	4 mg/kg	6 mg	20 mg/mL	0.3 mL
PROPOFOL		IV	3 mg/kg	4.5 mg	10 mg/mL	0.45 mL
ETOMIDATE	>10 y	IV	0.3 mg/kg	0.45 mg	2 mg/mL	0.225 mL
FENTANYL		IV	1 mcg/kg	1.5 mcg	50 mcg/mL	0.03 mL
FENTANYL		IN	2 mcg/kg	3 mcg	50 mcg/mL	0.06 mL
MORPHINE	<6 mo	IV/IM	0.05 mg/kg	0.075 mg	10 mg/mL	0.0075 mL
MORPHINE	>6 mo	IV/IM	0.1 mg/kg	0.15 mg	10 mg/mL	0.015 mL
TORADOL	>2-16 y	IV	0.5 mg/kg	0.75 mg	30 mg/mL	0.025 mL
TORADOL	>2-16 y	IM	1 mg/kg	1.5 mg	30 mg/mL	0.05 mL
ACETAMINOPHEN		PR	20 mg/kg	30 mg		
ACETAMINOPHEN	2-12 y	IV	15 mg/kg	22.5 mg	10 mg/mL	2.25 mL
CISATRACURIUM		IV	0.1 mg/kg	0.15 mg	2 mg/mL	0.075 mL
PANCURONIUM	<1 mo	IV	0.02 mg/kg	0.03 mg	1 mg/mL	0.03 mL
PANCURONIUM	>1 mo	IV	0.1 mg/kg	0.15 mg	1 mg/mL	0.15 mL
ROCURONIUM		IV	0.6 mg/kg	0.9 mg	10 mg/mL	0.09 mL
ROCURONIUM	RSI	IV	1.2 mg/kg	1.8 mg	10 mg/mL	0.18 mL
VECURONIUM		IV	0.1 mg/kg	0.15 mg	1 mg/mL	0.15 mL
GLYCOPYRROLATE	reversal	IV	0.007 mg/kg	0.0105 mg	0.2 mg/mL	0.0525 mL
NEOSTIGMINE		IV	0.07 mg/kg	0.105 mg	1 mg/mL	0.105 mL
DEXAMETHASONE		IV	0.25 mg/kg	0.375 mg	10 mg/mL	0.0375 mL
ONDANSETRON		IV	0.15 mg/kg	0.225 mg	2 mg/mL	0.1125 mL

additional pediatric drugs	route		dose	mg to pt	supplied	mL to give
PREMED/SEDATION; VAGOLYTIC/ANTISIALAGOGUE; GIVE IM 30-60 MIN PREOP						
ATROPINE	IM		0.02 mg/kg	0.4 mg	0.4 mg/mL	0.075 mL
GLYCOPYRROLATE	IM		0.004 mg/kg	0.006 mg	0.2 mg/mL	0.03
MIDAZOLAM	IM		0.1 mg/kg	0.15 mg	1 mg/mL	0.15 mL
DEXMEDETOMIDINE load dose	IV		0.5 mcg/kg	0.75 mcg	4 mcg/mL	0.1875 mL
INDUCTION						
KETAMINE	IV		2 mg/kg	3 mg	10 mg/mL	0.3 mL
KETAMINE	IM/PR		5 mg/kg	7.5 mg	10 mg/mL	0.75
OPIOIDS/NONOPIOIDS						
FENTANYL	IV	high dose	4 mcg/kg	6 mcg	50 mcg/mL	0.12 mL
FENTANYL	IV	cardiac	10 mcg/kg	15 mcg	50 mcg/mL	0.3
HYDROMORPHONE	IV/SQ	< 6 mo	0.005 mg/kg	0.0075 mg	10 mg/mL	0.00075 mL
HYDROMORPHONE	IV/SQ	> 6 mo	0.015 mg/kg	0.0225 mg	10 mg/mL	0.00225 mL
REMIFENTANIL	IV		0.5 mcg/kg	0.75 mcg	50 mcg/mL	0.015 mL
SUFENTANIL	IV		0.5 mcg/kg	0.75 mcg	50 mcg	0.015 mL
REVERSALS						
ATROPINE	IV		0.02 mg/kg	0.03 mg	0.4 mg/mL	0.075 mL
EDROPHONIUM	IV	neonate	0.1 mg single dose		10 mg/mL	0.01 mL
EDROPHONIUM	IV	> 2 mo	0.04 mg/kg	0.06 mg	10 mg/mL	0.006 mL
FLUMAZENIL	IV	> 1 y	0.01 mg/kg	0.015 mg	0.1 mg/mL	0.15
NALOXONE	IV/IM	< 5 y; < 20 kg	0.1 mg/kg	0.15 mg	0.4 mg/mL	0.375 mL
NALOXONE	IV/IM	> 5 y; > 20 kg	2 mg per dose		0.4 mg/mL	5 mL
NALOXONE	ETT		0.3 mg/kg	0.45 mg	0.4 mg/mL	1.125 mL

additional pediatric drugs		route	dose	mg to pt	supplied	mL to give
ANTIBIOTICS						
AMPICILLIN	<6 y	IV	50 mg/kg	75 mg		
AMPICILLIN	>6 y	IV	50 mg/kg	75 mg		
AMPICILLIN & SULBACTUM	>1 mo	IV	50 mg/kg	75 mg		
CEFAZOLIN		IV	25 mg/kg	37.5 mg		
CLINDAMYCIN		IV	10 mg/kg	15 mg		
ERTAPENEM	3 mo-12 y	IV	15 mg/kg	22.5 mg		
ERTAPENEM	>12 y	IV	1 Gm	per dose		
GENTAMICIN		IV	2 mg/kg	3 mg		
LEVOFLOXACIN		IV	10 mg/kg	15 mg		
METRONIDAZOLE		IV	10 mg/kg	15 mg		
PIPERACILLIN & TAZOBACTAM	<40 kg & 2-9 mo	IV	80 mg/kg	120 mg		
PIPERACILLIN & TAZOBACTAM	<40 kg & >9 mo	IV	100 mg/kg	150 mg		
PIPERACILLIN & TAZOBACTAM	>40 kg	IV	3.375 Gm per dose			
VANCOMYCIN		IV	15 mg/kg	22.5 mg		
ANTINAUSEA						
METOCLOPROMIDE		IV	0.2 mg/kg	0.3 mg	5 mg/mL	0.06 mL
DIPHENHYDRAMINE		IV/IM	1.25 mg/kg	1.875 mg	50 mg/mL	0.0375 mL
SCOPOLAMINE		IV/IM	6 mcg/kg	9 mcg	400 mcg/mL	0.0225 mL
MISCELLANEOUS MEDS						
AMINOCAPROIC ACID		IV	100 mg/kg	150 mg	250 mg/mL	0.6 mL
DESMOPRESSIN		IV/SQ	0.3 mcg/kg	0.45 mcg	4 mcg/mL	0.1125 mL
DEXAMETHASONE	croup	IV	0.6 mg/kg	0.9 mg	4 mg/mL	0.225 mL
HYDROCORTISONE		IV/IO	3 mg/kg	4.5 mg	100 mg/mL	0.045 mL

1.5 KG

Ventilation: trained rescuer	1 breath q 6-8 sec (8-10 breaths/minute) about 1 second/breath-visible chest rise; if intubated, continuous compressions without pause for ventilations
Pulse check	brachial/femoral
Compression	2-3 fingers–1 finger width below nipples *Wrap hands around chest if possible, compress with thumbs*
Depth	1.5 inch (4 cm) or at least 1/3 chest depth
Rate	at least 100 compressions per minute
Compress/vent ratio	30:2 with 1 or 2 rescuers
Foreign body obstruction	5 back blows at level of scapula, support head; alternate with 5 chest compressions
	Never perform a blind finger-sweep. Open the mouth and look for object; if you see it, remove it.

sync cardioversion	0.5 J/kg	0.75 J
repeat	1 J/kg	1.5 J
defibrillation	2 J/kg	3 J
repeat	4 J/kg	6 J

IV Bolus Drugs		dose	mg to pt	supplied	mL to give
ADENOSINE	IV	0.1 mg/kg	0.15 mg	3 mg/mL	0.05 mL
ADENOSINE repeat dose	IV	0.2 mg/kg	0.3 mg	3 mg/mL	0.10 mL
AMIODARONE	IV/IO	5 mg/kg	7.5 mg	50 mg/mL	0.15 mL
ATROPINE	IV/IM	0.02 mg/kg	0.03 mg	0.4 mg/mL	0.08 mL
ATROPINE	ETT	0.04 mg/kg	0.06 mg	0.4 mg/mL	0.15 mL
CALCIUM CHLORIDE	IV	20 mg/kg	30 mg	100 mg/mL	0.30 mL
CALCIUM GLUCONATE	IV/IO	60 mg/kg	90 mg	100 mg/mL	0.90 mL
DANTROLENE	IV	2.5 mg/kg	3.75 mg		
EPHEDRINE	IV	0.15 mg/kg	0.225 mg	10 mg/mL	0.02 mL
EPINEPHRINE (1:10,000)	IV/IO	0.01 mg/kg	0.015 mg	0.1 mg/mL	0.15 mL
EPINEPHRINE (1:1,000)	ETT	0.1 mg/kg	0.15 mg	1 mg/mL	0.15 mL
ESMOLOL	IV	0.5 mg/kg	0.75 mg	10 mg/mL	0.08 mL
LABETALOL	IV	0.2 mg/kg	0.3 mg	5 mg/mL	0.06 mL
LIDOCAINE	IV/IO	1 mg/kg	1.5 mg	20 mg/mL	0.08 mL
NEOSYNEPHRINE	IV	5 mcg/kg	7.5 mcg	100 mcg/mL	0.08 mL
ROMAZICON	IV	0.01 mg/kg	0.015 mg	0.1 mg/mL	0.15 mL
VASOPRESSIN	IV/IO	0.4 unit/kg	0.6 units	20 u/mL	0.03 mL

2 KG MAINTENANCE IV FLUIDS: 8 ML/HR

common pediatric drugs		route	dose	mg to pt	supplied	mL to give
ATROPINE	vagolytic	IV	0.02 mg/kg	0.04 mg	0.4 mg/mL	0.1 mL
GLYCOPYRROLATE	vagolytic	IV	0.004 mg/kg	0.008 mg	0.2 mg/mL	0.04 mL
MIDAZOLAM		IV	0.05 mg/kg	0.1 mg	1 mg/mL	0.1 mL
MIDAZOLAM		PO	0.5 mg/kg	1 mg	1 mg/mL	1 mL
MIDAZOLAM		IN	0.2 mg/kg	0.4 mg	1 mg/mL	0.4 mL
SUCCINYLCHOLINE		IV	2 mg/kg	4 mg	20 mg/mL	0.2 mL
SUCCINYLCHOLINE		IM	4 mg/kg	8 mg	20 mg/mL	0.4 mL
PROPOFOL		IV	3 mg/kg	6 mg	10 mg/mL	0.6 mL
ETOMIDATE	>10 y	IV	0.3 mg/kg	0.6 mg	2 mg/mL	0.3 mL
FENTANYL		IV	1 mcg/kg	2 mcg	50 mcg/mL	0.04 mL
FENTANYL		IN	2 mcg/kg	4 mcg	50 mcg/mL	0.08 mL
MORPHINE	<6 mo	IV/IM	0.05 mg/kg	0.1 mg	10 mg/mL	0.01 mL
MORPHINE	>6 mo	IV/IM	0.1 mg/kg	0.2 mg	10 mg/mL	0.02 mL
TORADOL	>2-16 y	IV	0.5 mg/kg	1 mg	30 mg/mL	0.033 mL
TORADOL	>2-16 y	IM	1 mg/kg	2 mg	30 mg/mL	0.067 mL
ACETAMINOPHEN		PR	20 mg/kg	40 mg		
ACETAMINOPHEN	2-12 y	IV	15 mg/kg	30 mg	10 mg/mL	3 mL
CISATRACURIUM		IV	0.1 mg/kg	0.2 mg	2 mg/mL	0.1 mL
PANCURONIUM	<1 mo	IV	0.02 mg/kg	0.04 mg	1 mg/mL	0.04 mL
PANCURONIUM	>1 mo	IV	0.1 mg/kg	0.2 mg	1 mg/mL	0.2 mL
ROCURONIUM		IV	0.6 mg/kg	1.2 mg	10 mg/mL	0.12 mL
ROCURONIUM	RSI	IV	1.2 mg/kg	2.4 mg	10 mg/mL	0.24 mL
VECURONIUM		IV	0.1 mg/kg	0.2 mg	1 mg/mL	0.2 mL
GLYCOPYRROLATE	reversal	IV	0.007 mg/kg	0.014 mg	0.2 mg/mL	0.07 mL
NEOSTIGMINE		IV	0.07 mg/kg	0.14 mg	1 mg/mL	0.14 mL
DEXAMETHASONE		IV	0.25 mg/kg	0.5 mg	10 mg/mL	0.05 mL
ONDANSETRON		IV	0.15 mg/kg	0.3 mg	2 mg/mL	0.15 mL

additional pediatric drugs	route	dose	mg to pt	supplied	mL to give
PREMED/SEDATION; VAGOLYTIC/ANTISIALAGOGUE; GIVE IM 30-60 MIN PREOP					
ATROPINE	IM	0.02 mg/kg	0.04 mg	0.4 mg/mL	0.1 mL
GLYCOPYRROLATE	IM	0.004 mg/kg	0.008 mg	0.2 mg/mL	0.04 mL
MIDAZOLAM	IM	0.1 mg/kg	0.2 mg	1 mg/mL	0.2 mL
DEXMEDETOMIDINE load dose	IV	0.5 mcg/kg	1 mcg	4 mcg/mL	0.25 mL
INDUCTION					
KETAMINE	IV	2 mg/kg	4 mg	10 mg/mL	0.4 mL
KETAMINE	IM/PR	5 mg/kg	10 mg	10 mg/mL	1 mL
OPIOIDS/NONOPIOIDS					
FENTANYL	IV	4 mcg/kg	8 mcg	50 mcg/mL	0.16 mL
FENTANYL high dose	cardiac	10 mcg/kg	20 mcg	50 mcg/mL	0.4 mL
HYDROMORPHONE	IV/SQ	0.005 mg/kg	0.01 mg	10 mg/mL	0.001 mL
HYDROMORPHONE > 6 mo	IV/SQ	0.015 mg/kg	0.03 mg	10 mg/mL	0.003 mL
REMIFENTANIL	IV	0.5 mcg/kg	1 mcg	50 mcg/mL	0.02 mL
SUFENTANIL	IV	0.5 mcg/kg	1 mcg	50 mcg/mL	0.02 mL
REVERSALS					
ATROPINE	IV	0.02 mg/kg	0.04 mg	0.4 mg/mL	0.1 mL
EDROPHONIUM neonate	IV	0.1 mg single dose		10 mg/mL	0.01 mL
EDROPHONIUM > 2 mo	IV	0.04 mg/kg	0.08 mg	10 mg/mL	0.008 mL
FLUMAZENIL < 1 y	IV	0.01 mg/kg	0.02 mg	0.1 mg/mL	0.2 mL
NALOXONE < 5 y; < 20 kg	IV/IM	0.1 mg/kg	0.2 mg	0.4 mg/mL	0.5 mL
NALOXONE > 5 y; > 20 kg	IV/IM	2 mg per dose		0.4 mg/mL	5 mL
NALOXONE	ETT	0.3 mg/kg	0.6 mg	0.4 mg/mL	1.5 mL

additional pediatric drugs		route	dose	mg to pt	supplied	mL to give
ANTIBIOTICS						
AMPICILLIN	<6 y	IV	50 mg/kg	100 mg		
AMPICILLIN	>6 y	IV	50 mg/kg	100 mg		
AMPICILLIN & SULBACTUM	>1 mo	IV	50 mg/kg	100 mg		
CEFAZOLIN		IV	25 mg/kg	50 mg		
CLINDAMYCIN		IV	10 mg/kg	20 mg		
ERTAPENEM	3 mo-12 y	IV	15 mg/kg	30 mg		
ERTAPENEM	>12 y	IV	1 Gm	per dose		
GENTAMICIN		IV	2 mg/kg	4 mg		
LEVOFLOXACIN		IV	10 mg/kg	20 mg		
METRONIDAZOLE		IV	10 mg/kg	20 mg		
PIPERACILLIN & TAZOBACTAM	<40 kg & 2-9 mo	IV	80 mg/kg	160 mg		
PIPERACILLIN & TAZOBACTAM	<40 kg & >9 mo	IV	100 mg/kg	200 mg		
PIPERACILLIN & TAZOBACTAM	>40 kg	IV	3.375 Gm per dose			
VANCOMYCIN		IV	15 mg/kg	30 mg		
ANTINAUSEA						
METOCLOPROMIDE		IV	0.2 mg/kg	0.4 mg	5 mg/mL	0.08 mL
DIPHENHYDRAMINE		IV/IM	1.25 mg/kg	2.5 mg	50 mg/mL	0.05 mL
SCOPOLAMINE		IV/IM	6 mcg/kg	12 mcg	400 mcg/mL	0.03 mL
MISCELLANEOUS MEDS						
AMINOCAPROIC ACID		IV	100 mg/kg	200 mg	250 mg/mL	0.8 mL
DESMOPRESSIN		IV/SQ	0.3 mcg/kg	0.6 mcg	4 mcg/mL	0.15 mL
DEXAMETHASONE	croup	IV	0.6 mg/kg	1.2 mg	4 mg/mL	0.3 mL
HYDROCORTISONE		IV/IO	3 mg/kg	6 mg	100 mg/mL	0.06 mL

2 KG

Ventilation: trained rescuer	1 breath q 6-8 sec (8-10 breaths/minute) about 1 second/breath-visible chest rise; if intubated, continuous compressions without pause for ventilations
Pulse check	brachial/femoral
Compression	2-3 fingers—1 finger width below nipples; Wrap hands around chest if possible, compress with thumbs
Depth	1.5 inch (4 cm) or at least 1/3 chest depth
Rate	at least 100 compressions per minute
Compress/vent ratio	30:2 with 1 or 2 rescuers
Foreign body obstruction	5 back blows at level of scapula, support head; alternate with 5 chest compressions. Never perform a blind finger-sweep. Open the mouth and look for object; if you see it, remove it.

	dose	J to pt
sync cardioversion	0.5 J/kg	1 J
defibrillation	2 J/kg	2 J
repeat	4 J/kg	4 J
repeat	4 J/kg	8 J

IV Bolus Drugs		dose	mg to pt	supplied	mL to give
ADENOSINE	IV	0.1 mg/kg	0.2 mg	3 mg/mL	0.07 mL
ADENOSINE repeat dose	IV	0.2 mg/kg	0.4 mg	3 mg/mL	0.13 mL
AMIODARONE	IV/IO	5 mg/kg	10 mg	50 mg/mL	0.20 mL
ATROPINE	IV/IM	0.02 mg/kg	0.04 mg	0.4 mg/mL	0.10 mL
ATROPINE	ETT	0.04 mg/kg	0.08 mg	0.4 mg/mL	0.20 mL
CALCIUM CHLORIDE	IV	20 mg/kg	40 mg	100 mg/mL	0.40 mL
CALCIUM GLUCONATE	IV/IO	60 mg/kg	120 mg	100 mg/mL	1.20 mL
DANTROLENE	IV	2.5 mg/kg	5 mg		
EPHEDRINE	IV	0.15 mg/kg	0.3 mg	10 mg/mL	0.03 mL
EPINEPHRINE (1:10,000)	IV/IO	0.01 mg/kg	0.02 mg	0.1 mg/mL	0.20 mL
EPINEPHRINE (1:1,000)	ETT	0.1 mg/kg	0.2 mg	1 mg/mL	0.20 mL
ESMOLOL	IV	0.5 mg/kg	1 mg	10 mg/mL	0.10 mL
LABETALOL	IV	0.2 mg/kg	0.4 mg	5 mg/mL	0.08 mL
LIDOCAINE	IV/IO	1 mg/kg	2 mg	20 mg/mL	0.10 mL
NEOSYNEPHRINE	IV	5 mcg/kg	10 mcg	100 mcg/mL	0.10 mL
ROMAZICON	IV	0.01 mg/kg	0.02 mg	0.1 mg/mL	0.20 mL
VASOPRESSIN	IV/IO	0.4 unit/kg	0.8 units	20 u/mL	0.04 mL

3 KG MAINTENANCE IV FLUIDS: 12 ML/HR

common pediatric drugs		route	dose	mg to pt	supplied	mL to give
ATROPINE	vagolytic	IV	0.02 mg/kg	0.06 mg	0.4 mg/mL	0.15 mL
GLYCOPYRROLATE	vagolytic	IV	0.004 mg/kg	0.012 mg	0.2 mg/mL	0.06 mL
MIDAZOLAM		IV	0.05 mg/kg	0.15 mg	1 mg/mL	0.15 mL
MIDAZOLAM		PO	0.5 mg/kg	1.5 mg	1 mg/mL	1.5 mL
MIDAZOLAM		IN	0.2 mg/kg	0.6 mg	1 mg/mL	0.6 mL
SUCCINYLCHOLINE		IV	2 mg/kg	6 mg	20 mg/mL	0.3 mL
SUCCINYLCHOLINE		IM	4 mg/kg	12 mg	20 mg/mL	0.6 mL
PROPOFOL		IV	3 mg/kg	9 mg	10 mg/mL	0.9 mL
ETOMIDATE	>10 y	IV	0.3 mg/kg	0.9 mg	2 mg/mL	0.45 mL
FENTANYL		IV	1 mcg/kg	3 mcg	50 mcg/mL	0.06 mL
FENTANYL		IN	2 mcg/kg	6 mcg	50 mcg/mL	0.12 mL
MORPHINE	<6 mo	IV/IM	0.05 mg/kg	0.15 mg	10 mg/mL	0.015 mL
MORPHINE	>6 mo	IV/IM	0.1 mg/kg	0.3 mg	10 mg/mL	0.03 mL
TORADOL	>2-16 y	IV	0.5 mg/kg	1.5 mg	30 mg/mL	0.05 mL
TORADOL	>2-16 y	IM	1 mg/kg	3 mg	30 mg/mL	0.1 mL
ACETAMINOPHEN		PR	20 mg/kg	60 mg		
ACETAMINOPHEN	2-12 y	IV	15 mg/kg	45 mg	10 mg/mL	4.5 mL
CISATRACURIUM		IV	0.1 mg/kg	0.3 mg	2 mg/mL	0.15 mL
PANCURONIUM	<1 mo	IV	0.02 mg/kg	0.06 mg	1 mg/mL	0.06 mL
PANCURONIUM	>1 mo	IV	0.1 mg/kg	0.3 mg	1 mg/mL	0.3 mL
ROCURONIUM		IV	0.6 mg/kg	1.8 mg	10 mg/mL	0.18 mL
ROCURONIUM	RSI	IV	1.2 mg/kg	3.6 mg	10 mg/mL	0.36 mL
VECURONIUM		IV	0.1 mg/kg	0.3 mg	1 mg/mL	0.3 mL
GLYCOPYRROLATE	reversal	IV	0.007 mg/kg	0.021 mg	0.2 mg/mL	0.105 mL
NEOSTIGMINE		IV	0.07 mg/kg	0.21 mg	1 mg/mL	0.21 mL
DEXAMETHASONE		IV	0.25 mg/kg	0.75 mg	10 mg/mL	0.075 mL
ONDANSETRON		IV	0.15 mg/kg	0.45 mg	2 mg/mL	0.225 mL

additional pediatric drugs	route	dose	mg to pt	supplied	mL to give
PREMED/SEDATION; VAGOLYTIC/ANTISIALAGOGUE; GIVE IM 30-60 MIN PREOP					
ATROPINE	IM	0.02 mg/kg	0.06 mg	0.4 mg/mL	0.15 mL
GLYCOPYRROLATE	IM	0.004 mg/kg	0.009 mg	0.2 mg/mL	0.045 mL
MIDAZOLAM	IM	0.1 mg/kg	0.3 mg	1 mg/mL	0.3 mL
DEXMEDETOMIDINE load dose	IV	0.5 mcg/kg	1 mcg	4 mcg/mL	0.25 mL
INDUCTION					
KETAMINE	IV	2 mg/kg	6 mg	10 mg/mL	0.6 mL
KETAMINE	IM/PR	5 mg/kg	15 mg	10 mg/mL	1.5 mL
OPIOIDS/NONOPIOIDS					
FENTANYL	IV	high dose	4 mcg/kg	12 mcg	50 mcg/mL	0.24 mL
FENTANYL	IV	cardiac	10 mcg/kg	30 mcg	50 mcg/mL	0.6 mL
HYDROMORPHONE	IV/SQ	< 6 mo	0.005 mg/kg	0.015 mg	10 mg/mL	0.0015 mL
HYDROMORPHONE	IV/SQ	> 6 mo	0.015 mg/kg	0.045 mg	10 mg/mL	0.0045 mL
REMIFENTANIL	IV	0.5 mcg/kg	1 mcg	50 mcg/mL	0.02 mL
SUFENTANIL	IV	0.5 mcg/kg	1.5 mcg	50 mcg/mL	0.03 mL
REVERSALS					
ATROPINE	IV	0.02 mg/kg	0.06 mg	0.4 mg/mL	0.15 mL
EDROPHONIUM	IV	neonate	0.1 mg single dose	10 mg/mL	0.01 mL
EDROPHONIUM	IV	> 2 mo	0.04 mg/kg	0.12 mg	10 mg/mL	0.012 mL
FLUMAZENIL	IV	>1 y	0.01 mg/kg	0.03 mg	0.1 mg/mL	0.3 mL
NALOXONE	IV/IM	< 5 y; < 20 kg	0.1 mg/kg	0.3 mg	0.4 mg/mL	0.75 mL
NALOXONE	IM	> 5 y; > 20 kg	2 mg per dose	0.4 mg/mL	5 mL
NALOXONE	ETT	0.3 mg/kg	0.9 mg	0.4 mg/mL	2.25 mL

additional pediatric drugs		route	dose	mg to pt	supplied	mL to give
ANTIBIOTICS						
AMPICILLIN	<6 y	IV	50 mg/kg	150 mg		
AMPICILLIN	>6 y	IV	50 mg/kg	150 mg		
AMPICILLIN & SULBACTUM	>1 mo	IV	50 mg/kg	150 mg		
CEFAZOLIN		IV	25 mg/kg	75 mg		
CLINDAMYCIN		IV	10 mg/kg	30 mg		
ERTAPENEM	3 mo-12 y	IV	15 mg/kg	45 mg		
ERTAPENEM	>12 y	IV	1 Gm	per dose		
GENTAMICIN		IV	2 mg/kg	6 mg		
LEVOFLOXACIN		IV	10 mg/kg	30 mg		
METRONIDAZOLE		IV	10 mg/kg	30 mg		
PIPERACILLIN & TAZOBACTAM	<40 kg & 2-9 mo	IV	80 mg/kg	240 mg		
PIPERACILLIN & TAZOBACTAM	<40 kg & >9 mo	IV	100 mg/kg	300 mg		
PIPERACILLIN & TAZOBACTAM	>40 kg	IV	3.375 Gm per dose			
VANCOMYCIN		IV	15 mg/kg	45 mg		
ANTINAUSEA						
METOCLOPROMIDE		IV	0.2 mg/kg	0.6 mg	5 mg/mL	0.12 mL
DIPHENHYDRAMINE		IV/IM	1.25 mg/kg	3.75 mg	50 mg/mL	0.075 mL
SCOPOLAMINE		IV/IM	6 mcg/kg	18 mcg	400 mcg/mL	0.045 mL
MISCELLANEOUS MEDS						
AMINOCAPROIC ACID		IV	100 mg/kg	300 mg	250 mg/mL	1.2 mL
DESMOPRESSIN		IV/SQ	0.3 mcg/kg	0.9 mcg	4 mcg/mL	0.225 mL
DEXAMETHASONE	croup	IV	0.6 mg/kg	1.8 mg	4 mg/mL	0.45 mL
HYDROCORTISONE		IV/IO	3 mg/kg	9 mg	100 mg/mL	0.09 mL

3 KG

Ventilation:	1 breath q 6-8 sec (8-10 breaths/minute) about 1 second/
trained rescuer	breath-visible chest rise; if intubated, continuous compressions without pause for ventilations
Pulse check	brachial/femoral
Compression	2-3 fingers—1 finger width below nipples
	Wrap hands around chest if possible, compress with thumbs
Depth	1.5 inch (4 cm) or at least 1/3 chest depth
Rate	at least 100 compressions per minute
Compress/vent ratio	30:2 with 1 or 2 rescuers
Foreign body obstruction	5 back blows at level of scapula, support head; alternate with 5 chest compressions
	Never perform a blind finger-sweep. Open the mouth and look for object; if you see it, remove it.

sync cardioversion	0.5 J/kg	1.5 J
	1 J/kg	3 J
defibrillation	2 J/kg	6 J
repeat	4 J/kg	12 J

IV Bolus Drugs	dose	mg to pt	supplied	mL to give
ADENOSINE	IV	0.1 mg/kg	0.3 mg	3 mg/mL	0.10 mL
ADENOSINE repeat dose	IV	0.2 mg/kg	0.6 mg	3 mg/mL	0.20 mL
AMIODARONE	IV/IO	5 mg/kg	15 mg	50 mg/mL	0.30 mL
ATROPINE	IV/IM	0.02 mg/kg	0.06 mg	0.4 mg/mL	0.15 mL
ATROPINE	ETT	0.04 mg/kg	0.12 mg	0.4 mg/mL	0.30 mL
CALCIUM CHLORIDE	IV	20 mg/kg	60 mg	100 mg/mL	0.60 mL
CALCIUM GLUCONATE	IV/IO	60 mg/kg	180 mg	100 mg/mL	1.80 mL
DANTROLENE	IV	2.5 mg/kg	7.5 mg		
EPHEDRINE	IV	0.15 mg/kg	0.45 mg	10 mg/mL	0.05 mL
EPINEPHRINE (1:10,000)	IV/IO	0.01 mg/kg	0.03 mg	0.1 mg/mL	0.30 mL
EPINEPHRINE (1:1,000)	ETT	0.1 mg/kg	0.3 mg	1 mg/mL	0.30 mL
ESMOLOL	IV	0.5 mg/kg	1.5 mg	10 mg/mL	0.15 mL
LABETALOL	IV	0.2 mg/kg	0.6 mg	5 mg/mL	0.12 mL
LIDOCAINE	IV/IO	1 mg/kg	3 mg	20 mg/mL	0.15 mL
NEOSYNEPHRINE	IV	5 mcg/kg	15 mcg	100 mcg/mL	0.15 mL
ROMAZICON	IV	0.01 mg/kg	0.03 mg	0.1 mg/mL	0.30 mL
VASOPRESSIN	IV/IO	0.4 unit/kg	1.2 units	20 u/mL	0.06 mL

4 KG MAINTENANCE IV FLUIDS: 16 ML/HR

common pediatric drugs		route	dose	mg to pt	supplied	mL to give
ATROPINE	vagolytic	IV	0.02 mg/kg	0.08 mg	0.4 mg/mL	0.2 mL
GLYCOPYRROLATE	vagolytic	IV	0.004 mg/kg	0.016 mg	0.2 mg/mL	0.08 mL
MIDAZOLAM		IV	0.05 mg/kg	0.2 mg	1 mg/mL	0.2 mL
MIDAZOLAM		PO	0.5 mg/kg	2 mg	1 mg/mL	2 mL
MIDAZOLAM		IN	0.2 mg/kg	0.8 mg	1 mg/mL	0.8 mL
SUCCINYLCHOLINE		IV	2 mg/kg	8 mg	20 mg/mL	0.4 mL
SUCCINYLCHOLINE		IM	4 mg/kg	16 mg	20 mg/mL	0.8 mL
PROPOFOL		IV	3 mg/kg	12 mg	10 mg/mL	1.2 mL
ETOMIDATE	>10 y	IV	0.3 mg/kg	1.2 mg	2 mg/mL	0.6 mL
FENTANYL		IV	1 mcg/kg	4 mcg	50 mcg/mL	0.08 mL
FENTANYL		IN	2 mcg/kg	8 mcg	50 mcg/mL	0.16 mL
MORPHINE	<6 mo	IV/IM	0.05 mg/kg	0.2 mg	10 mg/mL	0.02 mL
MORPHINE	>6 mo	IV/IM	0.1 mg/kg	0.4 mg	10 mg/mL	0.04 mL
TORADOL	>2-16 y	IV	0.5 mg/kg	2 mg	30 mg/mL	0.0667 mL
TORADOL	>2-16 y	IM	1 mg/kg	4 mg	30 mg/mL	0.1333 mL
ACETAMINOPHEN		PR	20 mg/kg	80 mg		
ACETAMINOPHEN	2-12 y	IV	15 mg/kg	60 mg	10 mg/mL	6 mL
CISATRACURIUM		IV	0.1 mg/kg	0.4 mg	2 mg/mL	0.2 mL
PANCURONIUM	<1 mo	IV	0.02 mg/kg	0.08 mg	1 mg/mL	0.08 mL
PANCURONIUM	>1 mo	IV	0.1 mg/kg	0.4 mg	1 mg/mL	0.4 mL
ROCURONIUM		IV	0.6 mg/kg	2.4 mg	10 mg/mL	0.24 mL
ROCURONIUM	RSI	IV	1.2 mg/kg	4.8 mg	10 mg/mL	0.48 mL
VECURONIUM		IV	0.1 mg/kg	0.4 mg	1 mg/mL	0.4 mL
GLYCOPYRROLATE	reversal	IV	0.007 mg/kg	0.028 mg	0.2 mg/mL	0.14 mL
NEOSTIGMINE		IV	0.07 mg/kg	0.28 mg	1 mg/mL	0.28 mL
DEXAMETHASONE		IV	0.25 mg/kg	1 mg	10 mg/mL	0.1 mL
ONDANSETRON		IV	0.15 mg/kg	0.6 mg	2 mg/mL	0.3 mL

additional pediatric drugs	route	dose	mg to pt	supplied	mL to give
PREMED/SEDATION; VAGOLYTIC/ANTISIALAGOGUE; GIVE IM 30-60 MIN PREOP					
ATROPINE	IV	0.02 mg/kg	0.08 mg	0.4 mg/mL	0.2 mL
GLYCOPYRROLATE	IM	0.004 mg/kg	0.000 600 mg	0.2 mg/mL	0.045 mL
MIDAZOLAM	IM	0.1 mg/kg	0.4 mg	1 mg/mL	0.4 mL
DEXMEDETOMIDINE load dose	IV	0.5 mcg/kg	1 mcg	4 mcg/mL	0.25 mL
INDUCTION					
KETAMINE	IV	2 mg/kg	8 mg	10 mg/mL	0.8 mL
KETAMINE	IM/PR	5 mg/kg	20 mg	10 mg/mL	2 mL
OPIOIDS/NONOPIOIDS					
FENTANYL	IV	4 mcg/kg	16 mcg	50 mcg/mL	0.32 mL
FENTANYL	IV cardiac	10 mcg/kg	40 mcg	50 mcg/mL	0.8 mL
HYDROMORPHONE	IV/SQ	< 6 mo 0.005 mg/kg	0.02 mg	10 mg/mL	0.002 mL
HYDROMORPHONE	IV/SQ	> 6 mo 0.015 mg/kg	0.06 mg	10 mg/mL	0.006 mL
REMIFENTANIL	IV	0.5 mcg/kg	1 mcg	50 mcg/mL	0.02 mL
SUFENTANIL	IV	0.5 mcg/kg	2 mcg	50 mcg/mL	0.04 mL
REVERSALS					
ATROPINE	IV	0.02 mg/kg	0.08 mg	0.4 mg/mL	0.2 mL
EDROPHONIUM	IV neonate	0.1 mg single dose		10 mg/mL	0.01 mL
EDROPHONIUM	IV > 2 mo	0.04 mg/kg	0.16 mg	10 mg/mL	0.016 mL
FLUMAZENIL	IV > 1 y	0.01 mg/kg	0.04 mg	0.1 mg/mL	0.4 mL
NALOXONE	IV/IM < 5 y; < 20 kg	0.1 mg/kg	0.4 mg	0.4 mg/mL	1 mL
NALOXONE	IV/IM > 5 y; > 20 kg	2 mg per dose		0.4 mg/mL	5 mL
NALOXONE	ETT	0.3 mg/kg	1.2 mg	0.4 mg/mL	3 mL

additional pediatric drugs		route	dose	mg to pt	supplied	mL to give
ANTIBIOTICS						
AMPICILLIN	<6 y	IV	50 mg/kg	200 mg		
AMPICILLIN	>6 y	IV	50 mg/kg	200 mg		
AMPICILLIN & SULBACTUM	>1 mo	IV	50 mg/kg	200 mg		
CEFAZOLIN		IV	25 mg/kg	100 mg		
CLINDAMYCIN		IV	10 mg/kg	40 mg		
ERTAPENEM	3 mo-12 y	IV	15 mg/kg	60 mg		
ERTAPENEM	>12 y	IV	1 Gm	per dose		
GENTAMICIN		IV	2 mg/kg	8 mg		
LEVOFLOXACIN		IV	10 mg/kg	40 mg		
METRONIDAZOLE		IV	10 mg/kg	40 mg		
PIPERACILLIN & TAZOBACTAM	<40 kg & 2-9 mo	IV	80 mg/kg	320 mg		
PIPERACILLIN & TAZOBACTAM	<40 kg & >9 mo	IV	100 mg/kg	400 mg		
PIPERACILLIN & TAZOBACTAM	>40 kg	IV	3.375 Gm per dose			
VANCOMYCIN		IV	15 mg/kg	60 mg		
ANTINAUSEA						
METOCLOPROMIDE		IV	0.2 mg/kg	0.8 mg	5 mg/mL	0.16 mL
DIPHENHYDRAMINE		IV/IM	1.25 mg/kg	5 mg	50 mg/mL	0.1 mL
SCOPOLAMINE		IV/IM	6 mcg/kg	24 mcg	400 mcg/mL	0.06 mL
MISCELLANEOUS MEDS						
AMINOCAPROIC ACID		IV	100 mg/kg	400 mg	250 mg/mL	1.6 mL
DESMOPRESSIN		IV/SQ	0.3 mcg/kg	1.2 mcg	4 mcg/mL	0.3 mL
DEXAMETHASONE	croup	IV	0.6 mg/kg	2.4 mg	4 mg/mL	0.6 mL
HYDROCORTISONE		IV/IO	3 mg/kg	12 mg	100 mg/mL	0.12 mL

4 KG

Ventilation: trained rescuer:	1 breath q 6-8 sec (8-10 breaths/minute) about 1 second/ breath-visible chest rise; if intubated, continuous compressions without pause for ventilations
Pulse check	brachial/femoral
Compression	2-3 fingers–1 finger width below nipples *Wrap hands around chest if possible, compress with thumbs*
Depth	1.5 inch (4 cm) or at least 1/3 chest depth
Rate	at least 100 compressions per minute
Compress/vent ratio	30:2 with 1 or 2 rescuers
Foreign body obstruction	5 back blows at level of scapula, support head; alternate with 5 chest compressions *Never perform a blind finger-sweep. Open the mouth and look for object; if you see it, remove it.*

sync cardioversion	0.5 J/kg	2 J
repeat	1 J/kg	4 J
defibrillation	2 J/kg	8 J
repeat	4 J/kg	16 J

IV Bolus Drugs		dose	mg to pt	supplied	mL to give
ADENOSINE	IV	0.1 mg/kg	0.4 mg	3 mg/mL	0.13 mL
repeat dose	IV	0.2 mg/kg	0.8 mg	3 mg/mL	0.27 mL
AMIODARONE	IV/IO	5 mg/kg	20 mg	50 mg/mL	0.40 mL
ATROPINE	ETT	0.04 mg/kg	0.16 mg	0.4 mg/mL	0.40 mL
	IV/IM	0.02 mg/kg	0.08 mg		0.20 mL
CALCIUM CHLORIDE	IV	20 mg/kg	80 mg	100 mg/mL	0.80 mL
CALCIUM GLUCONATE	IV/IO	60 mg/kg	240 mg	100 mg/mL	2.40 mL
DANTROLENE	IV	2.5 mg/kg	10 mg		
EPHEDRINE	IV	0.15 mg/kg	0.6 mg	10 mg/mL	0.06 mL
EPINEPHRINE (1:10,000)	IV/IO	0.01 mg/kg	0.04 mg	0.1 mg/mL	0.40 mL
EPINEPHRINE (1:1,000)	ETT	0.1 mg/kg	0.4 mg	1 mg/mL	0.40 mL
ESMOLOL	IV	0.5 mg/kg	2 mg	10 mg/mL	0.20 mL
LABETALOL	IV	0.2 mg/kg	0.8 mg	5 mg/mL	0.16 mL
LIDOCAINE	IV/IO	1 mg/kg	4 mg	20 mg/mL	0.20 mL
NEOSYNEPHRINE	IV	5 mcg/kg	20 mcg	100 mcg/mL	0.20 mL
ROMAZICON	IV	0.01 mg/kg	0.04 mg	0.1 mg/mL	0.40 mL
VASOPRESSIN	IV/IO	0.4 unit/kg	1.6 units	20 u/mL	0.08 mL

5 KG MAINTENANCE IV FLUIDS: 20 ML/HR

common pediatric drugs		route	dose	mg to pt	supplied	mL to give
ATROPINE	vagolytic	IV	0.02 mg/kg	0.1 mg	0.4 mg/mL	0.25 mL
GLYCOPYRROLATE	vagolytic	IV	0.004 mg/kg	0.02 mg	0.2 mg/mL	0.1 mL
MIDAZOLAM		IV	0.05 mg/kg	0.25 mg	1 mg/mL	0.25 mL
MIDAZOLAM		PO	0.5 mg/kg	2.5 mg	1 mg/mL	2.5 mL
MIDAZOLAM		IN	0.2 mg/kg	1 mg	1 mg/mL	1 mL
SUCCINYLCHOLINE		IV	2 mg/kg	10 mg	20 mg/mL	0.5 mL
SUCCINYLCHOLINE		IM	4 mg/kg	20 mg	20 mg/mL	1 mL
PROPOFOL		IV	3 mg/kg	15 mg	10 mg/mL	1.5 mL
ETOMIDATE	>10 y	IV	0.3 mg/kg	1.5 mg	2 mg/mL	0.75 mL
FENTANYL		IV	1 mcg/kg	5 mcg	50 mcg/mL	0.1 mL
FENTANYL		IN	2 mcg/kg	10 mcg	50 mcg/mL	0.2 mL
MORPHINE	<6 mo	IV/IM	0.05 mg/kg	0.25 mg	10 mg/mL	0.025 mL
MORPHINE	>6 mo	IV/IM	0.1 mg/kg	0.5 mg	10 mg/mL	0.05 mL
TORADOL	>2-16 y	IV	0.5 mg/kg	2.5 mg	30 mg/mL	0.0833 mL
TORADOL	>2-16 y	IM	1 mg/kg	5 mg	30 mg/mL	0.1667 mL
ACETAMINOPHEN		PR	20 mg/kg	100 mg		
ACETAMINOPHEN	2-12 y	IV	15 mg/kg	75 mg	10 mg/mL	7.5 mL
CISATRACURIUM		IV	0.1 mg/kg	0.5 mg	2 mg/mL	0.25 mL
PANCURONIUM	<1 mo	IV	0.02 mg/kg	0.1 mg	1 mg/mL	0.1 mL
PANCURONIUM	>1 mo	IV	0.1 mg/kg	0.5 mg	1 mg/mL	0.5 mL
ROCURONIUM		IV	0.6 mg/kg	3 mg	10 mg/mL	0.3 mL
ROCURONIUM	RSI	IV	1.2 mg/kg	6 mg	10 mg/mL	0.6 mL
VECURONIUM		IV	0.1 mg/kg	0.5 mg	1 mg/mL	0.5 mL
GLYCOPYRROLATE	reversal	IV	0.007 mg/kg	0.035 mg	0.2 mg/mL	0.175 mL
NEOSTIGMINE		IV	0.07 mg/kg	0.35 mg	1 mg/mL	0.35 mL
DEXAMETHASONE		IV	0.25 mg/kg	1.25 mg	10 mg/mL	0.125 mL
ONDANSETRON		IV	0.15 mg/kg	0.75 mg	2 mg/mL	0.375 mL

additional pediatric drugs	route	dose	mg to pt	supplied	mL to give
PREMED/SEDATION; VAGOLYTIC/ANTISIALAGOGUE; GIVE IM 30-60 MIN PREOP					
ATROPINE	IM	0.02 mg/kg	0.1 mg	0.4 mg/mL	0.25 mL
GLYCOPYRROLATE	IM	0.004 mg/kg	0.009 mg	0.2 mg/mL	0.045 mL
MIDAZOLAM	IM	0.1 mg/kg	0.5 mg	1 mg/mL	0.5 mL
DEXMEDETOMIDINE	IV load dose	0.5 mcg/kg	1 mcg	4 mcg/mL	0.25 mL
INDUCTION					
KETAMINE	IV	2 mg/kg	10 mg	10 mg/mL	1 mL
KETAMINE	IM/PR	5 mg/kg	25 mg	10 mg/mL	2.5 mL
OPIOIDS/NONOPIOIDS					
FENTANYL	IV high dose	4 mcg/kg	20 mcg	50 mcg/mL	0.4 mL
FENTANYL	IV cardiac	10 mcg/kg	50 mcg	50 mcg/mL	1 mL
HYDROMORPHONE	IV/SQ < 6 mo	0.005 mg/kg	0.025 mg	10 mg/mL	0.0025 mL
HYDROMORPHONE	IV/SQ > 6 mo	0.015 mg/kg	0.075 mg	10 mg/mL	0.0075 mL
REMIFENTANIL	IV	0.5 mcg/kg	1 mcg	50 mcg/mL	0.02 mL
SUFENTANIL	IV	0.5 mcg/kg	2.5 mcg	50 mcg/mL	0.05 mL
REVERSALS					
ATROPINE	IV	0.02 mg/kg	0.1 mg	0.4 mg/mL	0.25 mL
EDROPHONIUM	IV neonate		0.1 mg single dose	10 mg/mL	0.01 mL
EDROPHONIUM	IV > 2 mo	0.04 mg/kg	0.2 mg	10 mg/mL	0.02 mL
FLUMAZENIL	IV > 1 y	0.01 mg/kg	0.05 mg	0.1 mg/mL	0.5 mL
NALOXONE	IV/IM < 5 y; < 20 kg	0.1 mg/kg	0.5 mg	0.4 mg/mL	1.25 mL
NALOXONE	IV/IM > 5 y; > 20 kg		2 mg per dose	0.4 mg/mL	5 mL
NALOXONE	ETT	0.3 mg/kg	1.5 mg	0.4 mg/mL	3.75 mL

additional pediatric drugs		route	dose	mg to pt	supplied	mL to give
ANTIBIOTICS						
AMPICILLIN	<6 y	IV	50 mg/kg	250 mg		
AMPICILLIN	>6 y	IV	50 mg/kg	250 mg		
AMPICILLIN & SULBACTUM	>1 mo	IV	50 mg/kg	250 mg		
CEFAZOLIN		IV	25 mg/kg	125 mg		
CLINDAMYCIN		IV	10 mg/kg	50 mg		
ERTAPENEM	3 mo-12 y	IV	15 mg/kg	75 mg		
ERTAPENEM	>12 y	IV	1 Gm	per dose		
GENTAMICIN		IV	2 mg/kg	10 mg		
LEVOFLOXACIN		IV	10 mg/kg	50 mg		
METRONIDAZOLE		IV	10 mg/kg	50 mg		
PIPERACILLIN & TAZOBACTAM	<40 kg & 2-9 mo	IV	80 mg/kg	400 mg		
PIPERACILLIN & TAZOBACTAM	<40 kg & >9 mo	IV	100 mg/kg	500 mg		
PIPERACILLIN & TAZOBACTAM	>40 kg	IV	3.375 Gm per dose			
VANCOMYCIN		IV	15 mg/kg	75 mg		
ANTINAUSEA						
METOCLOPROMIDE		IV	0.2 mg/kg	1 mg	5 mg/mL	0.2 mL
DIPHENHYDRAMINE		IV/IM	1.25 mg/kg	6.25 mg	50 mg/mL	0.125 mL
SCOPOLAMINE		IV/IM	6 mcg/kg	30 mcg	400 mcg/mL	0.075 mL
MISCELLANEOUS MEDS						
AMINOCAPROIC ACID		IV	100 mg/kg	500 mg	250 mg/mL	2 mL
DESMOPRESSIN		IV/SQ	0.3 mcg/kg	1.5 mcg	4 mcg/mL	0.375 mL
DEXAMETHASONE	croup	IV	0.6 mg/kg	3 mg	4 mg/mL	0.75 mL
HYDROCORTISONE		IV/IO	3 mg/kg	15 mg	100 mg/mL	0.15 mL

5 KG

Ventilation: trained rescuer	1 breath q 6-8 sec (8-10 breaths/minute) about 1 second/ breath-visible chest rise; if intubated, continuous compressions without pause for ventilations
Pulse check	brachial/femoral
Compression	2-3 fingers-1 finger width below nipples *Wrap hands around chest if possible, compress with thumbs*
Depth	1.5 inch (4 cm) or at least 1/3 chest depth
Rate	at least 100 compressions per minute
Compress/vent ratio	30:2 with 1 or 2 rescuers
Foreign body obstruction	5 back blows at level of scapula, support head; alternate with 5 chest compressions Never perform a blind finger-sweep. Open the mouth and look for object; if you see it, remove it.

sync cardioversion	0.5 J/kg	2.5 J
repeat	1 J/kg	5 J
defibrillation	2 J/kg	10 J
repeat	4 J/kg	20 J

IV Bolus Drugs		dose	mg to pt	supplied	mL to give
ADENOSINE	IV	0.1 mg/kg	0.5 mg	3 mg/mL	0.17 mL
ADENOSINE repeat dose	IV	0.2 mg/kg	1 mg	3 mg/mL	0.33 mL
AMIODARONE	IV/IO	5 mg/kg	25 mg	50 mg/mL	0.50 mL
ATROPINE	IV/IM	0.02 mg/kg	0.1 mg	0.4 mg/mL	0.25 mL
ATROPINE	ETT	0.04 mg/kg	0.2 mg	0.4 mg/mL	0.50 mL
CALCIUM CHLORIDE	IV	20 mg/kg	100 mg	100 mg/mL	1.00 mL
CALCIUM GLUCONATE	IV/IO	60 mg/kg	300 mg	100 mg/mL	3.00 mL
DANTROLENE	IV	2.5 mg/kg	12.5 mg		
EPHEDRINE	IV	0.15 mg/kg	0.75 mg	10 mg/mL	0.08 mL
EPINEPHRINE (1:10,000)	IV/IO	0.01 mg/kg	0.05 mg	0.1 mg/mL	0.50 mL
EPINEPHRINE (1:1,000)	ETT	0.1 mg/kg	0.5 mg	1 mg/mL	0.50 mL
ESMOLOL	IV	0.5 mg/kg	2.5 mg	10 mg/mL	0.25 mL
LABETALOL	IV	0.2 mg/kg	1 mg	5 mg/mL	0.20 mL
LIDOCAINE	IV/IO	1 mg/kg	5 mcg	20 mg/mL	0.25 mL
NEOSYNEPHRINE	IV	5 mcg/kg	25 mcg	100 mcg/mL	0.25 mL
ROMAZICON	IV	0.01 mg/kg	0.05 mg	0.1 mg/mL	0.50 mL
VASOPRESSIN	IV/IO	0.4 unit/kg	2 units	20 u/mL	0.10 mL

6 KG MAINTENANCE IV FLUIDS: 24 ML/HR

common pediatric drugs		route	dose	mg to pt	supplied	mL to give
ATROPINE	vagolytic	IV	0.02 mg/kg	0.12 mg	0.4 mg/mL	0.3 mL
GLYCOPYRROLATE	vagolytic	IV	0.004 mg/kg	0.024 mg	0.2 mg/mL	0.12 mL
MIDAZOLAM		IV	0.05 mg/kg	0.3 mg	1 mg/mL	0.3 mL
MIDAZOLAM		PO	0.5 mg/kg	3 mg	1 mg/mL	3 mL
MIDAZOLAM		IN	0.2 mg/kg	1.2 mg	1 mg/mL	1.2 mL
SUCCINYLCHOLINE		IV	2 mg/kg	12 mg	20 mg/mL	0.6 mL
SUCCINYLCHOLINE		IM	4 mg/kg	24 mg	20 mg/mL	1.2 mL
PROPOFOL		IV	3 mg/kg	18 mg	10 mg/mL	1.8 mL
ETOMIDATE	>10 y	IV	0.3 mg/kg	1.8 mg	2 mg/mL	0.9 mL
FENTANYL		IV	1 mcg/kg	6 mcg	50 mcg/mL	0.12 mL
FENTANYL		IN	2 mcg/kg	12 mcg	50 mcg/mL	0.24 mL
MORPHINE	<6 mo	IV/IM	0.05 mg/kg	0.3 mg	10 mg/mL	0.03 mL
MORPHINE	>6 mo	IV/IM	0.1 mg/kg	0.6 mg	10 mg/mL	0.06 mL
TORADOL	>2-16 y	IV	0.5 mg/kg	3 mg	30 mg/mL	0.1 mL
TORADOL	>2-16 y	IM	1 mg/kg	6 mg	30 mg/mL	0.2 mL
ACETAMINOPHEN		PR	20 mg/kg	120 mg		
ACETAMINOPHEN	2-12 y	IV	15 mg/kg	90 mg	10 mg/mL	9 mL
CISATRACURIUM		IV	0.1 mg/kg	0.6 mg	2 mg/mL	0.3 mL
PANCURONIUM	<1 mo	IV	0.02 mg/kg	0.12 mg	1 mg/mL	0.12 mL
PANCURONIUM	>1 mo	IV	0.1 mg/kg	0.6 mg	1 mg/mL	0.6 mL
ROCURONIUM		IV	0.6 mg/kg	3.6 mg	10 mg/mL	0.36 mL
ROCURONIUM	RSI	IV	1.2 mg/kg	7.2 mg	10 mg/mL	0.72 mL
VECURONIUM		IV	0.1 mg/kg	0.6 mg	1 mg/mL	0.6 mL
GLYCOPYRROLATE	reversal	IV	0.007 mg/kg	0.042 mg	0.2 mg/mL	0.21 mL
NEOSTIGMINE		IV	0.07 mg/kg	0.42 mg	1 mg/mL	0.42 mL
DEXAMETHASONE		IV	0.25 mg/kg	1.5 mg	10 mg/mL	0.15 mL
ONDANSETRON		IV	0.15 mg/kg	0.9 mg	2 mg/mL	0.45 mL

6 Pediatric Pharmacology: Perioperative and Emergency Drugs

additional pediatric drugs	route		dose	mg to pt	supplied	mL to give
PREMED/SEDATION; VAGOLYTIC/ANTISIALAGOGUE; GIVE IM 30-60 MIN PREOP						
ATROPINE	IM		0.02 mg/kg	0.12 mg	0.4 mg/mL	0.3 mL
GLYCOPYRROLATE	IM		0.004 mg/kg	0.009 mg	0.2 mg/mL	0.045 mL
MIDAZOLAM	IM		0.1 mg/kg	0.5 mg	1 mg/mL	0.5 mL
DEXMEDETOMIDINE	IV	load dose	0.5 mcg/kg	1 mcg	4 mcg/mL	0.25 mL
INDUCTION						
KETAMINE	IV		2 mg/kg	12 mg	10 mg/mL	1.2 mL
KETAMINE	IM/PR		5 mg/kg	30 mg	10 mg/mL	3 mL
OPIOIDS/NONOPIOIDS						
FENTANYL	IV	high dose	4 mcg/kg	24 mcg	50 mcg/mL	0.48 mL
FENTANYL	IV	cardiac	10 mcg/kg	60 mcg	50 mcg/mL	1.2 mL
HYDROMORPHONE	IV/SQ	< 6 mo	0.005 mg/kg	0.03 mg	10 mg/mL	0.003 mL
HYDROMORPHONE	IV/SQ	> 6 mo	0.015 mg/kg	0.09 mg	10 mg/mL	0.009 mL
REMIFENTANIL	IV		0.5 mcg/kg	1 mcg	50 mcg/mL	0.02 mL
SUFENTANIL	IV		0.5 mcg/kg	3 mcg	50 mcg/mL	0.06 mL
REVERSALS						
ATROPINE	IV		0.02 mg/kg	0.12 mg	0.4 mg/mL	0.3 mL
EDROPHONIUM	IV	neonate	0.1 mg single dose		10 mg/mL	0.01 mL
EDROPHONIUM	IV	> 2 mo	0.04 mg/kg	0.24 mg	10 mg/mL	0.024 mL
FLUMAZENIL	IV	> 1 y	0.01 mg/kg	0.06 mg	0.1 mg/mL	0.6 mL
NALOXONE	IV/IM	< 5 y; < 20 kg	0.1 mg/kg	0.6 mg	0.4 mg/mL	1.5 mL
NALOXONE	IV/IM	> 5 y; < 20 kg		2 mg per dose	0.4 mg/mL	5 mL
NALOXONE	ETT		0.3 mg/kg	1.8 mg	0.4 mg/mL	4.5 mL

additional pediatric drugs		route	dose	mg to pt	supplied	mL to give
ANTIBIOTICS						
AMPICILLIN	<6 y	IV	50 mg/kg	300 mg		
AMPICILLIN	>6 y	IV	50 mg/kg	300 mg		
AMPICILLIN & SULBACTUM	>1 mo	IV	50 mg/kg	300 mg		
CEFAZOLIN		IV	25 mg/kg	150 mg		
CLINDAMYCIN		IV	10 mg/kg	60 mg		
ERTAPENEM	3 mo-12 y	IV	15 mg/kg	90 mg		
ERTAPENEM	>12 y	IV	1 Gm	per dose		
GENTAMICIN		IV	2 mg/kg	12 mg		
LEVOFLOXACIN		IV	10 mg/kg	60 mg		
METRONIDAZOLE		IV	10 mg/kg	60 mg		
PIPERACILLIN & TAZOBACTAM	<40 kg & 2-9 mo	IV	80 mg/kg	480 mg		
PIPERACILLIN & TAZOBACTAM	<40 kg & >9 mo	IV	100 mg/kg	600 mg		
PIPERACILLIN & TAZOBACTAM	>40 kg	IV	3.375 Gm per dose			
VANCOMYCIN		IV	15 mg/kg	90 mg		
ANTINAUSEA						
METOCLOPROMIDE		IV	0.2 mg/kg	1.2 mg	5 mg/mL	0.24 mL
DIPHENHYDRAMINE		IV/IM	1.25 mg/kg	7.5 mg	50 mg/mL	0.15 mL
SCOPOLAMINE		IV/IM	6 mcg/kg	36 mcg	400 mcg/mL	0.09 mL
MISCELLANEOUS MEDS						
AMINOCAPROIC ACID		IV	100 mg/kg	600 mg	250 mg/mL	2.4 mL
DESMOPRESSIN		IV/SQ	0.3 mcg/kg	1.8 mcg	4 mcg/mL	0.45 mL
DEXAMETHASONE	croup	IV	0.6 mg/kg	3.6 mg	4 mg/mL	0.9 mL
HYDROCORTISONE		IV/IO	3 mg/kg	18 mg	100 mg/mL	0.18 mL

6 KG

Ventilation: trained rescuer:	1 breath q 6-8 sec (8-10 breaths/minute) about 1 second/ breath-visible chest rise; if intubated, continuous compressions without pause for ventilations
Pulse check	brachial/femoral
Compression	2-3 fingers-1 finger width below nipples *Wrap hands around chest if possible, compress with thumbs*
Depth	1.5 inch (4 cm) or at least 1/3 chest depth
Rate	at least 100 compressions per minute
Compress/vent ratio	30:2 with 1 or 2 rescuers
Foreign body obstruction	5 back blows at level of scapula, support head; alternate with 5 chest compressions Never perform a blind finger-sweep. Open the mouth and look for object; if you see it, remove it.

sync cardioversion	0.5 J/kg	3 J
repeat	1 J/kg	6 J
defibrillation	2 J/kg	12 J
repeat	4 J/kg	24 J

IV Bolus Drugs		dose	mg to pt	supplied	mL to give
ADENOSINE	IV	0.1 mg/kg	0.6 mg	3 mg/mL	0.20 mL
ADENOSINE repeat dose	IV	0.2 mg/kg	1.2 mg	3 mg/mL	0.40 mL
AMIODARONE	IV/IO	5 mg/kg	30 mg	50 mg/mL	0.60 mL
ATROPINE	IV/IM	0.02 mg/kg	0.12 mg	0.4 mg/mL	0.30 mL
ATROPINE	ETT	0.04 mg/kg	0.24 mg	0.4 mg/mL	0.60 mL
CALCIUM CHLORIDE	IV	20 mg/kg	120 mg	100 mg/mL	1.20 mL
CALCIUM GLUCONATE	IV/IO	60 mg/kg	360 mg	100 mg/mL	3.60 mL
DANTROLENE	IV	2.5 mg/kg	15 mg		
EPHEDRINE	IV	0.15 mg/kg	0.9 mg	10 mg/mL	0.09 mL
EPINEPHRINE (1:10,000)	IV/IO	0.01 mg/kg	0.06 mg	0.1 mg/mL	0.60 mL
EPINEPHRINE (1:1,000)	ETT	0.1 mg/kg	0.6 mg	1 mg/mL	0.60 mL
ESMOLOL	IV	0.5 mg/kg	3 mg	10 mg/mL	0.30 mL
LABETALOL	IV	0.2 mg/kg	1.2 mg	5 mg/mL	0.24 mL
LIDOCAINE	IV/IO	1 mg/kg	6 mg	20 mg/mL	0.30 mL
NEOSYNEPHRINE	IV	5 mcg/kg	30 mcg	100 mcg/mL	0.30 mL
ROMAZICON	IV	0.01 mg/kg	0.06 mg	0.1 mg/mL	0.60 mL
VASOPRESSIN	IV/IO	0.4 unit/kg	2.4 units	20 u/mL	0.12 mL

7 KG MAINTENANCE IV FLUIDS: 28 ML/HR

common pediatric drugs		route	dose	mg to pt	supplied	mL to give
ATROPINE	vagolytic	IV	0.02 mg/kg	0.14 mg	0.4 mg/mL	0.35 mL
GLYCOPYRROLATE	vagolytic	IV	0.004 mg/kg	0.028 mg	0.2 mg/mL	0.14 mL
MIDAZOLAM		IV	0.05 mg/kg	0.35 mg	1 mg/mL	0.35 mL
MIDAZOLAM		PO	0.5 mg/kg	3.5 mg	1 mg/mL	3.5 mL
MIDAZOLAM		IN	0.2 mg/kg	1.4 mg	1 mg/mL	1.4 mL
SUCCINYLCHOLINE		IV	2 mg/kg	14 mg	20 mg/mL	0.7 mL
SUCCINYLCHOLINE		IM	4 mg/kg	28 mg	20 mg/mL	1.4 mL
PROPOFOL		IV	3 mg/kg	21 mg	10 mg/mL	2.1 mL
ETOMIDATE	>10 y	IV	0.3 mg/kg	2.1 mg	2 mg/mL	1.05 mL
FENTANYL		IV	1 mcg/kg	7 mcg	50 mcg/mL	0.14 mL
FENTANYL		IN	2 mcg/kg	14 mcg	50 mcg/mL	0.28 mL
MORPHINE	<6 mo	IV/IM	0.05 mg/kg	0.35 mg	10 mg/mL	0.035 mL
MORPHINE	>6 mo	IV/IM	0.1 mg/kg	0.7 mg	10 mg/mL	0.07 mL
TORADOL	>2-16 y	IV	0.5 mg/kg	3.5 mg	30 mg/mL	0.1167 mL
TORADOL	>2-16 y	IM	1 mg/kg	7 mg	30 mg/mL	0.2333 mL
ACETAMINOPHEN		PR	20 mg/kg	140 mg		
ACETAMINOPHEN	2-12 y	IV	15 mg/kg	105 mg	10 mg/mL	10.5 mL
CISATRACURIUM		IV	0.1 mg/kg	0.7 mg	2 mg/mL	0.35 mL
PANCURONIUM	<1 mo	IV	0.02 mg/kg	0.14 mg	1 mg/mL	0.14 mL
PANCURONIUM	>1 mo	IV	0.1 mg/kg	0.7 mg	1 mg/mL	0.7 mL
ROCURONIUM		IV	0.6 mg/kg	4.2 mg	10 mg/mL	0.42 mL
ROCURONIUM	RSI	IV	1.2 mg/kg	8.4 mg	10 mg/mL	0.84 mL
VECURONIUM		IV	0.1 mg/kg	0.7 mg	1 mg/mL	0.7 mL
GLYCOPYRROLATE	reversal	IV	0.007 mg/kg	0.049 mg	0.2 mg/mL	0.245 mL
NEOSTIGMINE		IV	0.07 mg/kg	0.49 mg	1 mg/mL	0.49 mL
DEXAMETHASONE		IV	0.25 mg/kg	1.75 mg	10 mg/mL	0.175 mL
ONDANSETRON		IV	0.15 mg/kg	1.05 mg	2 mg/mL	0.525 mL

additional pediatric drugs	route	dose	mg to pt	supplied	mL to give
PREMED/SEDATION; VAGOLYTIC/ANTISIALAGOGUE; GIVE IM 30–60 MIN PREOP					
ATROPINE	IV	0.02 mg/kg	0.14 mg	0.4 mg/mL	0.35 mL
GLYCOPYRROLATE	IM	0.004 mg/kg	0.000 600 mg	0.2 mg/mL	0.045 mL
MIDAZOLAM	IM	0.1 mg/kg	0.5 mg	1 mg/mL	0.5 mL
DEXMEDETOMIDINE load dose	IV	0.5 mcg/kg	1 mcg	4 mcg/mL	0.25 mL
INDUCTION					
KETAMINE	IV	2 mg/kg	14 mg	10 mg/mL	1.4 mL
KETAMINE	IM/PR	5 mg/kg	35 mg	10 mg/mL	3.5 mL
OPIOIDS/NONOPIOIDS					
FENTANYL high dose	IV	4 mcg/kg	28 mcg	50 mcg/mL	0.56 mL
FENTANYL cardiac	IV	10 mcg/kg	70 mcg	50 mcg/mL	1.4 mL
HYDROMORPHONE < 6 mo	IV/SQ	0.005 mg/kg	0.035 mg	10 mg/mL	0.0035 mL
HYDROMORPHONE > 6 mo	IV/SQ	0.015 mg/kg	0.105 mg	10 mg/mL	0.0105 mL
REMIFENTANIL	IV	0.5 mcg/kg	1 mcg	50 mcg/mL	0.02 mL
SUFENTANIL	IV	0.5 mcg/kg	3.5 mcg	50 mcg/mL	0.07 mL
REVERSALS					
ATROPINE	IV	0.02 mg/kg	0.14 mg	0.4 mg/mL	0.35 mL
EDROPHONIUM neonate	IV	0.1 mg single dose		10 mg/mL	0.01 mL
EDROPHONIUM > 2 mo	IV	0.04 mg/kg	0.28 mg	10 mg/mL	0.028 mL
FLUMAZENIL > 1 y	IV	0.01 mg/kg	0.07 mg	0.1 mg/mL	0.7 mL
NALOXONE < 5 y; < 20 kg	IM/IV	0.1 mg/kg	0.7 mg	0.4 mg/mL	1.75 mL
NALOXONE > 5 y; > 20 kg	IM/IV	2 mg per dose		0.4 mg/mL	5 mL
NALOXONE	ETT	0.3 mg/kg	2.1 mg	0.4 mg/mL	5.25 mL

additional pediatric drugs		route	dose	mg to pt	supplied	mL to give
ANTIBIOTICS						
AMPICILLIN	<6 y	IV	50 mg/kg	300 mg		
AMPICILLIN	>6 y	IV	50 mg/kg	350 mg		
AMPICILLIN & SULBACTUM	>1 mo	IV	50 mg/kg	350 mg		
CEFAZOLIN		IV	25 mg/kg	175 mg		
CLINDAMYCIN		IV	10 mg/kg	70 mg		
ERTAPENEM	3 mo-12 y	IV	15 mg/kg	105 mg		
ERTAPENEM	>12 y	IV	1 Gm	per dose		
GENTAMICIN		IV	2 mg/kg	14 mg		
LEVOFLOXACIN		IV	10 mg/kg	70 mg		
METRONIDAZOLE		IV	10 mg/kg	70 mg		
PIPERACILLIN & TAZOBACTAM	<40 kg & 2-9 mo	IV	80 mg/kg	560 mg		
PIPERACILLIN & TAZOBACTAM	<40 kg & >9 mo	IV	100 mg/kg	700 mg		
PIPERACILLIN & TAZOBACTAM	>40 kg	IV	3.375 Gm per dose			
VANCOMYCIN		IV	15 mg/kg	105 mg		
ANTINAUSEA						
METOCLOPROMIDE		IV	0.2 mg/kg	1.4 mg	5 mg/mL	0.28 mL
DIPHENHYDRAMINE		IV/IM	1.25 mg/kg	8.75 mg	50 mg/mL	0.175 mL
SCOPOLAMINE		IV/IM	6 mcg/kg	42 mcg	400 mcg/mL	0.105 mL
MISCELLANEOUS MEDS						
AMINOCAPROIC ACID		IV	100 mg/kg	700 mg	250 mg/mL	2.8 mL
DESMOPRESSIN		IV/SQ	0.3 mcg/kg	2.1 mcg	4 mcg/mL	0.525 mL
DEXAMETHASONE	croup	IV	0.6 mg/kg	4.2 mg	4 mg/mL	1.05 mL
HYDROCORTISONE		IV/IO	3 mg/kg	21 mg	100 mg/mL	0.21 mL

7 KG

Ventilation: trained rescuer	1 breath q 6-8 sec (8-10 breaths/minute) about 1 second/ breath–visible chest rise; if intubated, continuous compressions without pause for ventilations
Pulse check	brachial/femoral
Compression	2-3 fingers–1 finger width below nipples *Wrap hands around chest if possible, compress with thumbs*
Depth	1.5 inch (4 cm) or at least 1/3 chest depth
Rate	at least 100 compressions per minute
Compress/vent ratio	30:2 with 1 or 2 rescuers
Foreign body obstruction	5 back blows at level of scapula, support head; alternate with 5 chest compressions *Never perform a blind finger-sweep. Open the mouth and look for object; if you see it, remove it.*

sync cardioversion	0.5 J/kg	0.5 J	
	1 J/kg	1 J	repeat
defibrillation	2 J/kg	14 J	
	4 J/kg	28 J	repeat

IV Bolus Drugs		dose	mg to pt	supplied	mL to give
ADENOSINE	IV	0.1 mg/kg	0.7 mg	3 mg/mL	0.23 mL
ADENOSINE repeat dose	IV	0.2 mg/kg	1.4 mg	3 mg/mL	0.47 mL
AMIODARONE	IV/IO	5 mg/kg	35 mg	50 mg/mL	0.70 mL
ATROPINE	IV/IM	0.02 mg/kg	0.14 mg	0.4 mg/mL	0.35 mL
ATROPINE	ETT	0.04 mg/kg	0.28 mg	0.4 mg/mL	0.70 mL
CALCIUM CHLORIDE	IV	20 mg/kg	140 mg	100 mg/mL	1.40 mL
CALCIUM GLUCONATE	IV/IO	60 mg/kg	420 mg	100 mg/mL	4.20 mL
DANTROLENE	IV	2.5 mg/kg	17.5 mg		
EPHEDRINE	IV	0.15 mg/kg	1.05 mg	10 mg/mL	0.11 mL
EPINEPHRINE (1:10,000)	IV/IO	0.01 mg/kg	0.07 mg	0.1 mg/mL	0.70 mL
EPINEPHRINE (1:1,000)	ETT	0.1 mg/kg	1 mg	1 mg/mL	0.70 mL
ESMOLOL	IV	0.5 mg/kg	3.5 mg	10 mg/mL	0.35 mL
LABETALOL	IV	0.2 mg/kg	1.4 mg	5 mg/mL	0.28 mL
LIDOCAINE	IV/IO	1 mg/kg	7 mg	20 mg/mL	0.35 mL
NEOSYNEPHRINE	IV	5 mcg/kg	35 mcg	100 mcg/mL	0.35 mL
ROMAZICON	IV	0.01 mg/kg	0.07 mg	0.1 mg/mL	0.70 mL
VASOPRESSIN	IV/IO	0.4 unit/kg	2.8 units	20 u/mL	0.14 mL

8 KG MAINTENANCE IV FLUIDS: 32 ML/HR

common pediatric drugs		route	dose	mg to pt	supplied	mL to give
ATROPINE	vagolytic	IV	0.02 mg/kg	0.16 mg	0.4 mg/mL	0.4 mL
GLYCOPYRROLATE	vagolytic	IV	0.004 mg/kg	0.032 mg	0.2 mg/mL	0.16 mL
MIDAZOLAM		IV	0.05 mg/kg	0.4 mg	1 mg/mL	0.4 mL
MIDAZOLAM		PO	0.5 mg/kg	4 mg	1 mg/mL	4 mL
MIDAZOLAM		IN	0.2 mg/kg	1.6 mg	1 mg/mL	1.6 mL
SUCCINYLCHOLINE		IV	2 mg/kg	16 mg	20 mg/mL	0.8 mL
SUCCINYLCHOLINE		IM	4 mg/kg	32 mg	20 mg/mL	1.6 mL
PROPOFOL		IV	3 mg/kg	24 mg	10 mg/mL	2.4 mL
ETOMIDATE	>10 y	IV	0.3 mg/kg	2.4 mg	2 mg/mL	1.2 mL
FENTANYL		IV	1 mcg/kg	8 mcg	50 mcg/mL	0.16 mL
FENTANYL		IN	2 mcg/kg	16 mcg	50 mcg/mL	0.32 mL
MORPHINE	<6 mo	IV/IM	0.05 mg/kg	0.4 mg	10 mg/mL	0.04 mL
MORPHINE	>6 mo	IV/IM	0.1 mg/kg	0.8 mg	10 mg/mL	0.08 mL
TORADOL	>2-16 y	IV	0.5 mg/kg	4 mg	30 mg/mL	0.1333 mL
TORADOL	>2-16 y	IM	1 mg/kg	8 mg	30 mg/mL	0.2667 mL
ACETAMINOPHEN		PR	20 mg/kg	160 mg		
ACETAMINOPHEN	2-12 y	IV	15 mg/kg	120 mg	10 mg/mL	12 mL
CISATRACURIUM		IV	0.1 mg/kg	0.8 mg	2 mg/mL	0.4 mL
PANCURONIUM	<1 mo	IV	0.02 mg/kg	0.16 mg	1 mg/mL	0.16 mL
PANCURONIUM	>1 mo	IV	0.1 mg/kg	0.8 mg	1 mg/mL	0.8 mL
ROCURONIUM		IV	0.6 mg/kg	4.8 mg	10 mg/mL	0.48 mL
ROCURONIUM	RSI	IV	1.2 mg/kg	9.6 mg	10 mg/mL	0.96 mL
VECURONIUM		IV	0.1 mg/kg	0.8 mg	1 mg/mL	0.8 mL
GLYCOPYRROLATE	reversal	IV	0.007 mg/kg	0.056 mg	0.2 mg/mL	0.28 mL
NEOSTIGMINE		IV	0.07 mg/kg	0.56 mg	1 mg/mL	0.56 mL
DEXAMETHASONE		IV	0.25 mg/kg	2 mg	10 mg/mL	0.2 mL
ONDANSETRON		IV	0.15 mg/kg	1.2 mg	2 mg/mL	0.6 mL

additional pediatric drugs	route	dose	mg to pt	supplied	mL to give
PREMED/SEDATION; VAGOLYTIC/ANTISIALAGOGUE; GIVE IM 30–60 MIN PREOP					
ATROPINE	IV	0.02 mg/kg	0.16 mg	0.4 mg/mL	0.4 mL
GLYCOPYRROLATE	IM	0.004 mg/kg	0.009 mg	0.2 mg/mL	0.045 mL
MIDAZOLAM	IM	0.1 mg/kg	0.5 mg	1 mg/mL	0.5 mL
DEXMEDETOMIDINE	IV	load dose 0.5 mcg/kg	1 mcg	4 mcg/mL	0.25 mL
INDUCTION					
KETAMINE	IV	2 mg/kg	16 mg	10 mg/mL	1.6 mL
KETAMINE	IM/PR	5 mg/kg	40 mg	10 mg/mL	4 mL
OPIOIDS/NONOPIOIDS					
FENTANYL	IV	high dose 4 mcg/kg	32 mcg	50 mcg/mL	0.64 mL
FENTANYL	IV	cardiac 10 mcg/kg	80 mcg	50 mcg/mL	1.6 mL
HYDROMORPHONE	SQ/IV	< 6 mo 0.005 mg/kg	0.04 mg	10 mg/mL	0.004 mL
HYDROMORPHONE	SQ/IV	> 6 mo 0.015 mg/kg	0.12 mg	10 mg/mL	0.012 mL
REMIFENTANIL	IV	0.5 mcg/kg	1 mcg	50 mcg/mL	0.02 mL
SUFENTANIL	IV	0.5 mcg/kg	4 mcg	50 mcg/mL	0.08 mL
REVERSALS					
ATROPINE	IV	0.02 mg/kg	0.16 mg	0.4 mg/mL	0.4 mL
EDROPHONIUM	IV	neonate 0.1 mg single dose	1 mg single dose	10 mg/mL	0.10 mL
EDROPHONIUM	IV	> 2 mo 0.04 mg/kg	0.32 mg	10 mg/mL	0.032 mL
FLUMAZENIL	IV	> 1 y 0.01 mg/kg	0.08 mg	0.1 mg/mL	0.8 mL
NALOXONE	IV/IM	< 5 y; < 20 kg 0.1 mg/kg	0.8 mg	0.4 mg/mL	2 mL
NALOXONE	IV/IM	> 5 y; > 20 kg 2 mg per dose	2 mg per dose	0.4 mg/mL	5 mL
NALOXONE	ETT	0.3 mg/kg	2.4 mg	0.4 mg/mL	6 mL

additional pediatric drugs		route	dose	mg to pt	supplied	mL to give
ANTIBIOTICS						
AMPICILLIN	<6 y	IV	50 mg/kg	300 mg		
AMPICILLIN	>6 y	IV	50 mg/kg	400 mg		
AMPICILLIN & SULBACTUM	>1 mo	IV	50 mg/kg	400 mg		
CEFAZOLIN		IV	25 mg/kg	200 mg		
CLINDAMYCIN		IV	10 mg/kg	80 mg		
ERTAPENEM	3 mo-12 y	IV	15 mg/kg	120 mg		
ERTAPENEM	>12 y	IV	1 Gm	per dose		
GENTAMICIN		IV	2 mg/kg	16 mg		
LEVOFLOXACIN		IV	10 mg/kg	80 mg		
METRONIDAZOLE		IV	10 mg/kg	80 mg		
PIPERACILLIN & TAZOBACTAM	<40 kg & 2-9 mo	IV	80 mg/kg	640 mg		
PIPERACILLIN & TAZOBACTAM	<40 kg & >9 mo	IV	100 mg/kg	800 mg		
PIPERACILLIN & TAZOBACTAM	>40 kg	IV	3.375 Gm per dose			
VANCOMYCIN		IV	15 mg/kg	120 mg		
ANTINAUSEA						
METOCLOPROMIDE		IV	0.2 mg/kg	1.6 mg	5 mg/mL	0.32 mL
DIPHENHYDRAMINE		IV/IM	1.25 mg/kg	10 mg	50 mg/mL	0.2 mL
SCOPOLAMINE		IV/IM	6 mcg/kg	48 mcg	400 mcg/mL	0.12 mL
MISCELLANEOUS MEDS						
AMINOCAPROIC ACID		IV	100 mg/kg	800 mg	250 mg/mL	3.2 mL
DESMOPRESSIN		IV/SQ	0.3 mcg/kg	2.4 mcg	4 mcg/mL	0.6 mL
DEXAMETHASONE	croup	IV	0.6 mg/kg	4.8 mg	4 mg/mL	1.2 mL
HYDROCORTISONE		IV/IO	3 mg/kg	24 mg	100 mg/mL	0.24 mL

8 KG

Ventilation: trained rescuer	1 breath q 6-8 sec (8-10 breaths/minute) about 1 second/ breath-visible chest rise; if intubated, continuous compressions without pause for ventilations
Pulse check	brachial/femoral
Compression	2-3 fingers–1 finger width below nipples *Wrap hands around chest if possible, compress with thumbs*
Depth	1.5 inch (4 cm) or at least 1/3 chest depth
Rate	at least 100 compressions per minute
Compress/vent ratio	30:2 with 1 or 2 rescuers
Foreign body obstruction	5 back blows at level of scapula, support head; alternate with 5 chest compressions
	Never perform a blind finger-sweep. Open the mouth and look for object; if you see it, remove it.

sync cardioversion		0.5 J/kg	4 J
	repeat	1 J/kg	8 J
defibrillation		2 J/kg	16 J
	repeat	4 J/kg	32 J

IV Bolus Drugs		dose	mg to pt	supplied	mL to give
ADENOSINE	IV	0.1 mg/kg	0.8 mg	3 mg/mL	0.27 mL
ADENOSINE repeat dose	IV	0.2 mg/kg	1.6 mg	3 mg/mL	0.53 mL
AMIODARONE	IV/IO	5 mg/kg	40 mg	50 mg/mL	0.80 mL
ATROPINE	IV/IM	0.02 mg/kg	0.16 mg	0.4 mg/mL	0.40 mL
ATROPINE	ETT	0.04 mg/kg	0.32 mg	0.4 mg/mL	0.80 mL
CALCIUM CHLORIDE	IV	20 mg/kg	160 mg	100 mg/mL	1.60 mL
CALCIUM GLUCONATE	IV/IO	60 mg/kg	480 mg	100 mg/mL	4.80 mL
DANTROLENE	IV	2.5 mg/kg	20 mg		
EPHEDRINE	IV	0.15 mg/kg	1.2 mg	10 mg/mL	0.12 mL
EPINEPHRINE (1:10,000)	IV/IO	0.01 mg/kg	0.08 mg	0.1 mg/mL	0.80 mL
EPINEPHRINE (1:1,000)	ETT	0.1 mg/kg	0.8 mg	1 mg/mL	0.80 mL
ESMOLOL	IV	0.5 mg/kg	4 mg	10 mg/mL	0.40 mL
LABETALOL	IV	0.2 mg/kg	1.6 mg	5 mg/mL	0.32 mL
LIDOCAINE	IV/IO	1 mg/kg	8 mg	20 mg/mL	0.40 mL
NEOSYNEPHRINE	IV	5 mcg/kg	40 mcg	100 mcg/mL	0.40 mL
ROMAZICON	IV	0.01 mg/kg	0.08 mg	0.1 mg/mL	0.80 mL
VASOPRESSIN	IV/IO	0.4 unit/kg	3.2 units	20 u/mL	0.16 mL

9 KG MAINTENANCE IV FLUIDS: 36 ML/HR

common pediatric drugs		route	dose	mg to pt	supplied	mL to give
ATROPINE	vagolytic	IV	0.02 mg/kg	0.18 mg	0.4 mg/mL	0.45 mL
GLYCOPYRROLATE	vagolytic	IV	0.004 mg/kg	0.036 mg	0.2 mg/mL	0.18 mL
MIDAZOLAM		IV	0.05 mg/kg	0.45 mg	1 mg/mL	0.45 mL
MIDAZOLAM		PO	0.5 mg/kg	4.5 mg	1 mg/mL	4.5 mL
MIDAZOLAM		IN	0.2 mg/kg	1.8 mg	1 mg/mL	1.8 mL
SUCCINYLCHOLINE		IV	2 mg/kg	18 mg	20 mg/mL	0.9 mL
SUCCINYLCHOLINE		IM	4 mg/kg	36 mg	20 mg/mL	1.8 mL
PROPOFOL		IV	3 mg/kg	27 mg	10 mg/mL	2.7 mL
ETOMIDATE	>10 y	IV	0.3 mg/kg	2.7 mg	2 mg/mL	1.35 mL
FENTANYL		IV	1 mcg/kg	9 mcg	50 mcg/mL	0.18 mL
FENTANYL		IN	2 mcg/kg	18 mcg	50 mcg/mL	0.36 mL
MORPHINE	<6 mo	IV/IM	0.05 mg/kg	0.45 mg	10 mg/mL	0.045 mL
MORPHINE	>6 mo	IV/IM	0.1 mg/kg	0.9 mg	10 mg/mL	0.09 mL
TORADOL	>2-16 y	IV	0.5 mg/kg	4.5 mg	30 mg/mL	0.15 mL
TORADOL	>2-16 y	IM	1 mg/kg	9 mg	30 mg/mL	0.3 mL
ACETAMINOPHEN		PR	20 mg/kg	180 mg		
ACETAMINOPHEN	2-12 y	IV	15 mg/kg	135 mg	10 mg/mL	13.5 mL
CISATRACURIUM		IV	0.1 mg/kg	0.9 mg	2 mg/mL	0.45 mL
PANCURONIUM	<1 mo	IV	0.02 mg/kg	0.18 mg	1 mg/mL	0.18 mL
PANCURONIUM	>1 mo	IV	0.1 mg/kg	0.9 mg	1 mg/mL	0.9 mL
ROCURONIUM		IV	0.6 mg/kg	5.4 mg	10 mg/mL	0.54 mL
ROCURONIUM	RSI	IV	1.2 mg/kg	10.8 mg	10 mg/mL	1.08 mL
VECURONIUM		IV	0.1 mg/kg	0.9 mg	1 mg/mL	0.9 mL
GLYCOPYRROLATE	reversal	IV	0.007 mg/kg	0.063 mg	0.2 mg/mL	0.315 mL
NEOSTIGMINE		IV	0.07 mg/kg	0.63 mg	1 mg/mL	0.63 mL
DEXAMETHASONE		IV	0.25 mg/kg	2.25 mg	10 mg/mL	0.225 mL
ONDANSETRON		IV	0.15 mg/kg	1.35 mg	2 mg/mL	0.675 mL

additional pediatric drugs		route	dose	mg to pt	supplied	mL to give
PREMED/SEDATION; VAGOLYTIC/ANTISIALAGOGUE; GIVE IM 30-60 MIN PREOP						
ATROPINE		IV	0.02 mg/kg	0.18 mg	0.4 mg/mL	0.45 mL
GLYCOPYRROLATE		IM	0.004 mg/kg	0.009 mg	0.2 mg/mL	0.045 mL
MIDAZOLAM		IM	0.1 mg/kg	0.5 mg	1 mg/mL	0.5 mL
DEXMEDETOMIDINE	load dose	IV	0.5 mcg/kg	1 mcg	4 mcg/mL	0.25 mL
INDUCTION						
KETAMINE		IV	2 mg/kg	18 mg	10 mg/mL	1.8 mL
KETAMINE		IM/PR	5 mg/kg	45 mg	10 mg/mL	4.5 mL
OPIOIDS/NONOPIOIDS						
FENTANYL	high dose	IV	4 mcg/kg	36 mcg	50 mcg/mL	0.72 mL
FENTANYL	cardiac	IV	10 mcg/kg	90 mcg	50 mcg/mL	1.8 mL
HYDROMORPHONE	< 6 mo	IV/SQ	0.005 mg/kg	0.045 mg	10 mg/mL	0.005 mL
HYDROMORPHONE	> 6 mo	IV/SQ	0.015 mg/kg	0.135 mg	10 mg/mL	0.014 mL
REMIFENTANIL		IV	0.5 mcg/kg	1 mcg	50 mcg/mL	0.02 mL
SUFENTANIL		IV	0.5 mcg/kg	4.5 mcg	50 mcg/mL	0.09 mL
REVERSALS						
ATROPINE		IV	0.02 mg/kg	0.18 mg	0.4 mg/mL	0.45 mL
EDROPHONIUM	neonate	IV	0.1 mg single dose		10 mg/mL	0.01 mL
EDROPHONIUM	> 2 mo	IV	0.04 mg/kg	0.36 mg	10 mg/mL	0.036 mL
FLUMAZENIL	<1 y	IV	0.01 mg/kg	0.09 mg	0.1 mg/mL	0.9 mL
NALOXONE	<5 y; <20 kg	IV/IM	0.1 mg/kg	0.9 mg	0.4 mg/mL	2.25 mL
NALOXONE	>5 y; >20 kg	IV/IM	2 mg per dose		0.4 mg/mL	5 mL
NALOXONE		ETT	0.3 mg/kg	2.7 mg	0.4 mg/mL	6.75 mL

additional pediatric drugs		route	dose	mg to pt	supplied	mL to give
ANTIBIOTICS						
AMPICILLIN	<6 y	IV	50 mg/kg	300 mg		
AMPICILLIN	>6 y	IV	50 mg/kg	450 mg		
AMPICILLIN & SULBACTUM	>1 mo	IV	50 mg/kg	450 mg		
CEFAZOLIN		IV	25 mg/kg	225 mg		
CLINDAMYCIN		IV	10 mg/kg	90 mg		
ERTAPENEM	3 mo-12 y	IV	15 mg/kg	135 mg		
ERTAPENEM	>12 y	IV	1 Gm	per dose		
GENTAMICIN		IV	2 mg/kg	18 mg		
LEVOFLOXACIN		IV	10 mg/kg	90 mg		
METRONIDAZOLE		IV	10 mg/kg	90 mg		
PIPERACILLIN & TAZOBACTAM	<40 kg & 2-9 mo	IV	80 mg/kg	720 mg		
PIPERACILLIN & TAZOBACTAM	<40 kg & >9 mo	IV	100 mg/kg	900 mg		
PIPERACILLIN & TAZOBACTAM	>40 kg	IV	3.375 Gm per dose			
VANCOMYCIN		IV	15 mg/kg	135 mg		
ANTINAUSEA						
METOCLOPROMIDE		IV	0.2 mg/kg	1.8 mg	5 mg/mL	0.36 mL
DIPHENHYDRAMINE		IV/IM	1.25 mg/kg	11.25 mg	50 mg/mL	0.225 mL
SCOPOLAMINE		IV/IM	6 mcg/kg	54 mcg	400 mcg/mL	0.135 mL
MISCELLANEOUS MEDS						
AMINOCAPROIC ACID		IV	100 mg/kg	900 mg	250 mg/mL	3.6 mL
DESMOPRESSIN		IV/SQ	0.3 mcg/kg	2.7 mcg	4 mcg/mL	0.675 mL
DEXAMETHASONE	croup	IV	0.6 mg/kg	5.4 mg	4 mg/mL	1.35 mL
HYDROCORTISONE		IV/IO	3 mg/kg	27 mg	100 mg/mL	0.27 mL

9 KG

Ventilation: trained rescuer	1 breath q 6-8 sec (8-10 breaths/minute) about 1 second/ breath-visible chest rise; if intubated, continuous compressions without pause for ventilations
Pulse check	brachial/femoral
Compression	2-3 fingers–1 finger width below nipples *Wrap hands around chest if possible, compress with thumbs*
Depth	1.5 inch (4 cm) or at least 1/3 chest depth
Rate	at least 100 compressions per minute
Compress/vent ratio	30:2 with 1 or 2 rescuers
Foreign body obstruction	5 back blows at level of scapula, support head; alternate with 5 chest compressions *Never perform a blind finger-sweep. Open the mouth and look for object; if you see it, remove it.*

sync cardioversion	0.5 J/kg	4.5 J
defibrillation	1 J/kg	9 J
repeat	2 J/kg	18 J
repeat	4 J/kg	36 J

IV Bolus Drugs		dose		mg to pt	supplied	mL to give
ADENOSINE		IV	0.1 mg/kg	0.9 mg	3 mg/mL	0.30 mL
ADENOSINE repeat dose		IV	0.2 mg/kg	1.8 mg	3 mg/mL	0.60 mL
AMIODARONE		IV/IO	5 mg/kg	45 mg	50 mg/mL	0.90 mL
ATROPINE		IM/IV	0.02 mg/kg	0.18 mg	0.4 mg/mL	0.45 mL
ATROPINE		ETT	0.04 mg/kg	0.36 mg	0.4 mg/mL	0.90 mL
CALCIUM CHLORIDE		IV	20 mg/kg	180 mg	100 mg/mL	1.80 mL
CALCIUM GLUCONATE		IV/IO	60 mg/kg	540 mg	100 mg/mL	5.40 mL
DANTROLENE		IV	2.5 mg/kg	22.5 mg		
EPHEDRINE		IV	0.15 mg/kg	1.35 mg	10 mg/mL	0.14 mL
EPINEPHRINE (1:10,000)		IV/IO	0.01 mg/kg	0.09 mg	0.1 mg/mL	0.90 mL
EPINEPHRINE (1:1,000)		ETT	0.1 mg/kg	0.9 mg	1 mg/mL	0.90 mL
ESMOLOL		IV	0.5 mg/kg	4.5 mg	10 mg/mL	0.45 mL
LABETALOL		IV	0.2 mg/kg	1.8 mg	5 mg/mL	0.36 mL
LIDOCAINE		IV/IO	1 mg/kg	9 mg	20 mg/mL	0.45 mL
NEOSYNEPHRINE		IV	5 mcg/kg	45 mcg	100 mcg/mL	0.45 mL
ROMAZICON		IV	0.01 mg/kg	0.09 mg	0.1 mg/mL	0.90 mL
VASOPRESSIN		IV/IO	0.4 unit/kg	3.6 units	20 u/mL	0.18 mL

10 KG MAINTENANCE IV FLUIDS: 40 ML/HR

common pediatric drugs		route	dose	mg to pt	supplied	mL to give
ATROPINE	vagolytic	IV	0.02 mg/kg	0.2 mg	0.4 mg/mL	0.5 mL
GLYCOPYRROLATE	vagolytic	IV	0.004 mg/kg	0.04 mg	0.2 mg/mL	0.2 mL
MIDAZOLAM		IV	0.05 mg/kg	0.5 mg	1 mg/mL	0.5 mL
MIDAZOLAM		PO	0.5 mg/kg	5 mg	1 mg/mL	5 mL
MIDAZOLAM		IN	0.2 mg/kg	2 mg	1 mg/mL	2 mL
SUCCINYLCHOLINE		IV	2 mg/kg	20 mg	20 mg/mL	1 mL
SUCCINYLCHOLINE		IM	4 mg/kg	40 mg	20 mg/mL	2 mL
PROPOFOL		IV	3 mg/kg	30 mg	10 mg/mL	3 mL
ETOMIDATE	>10 y	IV	0.3 mg/kg	3 mg	2 mg/mL	1.5 mL
FENTANYL		IV	1 mcg/kg	10 mcg	50 mcg/mL	0.2 mL
FENTANYL		IN	2 mcg/kg	20 mcg	50 mcg/mL	0.4 mL
MORPHINE	<6 mo	IV/IM	0.05 mg/kg	0.5 mg	10 mg/mL	0.05 mL
MORPHINE	>6 mo	IV/IM	0.1 mg/kg	1 mg	10 mg/mL	0.1 mL
TORADOL	>2-16 y	IV	0.5 mg/kg	5 mg	30 mg/mL	0.167 mL
TORADOL	>2-16 y	IM	1 mg/kg	10 mg	30 mg/mL	0.333 mL
ACETAMINOPHEN		PR	20 mg/kg	200 mg		
ACETAMINOPHEN	2-12 y	IV	15 mg/kg	150 mg	10 mg/mL	15 mL
CISATRACURIUM		IV	0.1 mg/kg	1 mg	2 mg/mL	0.5 mL
PANCURONIUM	<1 mo	IV	0.02 mg/kg	0.2 mg	1 mg/mL	0.2 mL
PANCURONIUM	>1 mo	IV	0.1 mg/kg	1 mg	1 mg/mL	1 mL
ROCURONIUM		IV	0.6 mg/kg	6 mg	10 mg/mL	0.6 mL
ROCURONIUM	RSI	IV	1.2 mg/kg	12 mg	10 mg/mL	1.2 mL
VECURONIUM		IV	0.1 mg/kg	1 mg	1 mg/mL	1 mL
GLYCOPYRROLATE	reversal	IV	0.007 mg/kg	0.07 mg	0.2 mg/mL	0.35 mL
NEOSTIGMINE		IV	0.07 mg/kg	0.7 mg	1 mg/mL	0.7 mL
DEXAMETHASONE		IV	0.25 mg/kg	2.5 mg	10 mg/mL	0.25 mL
ONDANSETRON		IV	0.15 mg/kg	1.5 mg	2 mg/mL	0.75 mL

additional pediatric drugs		route	dose	mg to pt	supplied	mL to give
PREMED/SEDATION; VAGOLYTIC/ANTISIALAGOGUE; GIVE IM 30-60 MIN PREOP						
ATROPINE		IM	0.02 mg/kg	0.2 mg	0.4 mg/mL	0.5 mL
GLYCOPYRROLATE		IM	0.004 mg/kg	0.009 mg	0.2 mg/mL	0.045 mL
MIDAZOLAM		IM	0.1 mg/kg	0.5 mg	1 mg/mL	0.5 mL
DEXMEDETOMIDINE	load dose	IV	0.5 mcg/kg	1 mcg	4 mcg/mL	0.25 mL
INDUCTION						
KETAMINE		IV	2 mg/kg	20 mg	10 mg/mL	2 mL
KETAMINE		IM/PR	5 mg/kg	50 mg	10 mg/mL	5 mL
OPIOIDS/NONOPIOIDS						
FENTANYL	high dose	IV	4 mcg/kg	40 mcg	50 mcg/mL	0.8 mL
FENTANYL	cardiac	IV	10 mcg/kg	100 mcg	50 mcg/mL	2 mL
HYDROMORPHONE	< 6 mo	IV/SQ	0.005 mg/kg	0.05 mg	10 mg/mL	0.005 mL
HYDROMORPHONE	> 6 mo	IV/SQ	0.015 mg/kg	0.15 mg	10 mg/mL	0.015 mL
REMIFENTANIL		IV	0.5 mcg/kg	1 mcg	50 mcg/mL	0.02 mL
SUFENTANIL		IV	0.5 mcg/kg	5 mcg	50 mcg/mL	0.1 mL
REVERSALS						
ATROPINE		IV	0.02 mg/kg	0.2 mg	0.4 mg/mL	0.5 mL
EDROPHONIUM	neonate	IV	0.1 mg single dose		10 mg/mL	0.01 mL
EDROPHONIUM	> 2 mo	IV	0.04 mg/kg	0.4 mg	10 mg/mL	0.04 mL
FLUMAZENIL	< 1 y	IV	0.01 mg/kg	0.1 mg	0.1 mg/mL	1 mL
NALOXONE	< 5 y; < 20 kg	IV/IM	0.01 mg/kg	1 mg	0.4 mg/mL	2.5 mL
NALOXONE	> 5 y; > 20 kg	IV/IM	2 mg per dose		0.4 mg/mL	5 mL
NALOXONE		ETT	0.3 mg/kg	3 mg	0.4 mg/mL	7.5 mL

additional pediatric drugs		route	dose	mg to pt	supplied	mL to give
ANTIBIOTICS						
AMPICILLIN	<6 y	IV	50 mg/kg	300 mg		
AMPICILLIN	>6 y	IV	50 mg/kg	500 mg		
AMPICILLIN & SULBACTUM	>1 mo	IV	50 mg/kg	500 mg		
CEFAZOLIN		IV	25 mg/kg	250 mg		
CLINDAMYCIN		IV	10 mg/kg	100 mg		
ERTAPENEM	3 mo-12 y	IV	15 mg/kg	150 mg		
ERTAPENEM	>12 y	IV	1 Gm	per dose		
GENTAMICIN		IV	2 mg/kg	20 mg		
LEVOFLOXACIN		IV	10 mg/kg	100 mg		
METRONIDAZOLE		IV	10 mg/kg	100 mg		
PIPERACILLIN & TAZOBACTAM	<40 kg & 2-9 mo	IV	80 mg/kg	800 mg		
PIPERACILLIN & TAZOBACTAM	<40 kg & >9 mo	IV	100 mg/kg	1,000 mg		
PIPERACILLIN & TAZOBACTAM	>40 kg	IV	3.375 Gm per dose			
VANCOMYCIN		IV	15 mg/kg	150 mg		
ANTINAUSEA						
METOCLOPROMIDE		IV	0.2 mg/kg	2 mg	5 mg/mL	0.4 mL
DIPHENHYDRAMINE		IV/IM	1.25 mg/kg	12.5 mg	50 mg/mL	0.25 mL
SCOPOLAMINE		IV/IM	6 mcg/kg	60 mcg	400 mcg/mL	0.15 mL
MISCELLANEOUS MEDS						
AMINOCAPROIC ACID		IV	100 mg/kg	1,000 mg	250 mg/mL	4 mL
DESMOPRESSIN		IV/SQ	0.3 mcg/kg	3 mcg	4 mcg/mL	0.75 mL
DEXAMETHASONE	croup	IV	0.6 mg/kg	6 mg	4 mg/mL	1.5 mL
HYDROCORTISONE		IV/IO	3 mg/kg	30 mg	100 mg/mL	0.3 mL

10 KG

Ventilation: trained rescuer	1 breath q 6-8 sec (8-10 breaths/minute) about 1 second/ breath-visible chest rise; if intubated, continuous compressions without pause for ventilations
Pulse check	brachial/femoral
Compression	2-3 fingers-1 finger width below nipples *Wrap hands around chest if possible, compress with thumbs*
Depth	1.5 inch (4 cm) or at least 1/3 chest depth
Rate	at least 100 compressions per minute
Compress/vent ratio	30:2 with 1 or 2 rescuers
Foreign body obstruction	5 back blows at level of scapula, support head; alternate with 5 chest compressions *Never perform a blind finger-sweep. Open the mouth and look for object; if you see it, remove it.*

sync cardioversion	0.5 J/kg	5 J
repeat	1 J/kg	10 J
defibrillation	2 J/kg	20 J
repeat	4 J/kg	40 J

IV Bolus Drugs		dose	mg to pt	supplied	mL to give
ADENOSINE	IV	0.1 mg/kg	1 mg	3 mg/mL	0.33 mL
ADENOSINE repeat dose	IV	0.2 mg/kg	2 mg	3 mg/mL	0.67 mL
AMIODARONE	IV/IO	5 mg/kg	50 mg	50 mg/mL	1.00 mL
ATROPINE	IV/IM	0.02 mg/kg	0.2 mg	0.4 mg/mL	0.50 mL
ATROPINE	ETT	0.04 mg/kg	0.4 mg	0.4 mg/mL	1.00 mL
CALCIUM CHLORIDE	IV	20 mg/kg	200 mg	100 mg/mL	2.00 mL
CALCIUM GLUCONATE	IV/IO	60 mg/kg	600 mg	100 mg/mL	6.00 mL
DANTROLENE	IV	2.5 mg/kg	25 mg		
EPHEDRINE	IV	0.15 mg/kg	1.5 mg	10 mg/mL	0.15 mL
EPINEPHRINE (1:10,000)	IV/IO	0.01 mg/kg	0.1 mg	0.1 mg/mL	1.00 mL
EPINEPHRINE (1:1,000)	ETT	0.1 mg/kg	1 mg	1 mg/mL	1.00 mL
ESMOLOL	IV	0.5 mg/kg	5 mg	10 mg/mL	0.50 mL
LABETALOL	IV	0.2 mg/kg	2 mg	5 mg/mL	0.40 mL
LIDOCAINE	IV/IO	1 mg/kg	10 mg	20 mg/mL	0.50 mL
NEOSYNEPHRINE	IV	5 mcg/kg	50 mcg	100 mcg/mL	0.50 mL
ROMAZICON	IV	0.01 mg/kg	0.1 mg	0.1 mg/mL	1.00 mL
VASOPRESSIN	IV/IO	0.4 unit/kg	4 units	20 u/mL	0.20 mL

11 KG MAINTENANCE IV FLUIDS: 42 ML/HR

common pediatric drugs		route	dose	mg to pt	supplied	mL to give
ATROPINE	vagolytic	IV	0.02 mg/kg	0.22 mg	0.4 mg/mL	0.55 mL
GLYCOPYRROLATE	vagolytic	IV	0.004 mg/kg	0.044 mg	0.2 mg/mL	0.22 mL
MIDAZOLAM		IV	0.05 mg/kg	0.55 mg	1 mg/mL	0.55 mL
MIDAZOLAM		PO	0.5 mg/kg	5.5 mg	1 mg/mL	5.5 mL
MIDAZOLAM		IN	0.2 mg/kg	2.2 mg	1 mg/mL	2.2 mL
SUCCINYLCHOLINE		IV	2 mg/kg	22 mg	20 mg/mL	1.1 mL
SUCCINYLCHOLINE		IM	4 mg/kg	44 mg	20 mg/mL	2.2 mL
PROPOFOL		IV	3 mg/kg	33 mg	10 mg/mL	3.3 mL
ETOMIDATE	>10 y	IV	0.3 mg/kg	3.3 mg	2 mg/mL	1.65 mL
FENTANYL		IV	1 mcg/kg	11 mcg	50 mcg/mL	0.22 mL
FENTANYL		IN	2 mcg/kg	22 mcg	50 mcg/mL	0.44 mL
MORPHINE	<6 mo	IV/IM	0.05 mg/kg	0.55 mg	10 mg/mL	0.055 mL
MORPHINE	>6 mo	IV/IM	0.1 mg/kg	1.1 mg	10 mg/mL	0.11 mL
TORADOL	>2-16 y	IV	0.5 mg/kg	5.5 mg	30 mg/mL	0.183 mL
TORADOL	>2-16 y	IM	1 mg/kg	11 mg	30 mg/mL	0.367 mL
ACETAMINOPHEN		PR	20 mg/kg	220 mg		
ACETAMINOPHEN	2-12 y	IV	15 mg/kg	165 mg	10 mg/mL	16.5 mL
CISATRACURIUM		IV	0.1 mg/kg	1.1 mg	2 mg/mL	0.55 mL
PANCURONIUM	<1 mo	IV	0.02 mg/kg	0.22 mg	1 mg/mL	0.22 mL
PANCURONIUM	>1 mo	IV	0.1 mg/kg	1.1 mg	1 mg/mL	1.1 mL
ROCURONIUM		IV	0.6 mg/kg	6.6 mg	10 mg/mL	0.66 mL
ROCURONIUM	RSI	IV	1.2 mg/kg	13.2 mg	10 mg/mL	1.32 mL
VECURONIUM		IV	0.1 mg/kg	1.1 mg	1 mg/mL	1.1 mL
GLYCOPYRROLATE	reversal	IV	0.007 mg/kg	0.077 mg	0.2 mg/mL	0.385 mL
NEOSTIGMINE		IV	0.07 mg/kg	0.77 mg	1 mg/mL	0.77 mL
DEXAMETHASONE		IV	0.25 mg/kg	2.75 mg	10 mg/mL	0.275 mL
ONDANSETRON		IV	0.15 mg/kg	1.65 mg	2 mg/mL	0.825 mL

additional pediatric drugs	route	dose	mg to pt	supplied	mL to give
PREMED/SEDATION; VAGOLYTIC/ANTISIALAGOGUE; GIVE IM 30-60 MIN PREOP					
ATROPINE	IV	0.02 mg/kg	0.22 mg	0.4 mg/mL	0.55 mL
GLYCOPYRROLATE	IM	0.004 mg/kg	0.009 mg	0.2 mg/mL	0.045 mL
MIDAZOLAM	IM	0.1 mg/kg	0.5 mg	1 mg/mL	0.5 mL
INDUCTION					
DEXMEDETOMIDINE load dose	IV	1 mcg/kg	1 mcg	4 mcg/mL	0.25 mL
KETAMINE	IV	2 mg/kg	22 mg	10 mg/mL	2.2 mL
KETAMINE	IM/PR	5 mg/kg	55 mg	10 mg/mL	5.5 mL
OPIOIDS/NONOPIOIDS					
FENTANYL high dose	IV	4 mcg/kg	44 mcg	50 mcg/mL	0.88 mL
FENTANYL cardiac	IV	10 mcg/kg	110 mcg	50 mcg/mL	2.2 mL
HYDROMORPHONE < 6 mo	IV/SQ	0.005 mg/kg	0.055 mg	10 mg/mL	0.0055 mL
HYDROMORPHONE > 6 mo	IV/SQ	0.015 mg/kg	0.165 mg	10 mg/mL	0.0165 mL
REMIFENTANIL	IV	0.5 mcg/kg	1 mcg	50 mcg/mL	0.02 mL
SUFENTANIL	IV	0.5 mcg/kg	5.5 mcg	50 mcg/mL	0.11 mL
REVERSALS					
ATROPINE	IV	0.02 mg/kg	0.22 mg	0.4 mg/mL	0.55 mL
EDROPHONIUM neonate	IV	0.1 mg single dose		10 mg/mL	0.01 mL
EDROPHONIUM > 2 mo	IV	0.04 mg/kg	0.44 mg	10 mg/mL	0.044 mL
FLUMAZENIL	IV	> 1 y	0.01 mg/kg	0.11 mg	0.1 mg/mL	1.1 mL
NALOXONE < 5 y; < 20 kg	IM/IV	0.1 mg/kg	1.1 mg	0.4 mg/mL	2.75 mL
NALOXONE > 5 y; > 20 kg	IM/IV	2 mg per dose		0.4 mg/mL	5 mL
NALOXONE	ETT	0.3 mg/kg	3.3 mg	0.4 mg/mL	8.25 mL

additional pediatric drugs		route	dose	mg to pt	supplied	mL to give
ANTIBIOTICS						
AMPICILLIN	<6 y	IV	50 mg/kg	300 mg		
AMPICILLIN	>6 y	IV	50 mg/kg	550 mg		
AMPICILLIN & SULBACTUM	>1 mo	IV	50 mg/kg	550 mg		
CEFAZOLIN		IV	25 mg/kg	275 mg		
CLINDAMYCIN		IV	10 mg/kg	110 mg		
ERTAPENEM	3 mo-12 y	IV	15 mg/kg	165 mg		
ERTAPENEM	>12 y	IV	1 Gm	per dose		
GENTAMICIN		IV	2 mg/kg	22 mg		
LEVOFLOXACIN		IV	10 mg/kg	110 mg		
METRONIDAZOLE		IV	10 mg/kg	110 mg		
PIPERACILLIN & TAZOBACTAM	<40 kg & 2-9 mo	IV	80 mg/kg	880 mg		
PIPERACILLIN & TAZOBACTAM	<40 kg & >9 mo	IV	100 mg/kg	1,100 mg		
PIPERACILLIN & TAZOBACTAM	>40 kg	IV	3.375 Gm per dose			
VANCOMYCIN		IV	15 mg/kg	165 mg		
ANTINAUSEA						
METOCLOPROMIDE		IV	0.2 mg/kg	2.2 mg	5 mg/mL	0.44 mL
DIPHENHYDRAMINE		IV/IM	1.25 mg/kg	13.75 mg	50 mg/mL	0.275 mL
SCOPOLAMINE		IV/IM	6 mcg/kg	66 mcg	400 mcg/mL	0.165 mL
MISCELLANEOUS MEDS						
AMINOCAPROIC ACID		IV	100 mg/kg	1,100 mg	250 mg/mL	4.4 mL
DESMOPRESSIN		IV/SQ	0.3 mcg/kg	3.3 mcg	4 mcg/mL	0.825 mL
DEXAMETHASONE	croup	IV	0.6 mg/kg	6.6 mg	4 mg/mL	1.65 mL
HYDROCORTISONE		IV/IO	3 mg/kg	33 mg	100 mg/mL	0.33 mL

11 KG

Ventilation: trained rescuer	1 breath q 6-8 sec (8-10 breaths/minute) about 1 second/ breath-visible chest rise; if intubated, continuous compressions *without pause for ventilations*
Pulse check	brachial/femoral
Compression	2-3 fingers-1 finger width below nipples *Wrap hands around chest if possible, compress with thumbs*
Depth	1.5 inch (4 cm) or at least 1/3 chest depth
Rate	at least 100 compressions per minute
Compress/vent ratio	30:2 with 1 or 2 rescuers
Foreign body obstruction	5 back blows at level of scapula, support head; alternate with 5 chest compressions Never perform a blind finger-sweep. Open the mouth and look for object; if you see it, remove it.

sync cardioversion	0.5 J/kg	5.5 J
defibrillation	1 J/kg	11 J
repeat	2 J/kg	22 J
repeat	4 J/kg	44 J

IV Bolus Drugs		dose	mg to pt	supplied	mL to give
ADENOSINE	IV	0.1 mg/kg	1.1 mg	3 mg/mL	0.37 mL
ADENOSINE repeat dose	IV	0.2 mg/kg	2.2 mg	3 mg/mL	0.73 mL
AMIODARONE	IV/IO	5 mg/kg	55 mg	50 mg	1.10 mL
ATROPINE	IV/IM	0.02 mg/kg	0.22 mg	0.4 mg/mL	0.55 mL
ATROPINE	ETT	0.04 mg/kg	0.44 mg	0.4 mg/mL	1.10 mL
CALCIUM CHLORIDE	IV	20 mg/kg	220 mg	100 mg	2.20 mL
CALCIUM GLUCONATE	IV/IO	60 mg/kg	660 mg	100 mg/mL	6.60 mL
DANTROLENE	IV	2.5 mg/kg	27.5 mg		
EPHEDRINE	IV	0.15 mg/kg	1.65 mg	10 mg/mL	0.17 mL
EPINEPHRINE (1:10,000)	IV/IO	0.01 mg/kg	0.11 mg	0.1 mg/mL	1.10 mL
EPINEPHRINE (1:1,000)	ETT	0.1 mg/kg	1.1 mg	1 mg/mL	1.10 mL
ESMOLOL	IV	0.5 mg/kg	5.5 mg	10 mg/mL	0.55 mL
LABETALOL	IV	0.2 mg/kg	2.2 mg	5 mg/mL	0.44 mL
LIDOCAINE	IV/IO	1 mg/kg	11 mg	20 mg/mL	0.55 mL
NEOSYNEPHRINE	IV	5 mcg/kg	55 mcg	100 mcg/mL	0.55 mL
ROMAZICON	IV	0.01 mg/kg	0.11 mg	0.1 mg	1.10 mL
VASOPRESSIN	IV/IO	0.4 unit/kg	4.4 units	20 u/mL	0.22 mL

12 KG MAINTENANCE IV FLUIDS: 44 ML/HR

common pediatric drugs		route	dose	mg to pt	supplied	mL to give
ATROPINE	vagolytic	IV	0.02 mg/kg	0.24 mg	0.4 mg/mL	0.6 mL
GLYCOPYRROLATE	vagolytic	IV	0.004 mg/kg	0.048 mg	0.2 mg/mL	0.24 mL
MIDAZOLAM		IV	0.05 mg/kg	0.6 mg	1 mg/mL	0.6 mL
MIDAZOLAM		PO	0.5 mg/kg	6 mg	1 mg/mL	6 mL
MIDAZOLAM		IN	0.2 mg/kg	2.4 mg	1 mg/mL	2.4 mL
SUCCINYLCHOLINE		IV	2 mg/kg	24 mg	20 mg/mL	1.2 mL
SUCCINYLCHOLINE		IM	4 mg/kg	48 mg	20 mg/mL	2.4 mL
PROPOFOL		IV	3 mg/kg	36 mg	10 mg/mL	3.6 mL
ETOMIDATE	>10 y	IV	0.3 mg/kg	3.6 mg	2 mg/mL	1.8 mL
FENTANYL		IV	1 mcg/kg	12 mcg	50 mcg/mL	0.24 mL
FENTANYL		IN	2 mcg/kg	24 mcg	50 mcg/mL	0.48 mL
MORPHINE	<6 mo	IV/IM	0.05 mg/kg	0.6 mg	10 mg/mL	0.06 mL
MORPHINE	>6 mo	IV/IM	0.1 mg/kg	1.2 mg	10 mg/mL	0.12 mL
TORADOL	>2-16 y	IV	0.5 mg/kg	6 mg	30 mg/mL	0.2 mL
TORADOL	>2-16 y	IM	1 mg/kg	12 mg	30 mg/mL	0.4 mL
ACETAMINOPHEN		PR	20 mg/kg	240 mg		
ACETAMINOPHEN	2-12 y	IV	15 mg/kg	180 mg	10 mg/mL	18 mL
CISATRACURIUM		IV	0.1 mg/kg	1.2 mg	2 mg/mL	0.6 mL
PANCURONIUM	<1 mo	IV	0.02 mg/kg	0.24 mg	1 mg/mL	0.24 mL
PANCURONIUM	>1 mo	IV	0.1 mg/kg	1.2 mg	1 mg/mL	1.2 mL
ROCURONIUM		IV	0.6 mg/kg	7.2 mg	10 mg/mL	0.72 mL
ROCURONIUM	RSI	IV	1.2 mg/kg	14.4 mg	10 mg/mL	1.44 mL
VECURONIUM		IV	0.1 mg/kg	1.2 mg	1 mg/mL	1.2 mL
GLYCOPYRROLATE	reversal	IV	0.007 mg/kg	0.084 mg	0.2 mg/mL	0.42 mL
NEOSTIGMINE		IV	0.07 mg/kg	0.84 mg	1 mg/mL	0.84 mL
DEXAMETHASONE		IV	0.25 mg/kg	3 mg	10 mg/mL	0.3 mL
ONDANSETRON		IV	0.15 mg/kg	1.8 mg	2 mg/mL	0.9 mL

additional pediatric drugs	route	dose	mg to pt	supplied	mL to give
PREMED/SEDATION, VAGOLYTIC/ANTISIALAGOGUE; GIVE IM 30-60 MIN PREOP					
ATROPINE	IM	0.02 mg/kg	0.24 mg	0.4 mg/mL	0.6 mL
GLYCOPYRROLATE	IM	0.004 mg/kg	0.009 mg	0.2 mg/mL	0.045 mL
MIDAZOLAM	IM	0.1 mg/kg	0.5 mg	1 mg/mL	0.5 mL
DEXMEDETOMIDINE load dose	IV	0.5 mcg/kg	1 mcg	4 mcg/mL	0.25 mL
INDUCTION					
KETAMINE	IV	2 mg/kg	24 mg	10 mg/mL	2.4 mL
KETAMINE	IM/PR	5 mg/kg	60 mg	10 mg/mL	6 mL
OPIOIDS/NONOPIOIDS					
FENTANYL high dose	IV	4 mcg/kg	48 mcg	50 mcg/mL	0.96 mL
FENTANYL cardiac	IV	10 mcg/kg	120 mcg	50 mcg/mL	2.4 mL
HYDROMORPHONE <6 mo	IV/SQ	0.005 mg/kg	0.06 mg	10 mg/mL	0.006 mL
HYDROMORPHONE >6 mo	IV/SQ	0.015 mg/kg	0.18 mg	10 mg/mL	0.018 mL
REMIFENTANIL	IV	0.5 mcg/kg	1 mcg	50 mcg/mL	0.02 mL
SUFENTANIL	IV	0.5 mcg/kg	6 mcg	50 mcg/mL	0.12 mL
REVERSALS					
ATROPINE	IV	0.02 mg/kg	0.24 mg	0.4 mg/mL	0.6 mL
EDROPHONIUM neonate	IV	0.1 mg single dose		10 mg/mL	0.01 mL
EDROPHONIUM >2 mo	IV	0.04 mg/kg	0.48 mg	10 mg/mL	0.048 mL
FLUMAZENIL >1 y	IV	0.01 mg/kg	0.12 mg	0.1 mg/mL	1.2 mL
NALOXONE <5 y; <20 kg	IM/IV	0.1 mg/kg	1.2 mg	0.4 mg/mL	3 mL
NALOXONE >5 y; >20 kg	IM	2 mg per dose		0.4 mg/mL	5 mL
NALOXONE	ETT	0.3 mg/kg	3.6 mg	0.4 mg/mL	9 mL

additional pediatric drugs		route	dose	mg to pt	supplied	mL to give
ANTIBIOTICS						
AMPICILLIN	<6 y	IV	50 mg/kg	300 mg		
AMPICILLIN	>6 y	IV	50 mg/kg	600 mg		
AMPICILLIN & SULBACTUM	>1 mo	IV	50 mg/kg	600 mg		
CEFAZOLIN		IV	25 mg/kg	300 mg		
CLINDAMYCIN		IV	10 mg/kg	120 mg		
ERTAPENEM	3 mo-12 y	IV	15 mg/kg	180 mg		
ERTAPENEM	>12 y	IV	1 Gm	per dose		
GENTAMICIN		IV	2 mg/kg	24 mg		
LEVOFLOXACIN		IV	10 mg/kg	120 mg		
METRONIDAZOLE		IV	10 mg/kg	120 mg		
PIPERACILLIN & TAZOBACTAM	<40 kg & 2-9 mo	IV	80 mg/kg	960 mg		
PIPERACILLIN & TAZOBACTAM	<40 kg & >9 mo	IV	100 mg/kg	1,200 mg		
PIPERACILLIN & TAZOBACTAM	>40 kg	IV	3.375 Gm per dose			
VANCOMYCIN		IV	15 mg/kg	180 mg		
ANTINAUSEA						
METOCLOPROMIDE		IV	0.2 mg/kg	2.4 mg	5 mg/mL	0.48 mL
DIPHENHYDRAMINE		IV/IM	1.25 mg/kg	15 mg	50 mg/mL	0.3 mL
SCOPOLAMINE		IV/IM	6 mcg/kg	72 mcg	400 mcg/mL	0.18 mL
MISCELLANEOUS MEDS						
AMINOCAPROIC ACID		IV	100 mg/kg	1,200 mg	250 mg/mL	4.8 mL
DESMOPRESSIN		IV/SQ	0.3 mcg/kg	3.6 mcg	4 mcg/mL	0.9 mL
DEXAMETHASONE	croup	IV	0.6 mg/kg	7.2 mg	4 mg/mL	1.8 mL
HYDROCORTISONE		IV/IO	3 mg/kg	36 mg	100 mg/mL	0.36 mL

● Pediatric Pharmacology: Perioperative and Emergency Drugs

12 KG

Ventilation: trained rescuer	1 breath q 6-8 sec (8-10 breaths/minute) about 1 second/ breath-visible chest rise; if intubated, continuous compressions without pause for ventilations
Pulse check	brachial/femoral
Compression	2-3 fingers–1 finger width below nipples *Wrap hands around chest if possible, compress with thumbs*
Depth	1.5 inch (4 cm) or at least 1/3 chest depth
Rate	at least 100 compressions per minute
Compress/vent ratio	30:2 with 1 or 2 rescuers
Foreign body obstruction	5 back blows at level of scapula, support head; alternate with 5 chest compressions. Never perform a blind finger-sweep. Open the mouth and look for object; if you see it, remove it.

sync cardioversion		0.5 J/kg	6 J
defibrillation	repeat	1 J/kg	12 J
		2 J/kg	24 J
	repeat	4 J/kg	48 J

IV Bolus Drugs		dose	mg to pt	supplied	mL to give
ADENOSINE	IV	0.1 mg/kg	1.2 mg	3 mg/mL	0.40 mL
ADENOSINE repeat dose	IV	0.2 mg/kg	2.4 mg	3 mg/mL	0.80 mL
AMIODARONE	IV/IO	5 mg/kg	60 mg	50 mg/mL	1.20 mL
ATROPINE	IV/IM	0.02 mg/kg	0.24 mg	0.4 mg/mL	0.60 mL
ATROPINE	ETT	0.04 mg/kg	0.48 mg	0.4 mg/mL	1.20 mL
CALCIUM CHLORIDE	IV	20 mg/kg	240 mg	100 mg/mL	2.40 mL
CALCIUM GLUCONATE	IV/IO	60 mg/kg	720 mg	100 mg/mL	7.20 mL
DANTROLENE	IV	2.5 mg/kg	30 mg		
EPHEDRINE	IV	0.15 mg/kg	1.8 mg	10 mg/mL	0.18 mL
EPINEPHRINE (1:10,000)	IV/IO	0.01 mg/kg	0.12 mg	0.1 mg/mL	1.20 mL
EPINEPHRINE (1:1,000)	ETT	0.1 mg/kg	1.2 mg	1 mg/mL	1.20 mL
ESMOLOL	IV	0.5 mg/kg	6 mg	10 mg/mL	0.60 mL
LABETALOL	IV	0.2 mg/kg	2.4 mg	5 mg/mL	0.48 mL
LIDOCAINE	IV/IO	1 mg/kg	12 mg	20 mg/mL	0.60 mL
NEOSYNEPHRINE	IV	5 mcg/kg	60 mcg	100 mcg/mL	0.60 mL
ROMAZICON	IV	0.01 mg/kg	0.12 mg	0.1 mg/mL	1.20 mL
VASOPRESSIN	IV/IO	0.4 unit/kg	4.8 units	20 u/mL	0.24 mL

13 KG MAINTENANCE IV FLUIDS: 46 ML/HR

common pediatric drugs		route	dose	mg to pt	supplied	mL to give
ATROPINE	vagolytic	IV	0.02 mg/kg	0.26 mg	0.4 mg/mL	0.65 mL
GLYCOPYRROLATE	vagolytic	IV	0.004 mg/kg	0.052 mg	0.2 mg/mL	0.26 mL
MIDAZOLAM		IV	0.05 mg/kg	0.6 mg	1 mg/mL	0.6 mL
MIDAZOLAM		PO	0.5 mg/kg	6.5 mg	1 mg/mL	6.5 mL
MIDAZOLAM		IN	0.2 mg/kg	2.6 mg	1 mg/mL	2.6 mL
SUCCINYLCHOLINE		IV	2 mg/kg	26 mg	20 mg/mL	1.3 mL
SUCCINYLCHOLINE		IM	4 mg/kg	52 mg	20 mg/mL	2.6 mL
PROPOFOL		IV	3 mg/kg	39 mg	10 mg/mL	3.9 mL
ETOMIDATE	>10 y	IV	0.3 mg/kg	3.9 mg	2 mg/mL	1.95 mL
FENTANYL		IV	1 mcg/kg	13 mcg	50 mcg/mL	0.26 mL
FENTANYL		IN	2 mcg/kg	26 mcg	50 mcg/mL	0.52 mL
MORPHINE	<6 mo	IV/IM	0.05 mg/kg	0.65 mg	10 mg/mL	0.065 mL
MORPHINE	>6 mo	IV/IM	0.1 mg/kg	1.3 mg	10 mg/mL	0.13 mL
TORADOL	>2-16 y	IV	0.5 mg/kg	6.5 mg	30 mg/mL	0.217 mL
TORADOL	>2-16 y	IM	1 mg/kg	13 mg	30 mg/mL	0.433 mL
ACETAMINOPHEN		PR	20 mg/kg	260 mg		
ACETAMINOPHEN	2-12 y	IV	15 mg/kg	195 mg	10 mg/mL	19.5 mL
CISATRACURIUM		IV	0.1 mg/kg	1.3 mg	2 mg/mL	0.65 mL
PANCURONIUM	<1 mo	IV	0.02 mg/kg	0.26 mg	1 mg/mL	0.26 mL
PANCURONIUM	>1 mo	IV	0.1 mg/kg	1.3 mg	1 mg/mL	1.3 mL
ROCURONIUM		IV	0.6 mg/kg	7.8 mg	10 mg/mL	0.78 mL
ROCURONIUM	RSI	IV	1.2 mg/kg	15.6 mg	10 mg/mL	1.56 mL
VECURONIUM		IV	0.1 mg/kg	1.3 mg	1 mg/mL	1.3 mL
GLYCOPYRROLATE	reversal	IV	0.007 mg/kg	0.091 mg	0.2 mg/mL	0.455 mL
NEOSTIGMINE		IV	0.07 mg/kg	0.91 mg	1 mg/mL	0.91 mL
DEXAMETHASONE		IV	0.25 mg/kg	3.25 mg	10 mg/mL	0.325 mL
ONDANSETRON		IV	0.15 mg/kg	1.95 mg	2 mg/mL	0.975 mL

additional pediatric drugs	route	dose	mg to pt	supplied	mL to give
PREMED/SEDATION; VAGOLYTIC/ANTISIALAGOGUE; GIVE IM 30–60 MIN PREOP					
ATROPINE	IV	0.02 mg/kg	0.26 mg	0.4 mg/mL	0.65 mL
GLYCOPYRROLATE	IM	0.004 mg/kg	0.009 mg	0.2 mg/mL	0.045 mL
MIDAZOLAM	IM	0.1 mg/kg	0.5 mg	1 mg/mL	0.5 mL
DEXMEDETOMIDINE	IV	load dose 0.5 mcg/kg	1 mcg	4 mcg/mL	0.25 mL
INDUCTION					
KETAMINE	IV	2 mg/kg	26 mg	10 mg/mL	2.6 mL
KETAMINE	IM/PR	5 mg/kg	65 mg	10 mg/mL	6.5 mL
OPIOIDS/NONOPIOIDS					
FENTANYL	IV	high dose 4 mcg/kg	52 mcg	50 mcg/mL	1.04 mL
FENTANYL	IV	cardiac 10 mcg/kg	130 mcg	50 mcg/mL	2.6 mL
HYDROMORPHONE	IV/SQ	< 6 mo 0.005 mg/kg	0.065 mg	10 mg/mL	0.0065 mL
HYDROMORPHONE	IV/SQ	> 6 mo 0.015 mg/kg	0.195 mg	10 mg/mL	0.0195 mL
REMIFENTANIL	IV	0.5 mcg/kg	1 mcg	50 mcg/mL	0.02 mL
SUFENTANIL	IV	0.5 mcg/kg	6.5 mcg	50 mcg/mL	0.13 mL
REVERSALS					
ATROPINE	IV	0.02 mg/kg	0.26 mg	0.4 mg/mL	0.65 mL
EDROPHONIUM	IV	neonate	0.1 mg single dose	10 mg/mL	0.01 mL
EDROPHONIUM	IV	> 2 mo 0.04 mg/kg	0.52 mg	10 mg/mL	0.052 mL
FLUMAZENIL	IV	> 1 y 0.01 mg/kg	0.13 mg	0.1 mg/mL	1.3 mL
NALOXONE	IV/IM	< 20 kg; < 5 y 0.1 mg/kg	1.3 mg	0.4 mg/mL	3.25 mL
NALOXONE	IV/IM	> 20 kg; > 5 y	2 mg per dose	0.4 mg/mL	5 mL
NALOXONE	ETT	0.3 mg/kg	3.9 mg	0.4 mg/mL	9.75 mL

additional pediatric drugs		route	dose	mg to pt	supplied	mL to give
ANTIBIOTICS						
AMPICILLIN	<6 y	IV	50 mg/kg	300 mg		
AMPICILLIN	>6 y	IV	50 mg/kg	650 mg		
AMPICILLIN & SULBACTUM	>1 mo	IV	50 mg/kg	650 mg		
CEFAZOLIN		IV	25 mg/kg	325 mg		
CLINDAMYCIN		IV	10 mg/kg	130 mg		
ERTAPENEM	3 mo-12 y	IV	15 mg/kg	195 mg		
ERTAPENEM	>12 y	IV	1 Gm	per dose		
GENTAMICIN		IV	2 mg/kg	26 mg		
LEVOFLOXACIN		IV	10 mg/kg	130 mg		
METRONIDAZOLE		IV	10 mg/kg	130 mg		
PIPERACILLIN & TAZOBACTAM	<40 kg & 2-9 mo	IV	80 mg/kg	1,040 mg		
PIPERACILLIN & TAZOBACTAM	<40 kg & >9 mo	IV	100 mg/kg	1,300 mg		
PIPERACILLIN & TAZOBACTAM	>40 kg	IV	3.375 Gm per dose			
VANCOMYCIN		IV	15 mg/kg	195 mg		
ANTINAUSEA						
METOCLOPROMIDE		IV	0.2 mg/kg	2.6 mg	5 mg/mL	0.52 mL
DIPHENHYDRAMINE		IV/IM	1.25 mg/kg	16.25 mg	50 mg/mL	0.325 mL
SCOPOLAMINE		IV/IM	6 mcg/kg	78 mcg	400 mcg/mL	0.195 mL
MISCELLANEOUS MEDS						
AMINOCAPROIC ACID		IV	100 mg/kg	1,300 mg	250 mg/mL	5.2 mL
DESMOPRESSIN		IV/SQ	0.3 mcg/kg	3.9 mcg	4 mcg/mL	0.975 mL
DEXAMETHASONE	croup	IV	0.6 mg/kg	7.8 mg	4 mg/mL	1.95 mL
HYDROCORTISONE		IV/IO	3 mg/kg	39 mg	100 mg/mL	0.39 mL

13 KG

Ventilation: trained rescuer	1 breath q 6-8 sec (8-10 breaths/minute) about 1 second/breath-visible chest rise; if intubated, continuous compressions without pause for ventilations
Pulse check	carotid or femoral
Compression	heel of 1 hand or both hands one atop the other-lower half of sternum between nipples
Depth	2 inches (5 cm) or at least 1/3 chest depth
Rate	at least 100 compressions per minute
Compress/vent ratio	30:2 single rescuer; 15:2 2 healthcare providers
Foreign body obstruction	Heimlich maneuver; Never perform a blind finger-sweep. Open the mouth and look for object; if you see it, remove it.

sync cardioversion	0.5 J/kg	6.5 J
defibrillation	1 J/kg	13 J
repeat	2 J/kg	26 J
repeat	4 J/kg	52 J

IV Bolus Drugs		dose	mg to pt	supplied	mL to give
ADENOSINE	IV	0.1 mg/kg	1.3 mg	3 mg/mL	0.43 mL
ADENOSINE repeat dose	IV	0.2 mg/kg	2.6 mg	3 mg/mL	0.87 mL
AMIODARONE	IV/IO	5 mg/kg	65 mg	50 mg/mL	1.30 mL
ATROPINE	IV/IM	0.02 mg/kg	0.26 mg	0.4 mg/mL	0.65 mL
ATROPINE	ETT	0.04 mg/kg	0.52 mg	0.4 mg/mL	1.30 mL
CALCIUM CHLORIDE	IV	20 mg/kg	260 mg	100 mg/mL	2.60 mL
CALCIUM GLUCONATE	IV/IO	60 mg/kg	780 mg	100 mg/mL	7.80 mL
DANTROLENE	IV	2.5 mg/kg	30 mg		
EPHEDRINE	IV	0.15 mg/kg	1.95 mg	10 mg/mL	0.20 mL
EPINEPHRINE (1:10,000)	IV/IO	0.01 mg/kg	0.13 mg	0.1 mg/mL	1.30 mL
EPINEPHRINE (1:1,000)	ETT	0.1 mg/kg	1.3 mg	1 mg/mL	1.30 mL
ESMOLOL	IV	0.5 mg/kg	6.5 mg	10 mg/mL	0.65 mL
LABETALOL	IV	0.2 mg/kg	2.6 mg	5 mg/mL	0.52 mL
LIDOCAINE	IV/IO	1 mg/kg	13 mg	20 mg/mL	0.65 mL
NEOSYNEPHRINE	IV	5 mcg/kg	65 mcg	100 mcg/mL	0.65 mL
ROMAZICON	IV	0.01 mg/kg	0.13 mg	0.1 mg/mL	1.30 mL
VASOPRESSIN	IV/IO	0.4 unit/kg	5.2 units	20 u/mL	0.26 mL

14 KG MAINTENANCE IV FLUIDS: 48 ML/HR

common pediatric drugs		route	dose	mg to pt	supplied	mL to give
ATROPINE	vagolytic	IV	0.02 mg/kg	0.28 mg	0.4 mg/mL	0.7 mL
GLYCOPYRROLATE	vagolytic	IV	0.004 mg/kg	0.056 mg	0.2 mg/mL	0.28 mL
MIDAZOLAM		IV	0.05 mg/kg	0.6 mg	1 mg/mL	0.6 mL
MIDAZOLAM		PO	0.5 mg/kg	7 mg	1 mg/mL	7 mL
MIDAZOLAM		IN	0.2 mg/kg	2.8 mg	1 mg/mL	2.8 mL
SUCCINYLCHOLINE		IV	2 mg/kg	28 mg	20 mg/mL	1.4 mL
SUCCINYLCHOLINE		IM	4 mg/kg	56 mg	20 mg/mL	2.8 mL
PROPOFOL		IV	3 mg/kg	42 mg	10 mg/mL	4.2 mL
ETOMIDATE	>10 y	IV	0.3 mg/kg	4.2 mg	2 mg/mL	2.1 mL
FENTANYL		IV	1 mcg/kg	14 mcg	50 mcg/mL	0.28 mL
FENTANYL		IN	2 mcg/kg	28 mcg	50 mcg/mL	0.56 mL
MORPHINE	<6 mo	IV/IM	0.05 mg/kg	0.7 mg	10 mg/mL	0.07 mL
MORPHINE	>6 mo	IV/IM	0.1 mg/kg	1.4 mg	10 mg/mL	0.14 mL
TORADOL	>2-16 y	IV	0.5 mg/kg	7 mg	30 mg/mL	0.233 mL
TORADOL	>2-16 y	IM	1 mg/kg	14 mg	30 mg/mL	0.467 mL
ACETAMINOPHEN		PR	20 mg/kg	280 mg		
ACETAMINOPHEN	2-12 y	IV	15 mg/kg	210 mg	10 mg/mL	21 mL
CISATRACURIUM		IV	0.1 mg/kg	1.4 mg	2 mg/mL	0.7 mL
PANCURONIUM	<1 mo	IV	0.02 mg/kg	0.28 mg	1 mg/mL	0.28 mL
PANCURONIUM	>1 mo	IV	0.1 mg/kg	1.4 mg	1 mg/mL	1.4 mL
ROCURONIUM		IV	0.6 mg/kg	8.4 mg	10 mg/mL	0.84 mL
ROCURONIUM	RSI	IV	1.2 mg/kg	16.8 mg	10 mg/mL	1.68 mL
VECURONIUM		IV	0.1 mg/kg	1.4 mg	1 mg/mL	1.4 mL
GLYCOPYRROLATE	reversal	IV	0.007 mg/kg	0.098 mg	0.2 mg/mL	0.49 mL
NEOSTIGMINE		IV	0.07 mg/kg	0.98 mg	1 mg/mL	0.98 mL
DEXAMETHASONE		IV	0.25 mg/kg	3.5 mg	10 mg/mL	0.35 mL
ONDANSETRON		IV	0.15 mg/kg	2.1 mg	2 mg/mL	1.05 mL

Pediatric Pharmacology: Perioperative and Emergency Drugs   138

additional pediatric drugs		route	dose	mg to pt	supplied	mL to give
PREMED/SEDATION, VAGOLYTIC/ANTISIALAGOGUE; GIVE IM 30-60 MIN PREOP						
ATROPINE		IM	0.02 mg/kg	0.28 mg	0.4 mg/mL	0.7 mL
GLYCOPYRROLATE		IM	0.004 mg/kg	0.009 mg	0.2 mg/mL	0.045 mL
MIDAZOLAM		IM	0.1 mg/kg	0.5 mg	1 mg/mL	0.5 mL
DEXMEDETOMIDINE load dose		IV	0.5 mcg/kg	1 mcg	4 mcg/mL	0.25 mL
INDUCTION						
KETAMINE		IV	2 mg/kg	28 mg	10 mg/mL	2.8 mL
KETAMINE		IM/PR	5 mg/kg	70 mg	10 mg/mL	7 mL
OPIOIDS/NONOPIOIDS						
FENTANYL		IV	4 mcg/kg	56 mcg	50 mcg/mL	1.12 mL
FENTANYL	cardiac	IV	10 mcg/kg	140 mcg	50 mcg/mL	2.8 mL
HYDROMORPHONE	< 6 mo	IV/SQ	0.005 mg/kg	0.07 mg	10 mg/mL	0.007 mL
HYDROMORPHONE	> 6 mo	IV/SQ	0.015 mg/kg	0.21 mg	10 mg/mL	0.021 mL
REMIFENTANIL		IV	0.5 mcg/kg	1 mcg	50 mcg/mL	0.02 mL
SUFENTANIL		IV	0.5 mcg/kg	7 mcg	50 mcg/mL	0.14 mL
REVERSALS						
ATROPINE		IV	0.02 mg/kg	0.28 mg	0.4 mg/mL	0.7 mL
EDROPHONIUM	neonate	IV	0.1 mg single dose		10 mg/mL	0.01 mL
EDROPHONIUM	> 2 mo	IV	0.04 mg/kg	0.56 mg	10 mg/mL	0.056 mL
FLUMAZENIL	> 1 y	IV	0.01 mg/kg	0.14 mg	0.1 mg/mL	1.4 mL
NALOXONE	< 5 y; < 20 kg	IV/IM	0.1 mg/kg	1.4 mg	0.4 mg/mL	3.5 mL
NALOXONE	< 5 y; > 20 kg	IV/IM	2 mg per dose		0.4 mg/mL	5 mL
NALOXONE	ETT		0.3 mg/kg	4.2 mg	0.4 mg/mL	10.5 mL

additional pediatric drugs		route	dose	mg to pt	supplied	mL to give
ANTIBIOTICS						
AMPICILLIN	<6 y	IV	50 mg/kg	300 mg		
AMPICILLIN	>6 y	IV	50 mg/kg	700 mg		
AMPICILLIN & SULBACTUM	>1 mo	IV	50 mg/kg	700 mg		
CEFAZOLIN		IV	25 mg/kg	350 mg		
CLINDAMYCIN		IV	10 mg/kg	140 mg		
ERTAPENEM	3 mo-12 y	IV	15 mg/kg	210 mg		
ERTAPENEM	>12 y	IV	1 Gm	per dose		
GENTAMICIN		IV	2 mg/kg	28 mg		
LEVOFLOXACIN		IV	10 mg/kg	140 mg		
METRONIDAZOLE		IV	10 mg/kg	140 mg		
PIPERACILLIN & TAZOBACTAM	<40 kg & 2-9 mo	IV	80 mg/kg	1,120 mg		
PIPERACILLIN & TAZOBACTAM	<40 kg & >9 mo	IV	100 mg/kg	1,400 mg		
PIPERACILLIN & TAZOBACTAM	>40 kg	IV	3.375 Gm per dose			
VANCOMYCIN		IV	15 mg/kg	210 mg		
ANTINAUSEA						
METOCLOPROMIDE		IV	0.2 mg/kg	2.8 mg	5 mg/mL	0.56 mL
DIPHENHYDRAMINE		IV/IM	1.25 mg/kg	17.5 mg	50 mg/mL	0.35 mL
SCOPOLAMINE		IV/IM	6 mcg/kg	84 mcg	400 mcg/mL	0.21 mL
MISCELLANEOUS MEDS						
AMINOCAPROIC ACID		IV	100 mg/kg	1,400 mg	250 mg/mL	5.6 mL
DESMOPRESSIN		IV/SQ	0.3 mcg/kg	4.2 mcg	4 mcg/mL	1.05 mL
DEXAMETHASONE	croup	IV	0.6 mg/kg	8.4 mg	4 mg/mL	2.1 mL
HYDROCORTISONE		IV/IO	3 mg/kg	42 mg	100 mg/mL	0.42 mL

14 KG

1 year → 13 kg and up

Ventilation: trained rescuer	1 breath q 6-8 sec (8-10 breaths/minute) about 1 second/ breath-visible chest rise; if intubated, continuous compressions
Pulse check	carotid or femoral without pause for ventilations
Compression	heel of 1 hand or both hands one atop the other-lower half of sternum between nipples
Depth	2 inches (5 cm) or at least 1/3 chest depth
Rate	at least 100 compressions per minute
Compress/vent ratio	30:2 single rescuer 15:2 healthcare providers
Foreign body obstruction	Heimlich maneuver Never perform a blind finger-sweep. Open the mouth and look for object; if you see it, remove it.

sync cardioversion	0.5 J/kg	7 J	
defibrillation	1 J/kg	14 J	repeat
	2 J/kg	28 J	
	4 J/kg	56 J	repeat

IV Bolus Drugs		dose	mg to pt	supplied	mL to give
ADENOSINE	IV	0.1 mg/kg	1.4 mg	3 mg/mL	0.47 mL
ADENOSINE repeat dose	IV	0.2 mg/kg	2.8 mg	3 mg/mL	0.93 mL
AMIODARONE	IV/IO	5 mg/kg	70 mg	50 mg/mL	1.40 mL
ATROPINE	IM/IV	0.02 mg/kg	0.28 mg	0.4 mg/mL	0.70 mL
ATROPINE	ETT	0.04 mg/kg	0.56 mg	0.4 mg/mL	1.40 mL
CALCIUM CHLORIDE	IV	20 mg/kg	280 mg	100 mg/mL	2.80 mL
CALCIUM GLUCONATE	IV/IO	60 mg/kg	800 mg	100 mg/mL	8.00 mL
DANTROLENE	IV	2.5 mg/kg	30 mg		
EPHEDRINE	IV	0.15 mg/kg	2.1 mg	10 mg/mL	0.21 mL
EPINEPHRINE (1:10,000)	IV/IO	0.01 mg/kg	0.14 mg	0.1 mg/mL	1.40 mL
EPINEPHRINE (1:1,000)	ETT	0.1 mg/kg	1.4 mg	1 mg/mL	1.40 mL
ESMOLOL	IV	0.5 mg/kg	7 mg	10 mg/mL	0.70 mL
LABETALOL	IV	0.2 mg/kg	2.8 mg	5 mg/mL	0.56 mL
LIDOCAINE	IV/IO	1 mg/kg	14 mg	20 mg/mL	0.70 mL
NEOSYNEPHRINE	IV	5 mcg/kg	70 mcg	100 mcg/mL	0.70 mL
ROMAZICON	IV	0.01 mg/kg	0.14 mg	0.1 mg/mL	1.40 mL
VASOPRESSIN	IV/IO	0.4 unit/kg	5.6 units	20 u/mL	0.28 mL

15 KG MAINTENANCE IV FLUIDS: 50 ML/HR

common pediatric drugs		route	dose	mg to pt	supplied	mL to give
ATROPINE	vagolytic	IV	0.02 mg/kg	0.3 mg	0.4 mg/mL	0.75 mL
GLYCOPYRROLATE	vagolytic	IV	0.004 mg/kg	0.06 mg	0.2 mg/mL	0.3 mL
MIDAZOLAM		IV	0.05 mg/kg	0.6 mg	1 mg/mL	0.6 mL
MIDAZOLAM		PO	0.5 mg/kg	7.5 mg	1 mg/mL	7.5 mL
MIDAZOLAM		IN	0.2 mg/kg	3 mg	1 mg/mL	3 mL
SUCCINYLCHOLINE		IV	2 mg/kg	30 mg	20 mg/mL	1.5 mL
SUCCINYLCHOLINE		IM	4 mg/kg	60 mg	20 mg/mL	3 mL
PROPOFOL		IV	3 mg/kg	45 mg	10 mg/mL	4.5 mL
ETOMIDATE	>10 y	IV	0.3 mg/kg	4.5 mg	2 mg/mL	2.25 mL
FENTANYL		IV	1 mcg/kg	15 mcg	50 mcg/mL	0.3 mL
FENTANYL		IN	2 mcg/kg	30 mcg	50 mcg/mL	0.6 mL
MORPHINE	<6 mo	IV/IM	0.05 mg/kg	0.75 mg	10 mg/mL	0.075 mL
MORPHINE	>6 mo	IV/IM	0.1 mg/kg	1.5 mg	10 mg/mL	0.15 mL
TORADOL	>2-16 y	IV	0.5 mg/kg	7.5 mg	30 mg/mL	0.25 mL
TORADOL	>2-16 y	IM	1 mg/kg	15 mg	30 mg/mL	0.5 mL
ACETAMINOPHEN		PR	20 mg/kg	300 mg		
ACETAMINOPHEN	2-12 y	IV	15 mg/kg	225 mg	10 mg/mL	22.5 mL
CISATRACURIUM		IV	0.1 mg/kg	1.5 mg	2 mg/mL	0.75 mL
PANCURONIUM	<1 mo	IV	0.02 mg/kg	0.3 mg	1 mg/mL	0.3 mL
PANCURONIUM	>1 mo	IV	0.1 mg/kg	1.5 mg	1 mg/mL	1.5 mL
ROCURONIUM		IV	0.6 mg/kg	9 mg	10 mg/mL	0.9 mL
ROCURONIUM	RSI	IV	1.2 mg/kg	18 mg	10 mg/mL	1.8 mL
VECURONIUM		IV	0.1 mg/kg	1.5 mg	1 mg/mL	1.5 mL
GLYCOPYRROLATE	reversal	IV	0.007 mg/kg	0.105 mg	0.2 mg/mL	0.525 mL
NEOSTIGMINE		IV	0.07 mg/kg	1.05 mg	1 mg/mL	1.05 mL
DEXAMETHASONE		IV	0.25 mg/kg	3.75 mg	10 mg/mL	0.375 mL
ONDANSETRON		IV	0.15 mg/kg	2.25 mg	2 mg/mL	1.125 mL

additional pediatric drugs	route	dose	mg to pt	supplied	mL to give
PREMED/SEDATION; VAGOLYTIC/ANTISIALAGOGUE; GIVE IM 30–60 MIN PREOP					
ATROPINE	IV	0.02 mg/kg	0.3 mg	0.4 mg/mL	0.75 mL
GLYCOPYRROLATE	IM	0.004 mg/kg	0.009 mg	0.2 mg/mL	0.045 mL
MIDAZOLAM	IM	0.1 mg/kg	0.5 mg	1 mg/mL	0.5 mL
DEXMEDETOMIDINE	IV	load dose 0.5 mcg/kg	1 mcg	4 mcg/mL	0.25 mL
INDUCTION					
KETAMINE	IV	2 mg/kg	30 mg	10 mg/mL	3 mL
KETAMINE	IM/PR	5 mg/kg	75 mg	10 mg/mL	7.5 mL
OPIOIDS/NONOPIOIDS					
FENTANYL	IV	high dose 4 mcg/kg	60 mcg	50 mcg/mL	1.2 mL
FENTANYL	IV	cardiac 10 mcg/kg	150 mcg	50 mcg/mL	3 mL
HYDROMORPHONE	SQ/IV	< 6 mo 0.005 mg/kg	0.075 mg	10 mg/mL	0.0075 mL
HYDROMORPHONE	SQ/IV	> 6 mo 0.015 mg/kg	0.225 mg	10 mg/mL	0.0225 mL
REMIFENTANIL	IV	0.5 mcg/kg	1 mcg	50 mcg/mL	0.02 mL
SUFENTANIL	IV	0.5 mcg/kg	7.5 mcg	50 mcg/mL	0.15 mL
REVERSALS					
ATROPINE	IV	0.02 mg/kg	0.3 mg	0.4 mg/mL	0.75 mL
EDROPHONIUM	IV	neonate	0.1 mg single dose	10 mg/mL	0.01 mL
EDROPHONIUM	IV	> 2 mo 0.04 mg/kg	0.6 mg	10 mg/mL	0.06 mL
FLUMAZENIL	IV	> 1 y 0.01 mg/kg	0.15 mg	0.1 mg/mL	1.5 mL
NALOXONE	IM/IV	< 5 y; < 20 kg 0.1 mg/kg	1.5 mg	0.4 mg/mL	3.75 mL
NALOXONE	IM/IV	< 5 y; > 20 kg	2 mg per dose	0.4 mg/mL	5 mL
NALOXONE	ETT	0.3 mg/kg	4.5 mg	0.4 mg/mL	11.25 mL

additional pediatric drugs		route	dose	mg to pt	supplied	mL to give
ANTIBIOTICS						
AMPICILLIN	<6 y	IV	50 mg/kg	300 mg		
AMPICILLIN	>6 y	IV	50 mg/kg	750 mg		
AMPICILLIN & SULBACTUM	>1 mo	IV	50 mg/kg	750 mg		
CEFAZOLIN		IV	25 mg/kg	375 mg		
CLINDAMYCIN		IV	10 mg/kg	150 mg		
ERTAPENEM	3 mo-12 y	IV	15 mg/kg	225 mg		
ERTAPENEM	>12 y	IV	1 Gm	per dose		
GENTAMICIN		IV	2 mg/kg	30 mg		
LEVOFLOXACIN		IV	10 mg/kg	150 mg		
METRONIDAZOLE		IV	10 mg/kg	150 mg		
PIPERACILLIN & TAZOBACTAM	<40 kg & 2-9 mo	IV	80 mg/kg	1,200 mg		
PIPERACILLIN & TAZOBACTAM	<40 kg & >9 mo	IV	100 mg/kg	1,500 mg		
PIPERACILLIN & TAZOBACTAM	>40 kg	IV	3.375 Gm per dose			
VANCOMYCIN		IV	15 mg/kg	225 mg		
ANTINAUSEA						
METOCLOPROMIDE		IV	0.2 mg/kg	3 mg	5 mg/mL	0.6 mL
DIPHENHYDRAMINE		IV/IM	1.25 mg/kg	18.75 mg	50 mg/mL	0.375 mL
SCOPOLAMINE		IV/IM	6 mcg/kg	90 mcg	400 mcg/mL	0.225 mL
MISCELLANEOUS MEDS						
AMINOCAPROIC ACID		IV	100 mg/kg	1,500 mg	250 mg/mL	6 mL
DESMOPRESSIN		IV/SQ	0.3 mcg/kg	4.5 mcg	4 mcg/mL	1.125 mL
DEXAMETHASONE	croup	IV	0.6 mg/kg	9 mg	4 mg/mL	2.25 mL
HYDROCORTISONE		IV/IO	3 mg/kg	45 mg	100 mg/mL	0.45 mL

15 KG

1 year → 13 kg and up

Ventilation:	
trained rescuer	1 breath q 6-8 sec (8-10 breaths/minute) about 1 second/breath-visible chest rise; if intubated, continuous compressions without pause for ventilations
Pulse check	carotid or femoral
Compression	heel of 1 hand or both hands one atop the other-lower half of sternum between nipples
Depth	2 inches (5 cm) or at least 1/3 chest depth
Rate	at least 100 compressions per minute
Compress/vent ratio	30:2 single rescuer / 15:2 healthcare providers
Foreign body obstruction	Heimlich maneuver / Never perform a blind finger-sweep. Open the mouth and look for object; if you see it, remove it.

sync cardioversion	0.5 J/kg	7.5 J
repeat	1 J/kg	15 J
defibrillation	2 J/kg	30 J
repeat	4 J/kg	60 J

IV Bolus Drugs		dose	mg to pt	supplied	mL to give
ADENOSINE	IV	0.1 mg/kg	1.5 mg	3 mg/mL	0.50 mL
ADENOSINE repeat dose	IV	0.2 mg/kg	3 mg	3 mg/mL	1.00 mL
AMIODARONE	IV/IO	5 mg/kg	75 mg	50 mg/mL	1.50 mL
ATROPINE	IM/IV	0.02 mg/kg	0.3 mg	0.4 mg/mL	0.75 mL
ATROPINE	ETT	0.04 mg/kg	0.6 mg	0.4 mg/mL	1.50 mL
CALCIUM CHLORIDE	IV	20 mg/kg	300 mg	100 mg/mL	3.00 mL
CALCIUM GLUCONATE	IV/IO	60 mg/kg	800 mg	100 mg/mL	8.00 mL
DANTROLENE	IV	2.5 mg/kg	30 mg		
EPHEDRINE	IV	0.15 mg/kg	2.25 mg	10 mg/mL	0.23 mL
EPINEPHRINE (1:10,000)	IV/IO	0.01 mg/kg	0.15 mg	0.1 mg/mL	1.50 mL
EPINEPHRINE (1:1,000)	ETT	0.1 mg/kg	1.5 mg	1 mg/mL	1.50 mL
ESMOLOL	IV	0.5 mg/kg	7.5 mg	10 mg/mL	0.75 mL
LABETALOL	IV	0.2 mg/kg	3 mg	5 mg/mL	0.60 mL
LIDOCAINE	IV/IO	1 mg/kg	15 mg	20 mg/mL	0.75 mL
NEOSYNEPHRINE	IV	5 mcg/kg	75 mcg	100 mcg/mL	0.75 mL
ROMAZICON	IV	0.01 mg/kg	0.15 mg	0.1 mg/mL	1.50 mL
VASOPRESSIN	IV/IO	0.4 unit/kg	6 units	20 u/mL	0.30 mL

16 KG MAINTENANCE IV FLUIDS: 52 ML/HR

common pediatric drugs		route	dose	mg to pt	supplied	mL to give
ATROPINE	vagolytic	IV	0.02 mg/kg	0.32 mg	0.4 mg/mL	0.8 mL
GLYCOPYRROLATE	vagolytic	IV	0.004 mg/kg	0.064 mg	0.2 mg/mL	0.32 mL
MIDAZOLAM		IV	0.05 mg/kg	0.6 mg	1 mg/mL	0.6 mL
MIDAZOLAM		PO	0.5 mg/kg	8 mg	1 mg/mL	8 mL
MIDAZOLAM		IN	0.2 mg/kg	3.2 mg	1 mg/mL	3.2 mL
SUCCINYLCHOLINE		IV	2 mg/kg	32 mg	20 mg/mL	1.6 mL
SUCCINYLCHOLINE		IM	4 mg/kg	64 mg	20 mg/mL	3.2 mL
PROPOFOL		IV	3 mg/kg	48 mg	10 mg/mL	4.8 mL
ETOMIDATE	>10 y	IV	0.3 mg/kg	4.8 mg	2 mg/mL	2.4 mL
FENTANYL		IV	1 mcg/kg	16 mcg	50 mcg/mL	0.32 mL
FENTANYL		IN	2 mcg/kg	32 mcg	50 mcg/mL	0.64 mL
MORPHINE	<6 mo	IV/IM	0.05 mg/kg	0.8 mg	10 mg/mL	0.08 mL
MORPHINE	>6 mo	IV/IM	0.1 mg/kg	1.6 mg	10 mg/mL	0.16 mL
TORADOL	>2-16 y	IV	0.5 mg/kg	8 mg	30 mg/mL	0.267 mL
TORADOL	>2-16 y	IM	1 mg/kg	16 mg	30 mg/mL	0.533 mL
ACETAMINOPHEN		PR	20 mg/kg	320 mg		
ACETAMINOPHEN	2-12 y	IV	15 mg/kg	240 mg	10 mg/mL	24 mL
CISATRACURIUM		IV	0.1 mg/kg	1.6 mg	2 mg/mL	0.8 mL
PANCURONIUM	<1 mo	IV	0.02 mg/kg	0.32 mg	1 mg/mL	0.32 mL
PANCURONIUM	>1 mo	IV	0.1 mg/kg	1.6 mg	1 mg/mL	1.6 mL
ROCURONIUM		IV	0.6 mg/kg	9.6 mg	10 mg/mL	0.96 mL
ROCURONIUM	RSI	IV	1.2 mg/kg	19.2 mg	10 mg/mL	1.92 mL
VECURONIUM		IV	0.1 mg/kg	1.6 mg	1 mg/mL	1.6 mL
GLYCOPYRROLATE	reversal	IV	0.007 mg/kg	0.112 mg	0.2 mg/mL	0.56 mL
NEOSTIGMINE		IV	0.07 mg/kg	1.12 mg	1 mg/mL	1.12 mL
DEXAMETHASONE		IV	0.25 mg/kg	4 mg	10 mg/mL	0.4 mL
ONDANSETRON		IV	0.15 mg/kg	2.4 mg	2 mg/mL	1.2 mL

6 Pediatric Pharmacology: Perioperative and Emergency Drugs   145

additional pediatric drugs	route	dose	mg to pt	supplied	mL to give
PREMED/SEDATION; VAGOLYTIC/ANTISIALAGOGUE; GIVE IM 30-60 MIN PREOP					
ATROPINE	IM	0.02 mg/kg	0.32 mg	0.4 mg/mL	0.8 mL
GLYCOPYRROLATE	IM	0.004 mg/kg	0.009 mg	0.2 mg/mL	0.045 mL
MIDAZOLAM	IM	0.1 mg/kg	0.5 mg	1 mg/mL	0.5 mL
DEXMEDETOMIDINE load dose	IV	0.5 mcg/kg	1 mcg	4 mcg/mL	0.25 mL
INDUCTION					
KETAMINE	IV	2 mg/kg	32 mg	10 mg/mL	3.2 mL
KETAMINE	IM/PR	5 mg/kg	80 mg	10 mg/mL	8 mL
OPIOIDS/NONOPIOIDS					
FENTANYL high dose	IV	4 mcg/kg	64 mcg	50 mcg/mL	1.28 mL
FENTANYL cardiac	IV	10 mcg/kg	160 mcg	50 mcg/mL	3.2 mL
HYDROMORPHONE < 6 mo	IV/SQ	0.005 mg/kg	0.08 mg	10 mg/mL	0.008 mL
HYDROMORPHONE > 6 mo	IV/SQ	0.015 mg/kg	0.24 mg	10 mg/mL	0.024 mL
REMIFENTANIL	IV	0.5 mcg/kg	1 mcg	50 mcg/mL	0.02 mL
SUFENTANIL	IV	0.5 mcg/kg	8 mcg	50 mcg/mL	0.16 mL
REVERSALS					
ATROPINE	IV	0.02 mg/kg	0.32 mg	0.4 mg/mL	0.8 mL
EDROPHONIUM	neonate	IV	0.1 mg single dose	10 mg/mL	0.01 mL
EDROPHONIUM	> 2 mo	IV	0.04 mg/kg	0.64 mg	10 mg/mL	0.064 mL
FLUMAZENIL	> 1 y	IV	0.01 mg/kg	0.16 mg	0.1 mg/mL	1.6 mL
NALOXONE	< 5 y; < 20 kg	IV/IM	0.1 mg/kg	1.6 mg	0.4 mg/mL	4 mL
NALOXONE	< 5 y; > 20 kg	IV/IM	2 mg per dose	0.4 mg/mL	5 mL
NALOXONE	ETT	0.3 mg/kg	4.8 mg	0.4 mg/mL	12 mL

additional pediatric drugs		route	dose	mg to pt	supplied	mL to give
ANTIBIOTICS						
AMPICILLIN	<6 y	IV	50 mg/kg	300 mg		
AMPICILLIN	>6 y	IV	50 mg/kg	800 mg		
AMPICILLIN & SULBACTUM	>1 mo	IV	50 mg/kg	800 mg		
CEFAZOLIN		IV	25 mg/kg	400 mg		
CLINDAMYCIN		IV	10 mg/kg	160 mg		
ERTAPENEM	3 mo-12 y	IV	15 mg/kg	240 mg		
ERTAPENEM	>12 y	IV	1 Gm	per dose		
GENTAMICIN		IV	2 mg/kg	32 mg		
LEVOFLOXACIN		IV	10 mg/kg	160 mg		
METRONIDAZOLE		IV	10 mg/kg	160 mg		
PIPERACILLIN & TAZOBACTAM	<40 kg & 2-9 mo	IV	80 mg/kg	1,200 mg		
PIPERACILLIN & TAZOBACTAM	<40 kg & >9 mo	IV	100 mg/kg	1,600 mg		
PIPERACILLIN & TAZOBACTAM	>40 kg	IV	3.375 Gm per dose			
VANCOMYCIN		IV	15 mg/kg	240 mg		
ANTINAUSEA						
METOCLOPROMIDE		IV	0.2 mg/kg	3.2 mg	5 mg/mL	0.64 mL
DIPHENHYDRAMINE		IV/IM	1.25 mg/kg	20 mg	50 mg/mL	0.4 mL
SCOPOLAMINE		IV/IM	6 mcg/kg	96 mcg	400 mcg/mL	0.24 mL
MISCELLANEOUS MEDS						
AMINOCAPROIC ACID		IV	100 mg/kg	1,600 mg	250 mg/mL	6.4 mL
DESMOPRESSIN		IV/SQ	0.3 mcg/kg	4.8 mcg	4 mcg/mL	1.2 mL
DEXAMETHASONE	croup	IV	0.6 mg/kg	9.6 mg	4 mg/mL	2.4 mL
HYDROCORTISONE		IV/IO	3 mg/kg	48 mg	100 mg/mL	0.48 mL

16 KG

1 year → 13 kg and up

Ventilation: trained rescuer	1 breath q 6-8 sec (8-10 breaths/minute) about 1 second/ breath-visible chest rise; if intubated, continuous compressions without pause for ventilations
Pulse check	carotid or femoral
Compression	heel of 1 hand or both hands one atop the other–lower half of sternum between nipples
Depth	2 inches (5 cm) or at least 1/3 chest depth
Rate	at least 100 compressions per minute
Compress/vent ratio	30:2 single rescuer / 15:2 healthcare providers
Foreign body obstruction	Heimlich maneuver / Never perform a blind finger-sweep. Open the mouth and look for object; if you see it, remove it.

sync cardioversion	0.5 J/kg	8 J
repeat	1 J/kg	16 J
defibrillation	2 J/kg	32 J
repeat	4 J/kg	64 J

IV Bolus Drugs		dose	mg to pt	supplied	mL to give
ADENOSINE	IV	0.1 mg/kg	1.6 mg	3 mg/mL	0.53 mL
ADENOSINE repeat dose	IV	0.2 mg/kg	3.2 mg	3 mg/mL	1.07 mL
AMIODARONE	IV/IO	5 mg/kg	80 mg	50 mg/mL	1.60 mL
ATROPINE	IM/IV	0.02 mg/kg	0.32 mg	0.4 mg/mL	0.80 mL
ATROPINE	ETT	0.04 mg/kg	0.64 mg	0.4 mg/mL	1.60 mL
CALCIUM CHLORIDE	IV	20 mg/kg	320 mg	100 mg/mL	3.20 mL
CALCIUM GLUCONATE	IV/IO	60 mg/kg	800 mg	100 mg/mL	8.00 mL
DANTROLENE	IV	2.5 mg/kg	30 mg		
EPHEDRINE	IV	0.15 mg/kg	2.4 mg	10 mg/mL	0.24 mL
EPINEPHRINE (1:10,000)	IV/IO	0.01 mg/kg	0.16 mg	0.1 mg/mL	1.60 mL
EPINEPHRINE (1:1,000)	ETT	0.1 mg/kg	1.6 mg	1 mg/mL	1.60 mL
ESMOLOL	IV	0.5 mg/kg	8 mg	10 mg/mL	0.80 mL
LABETALOL	IV	0.2 mg/kg	3.2 mg	5 mg/mL	0.64 mL
LIDOCAINE	IV/IO	1 mg/kg	16 mg	20 mg/mL	0.80 mL
NEOSYNEPHRINE	IV	5 mcg/kg	80 mcg	100 mcg/mL	0.80 mL
ROMAZICON	IV	0.01 mg/kg	0.16 mg	0.1 mg/mL	1.60 mL
VASOPRESSIN	IV/IO	0.4 unit/kg	6.4 units	20 u/mL	0.32 mL

17 KG MAINTENANCE IV FLUIDS: 54 ML/HR

common pediatric drugs		route	dose	mg to pt	supplied	mL to give
ATROPINE	vagolytic	IV	0.02 mg/kg	0.34 mg	0.4 mg/mL	0.85 mL
GLYCOPYRROLATE	vagolytic	IV	0.004 mg/kg	0.068 mg	0.2 mg/mL	0.34 mL
MIDAZOLAM		IV	0.05 mg/kg	0.6 mg	1 mg/mL	0.6 mL
MIDAZOLAM		PO	0.5 mg/kg	8.5 mg	1 mg/mL	8.5 mL
MIDAZOLAM		IN	0.2 mg/kg	3.4 mg	1 mg/mL	3.4 mL
SUCCINYLCHOLINE		IV	2 mg/kg	34 mg	20 mg/mL	1.7 mL
SUCCINYLCHOLINE		IM	4 mg/kg	68 mg	20 mg/mL	3.4 mL
PROPOFOL		IV	3 mg/kg	51 mg	10 mg/mL	5.1 mL
ETOMIDATE	>10 y	IV	0.3 mg/kg	5.1 mg	2 mg/mL	2.55 mL
FENTANYL		IV	1 mcg/kg	17 mcg	50 mcg/mL	0.34 mL
FENTANYL		IN	2 mcg/kg	34 mcg	50 mcg/mL	0.68 mL
MORPHINE	<6 mo	IV/IM	0.05 mg/kg	0.85 mg	10 mg/mL	0.085 mL
MORPHINE	>6 mo	IV/IM	0.1 mg/kg	1.7 mg	10 mg/mL	0.17 mL
TORADOL	>2-16 y	IV	0.5 mg/kg	8.5 mg	30 mg/mL	0.283 mL
TORADOL	>2-16 y	IM	1 mg/kg	17 mg	30 mg/mL	0.567 mL
ACETAMINOPHEN		PR	20 mg/kg	340 mg		
ACETAMINOPHEN	2-12 y	IV	15 mg/kg	255 mg	10 mg/mL	25.5 mL
CISATRACURIUM		IV	0.1 mg/kg	1.7 mg	2 mg/mL	0.85 mL
PANCURONIUM	<1 mo	IV	0.02 mg/kg	0.34 mg	1 mg/mL	0.34 mL
PANCURONIUM	>1 mo	IV	0.1 mg/kg	1.7 mg	1 mg/mL	1.7 mL
ROCURONIUM		IV	0.6 mg/kg	10.2 mg	10 mg/mL	1.02 mL
ROCURONIUM	RSI	IV	1.2 mg/kg	20.4 mg	10 mg/mL	2.04 mL
VECURONIUM		IV	0.1 mg/kg	1.7 mg	1 mg/mL	1.7 mL
GLYCOPYRROLATE	reversal	IV	0.007 mg/kg	0.119 mg	0.2 mg/mL	0.595 mL
NEOSTIGMINE		IV	0.07 mg/kg	1.19 mg	1 mg/mL	1.19 mL
DEXAMETHASONE		IV	0.25 mg/kg	4.25 mg	10 mg/mL	0.425 mL
ONDANSETRON		IV	0.15 mg/kg	2.55 mg	2 mg/mL	1.275 mL

additional pediatric drugs	route	dose	mg to pt	supplied	mL to give
PREMED/SEDATION; VAGOLYTIC/ANTISIALAGOGUE; GIVE IM 30–60 MIN PREOP					
ATROPINE	IV	0.02 mg/kg	0.34 mg	0.4 mg/mL	0.85 mL
GLYCOPYRROLATE	IM	0.004 mg/kg	0.009 mg	0.2 mg/mL	0.045 mL
MIDAZOLAM	IM	0.1 mg/kg	0.5 mg	1 mg/mL	0.5 mL
DEXMEDETOMIDINE load dose	IV	0.5 mcg/kg	1 mcg	4 mcg/mL	0.25 mL
INDUCTION					
KETAMINE	IV	2 mg/kg	34 mg	10 mg/mL	3.4 mL
KETAMINE	IM/PR	5 mg/kg	85 mg	10 mg/mL	8.5 mL
OPIOIDS/NONOPIOIDS					
FENTANYL	IV	4 mcg/kg	68 mcg	50 mcg/mL	1.36 mL
FENTANYL cardiac	IV	10 mcg/kg	170 mcg	50 mcg/mL	3.4 mL
HYDROMORPHONE <6 mo	IV/SQ	0.005 mg/kg	0.085 mg	10 mg/mL	0.0085 mL
HYDROMORPHONE >6 mo	IV/SQ	0.015 mg/kg	0.255 mg	10 mg/mL	0.0255 mL
REMIFENTANIL	IV	0.5 mcg/kg	1 mcg	50 mcg/mL	0.20 mL
SUFENTANIL	IV	0.5 mcg/kg	8.5 mcg	50 mcg/mL	0.17 mL
REVERSALS					
ATROPINE	IV	0.02 mg/kg	0.34 mg	0.4 mg/mL	0.85 mL
EDROPHONIUM neonate	IV	0.1 mg single dose		10 mg/mL	0.01 mL
EDROPHONIUM >2 mo	IV	0.04 mg/kg	0.68 mg	10 mg/mL	0.068 mL
FLUMAZENIL <1 y	IV	0.01 mg/kg	0.17 mg	0.1 mg/mL	1.7 mL
NALOXONE <5 y; <20 kg	IV/IM		1.7 mg	0.4 mg/mL	4.25 mL
NALOXONE >5 y; >20 kg	IV/IM	2 mg per dose		0.4 mg/mL	5 mL
NALOXONE	ETT	0.3 mg/kg	5.1 mg	0.4 mg/mL	12.75 mL

additional pediatric drugs		route	dose	mg to pt	supplied	mL to give
ANTIBIOTICS						
AMPICILLIN	<6 y	IV	50 mg/kg	300 mg		
AMPICILLIN	>6 y	IV	50 mg/kg	850 mg		
AMPICILLIN & SULBACTUM	>1 mo	IV	50 mg/kg	850 mg		
CEFAZOLIN		IV	25 mg/kg	425 mg		
CLINDAMYCIN		IV	10 mg/kg	170 mg		
ERTAPENEM	3 mo-12 y	IV	15 mg/kg	255 mg		
ERTAPENEM	>12 y	IV	1 Gm	per dose		
GENTAMICIN		IV	2 mg/kg	34 mg		
LEVOFLOXACIN		IV	10 mg/kg	170 mg		
METRONIDAZOLE		IV	10 mg/kg	170 mg		
PIPERACILLIN & TAZOBACTAM	<40 kg & 2-9 mo	IV	80 mg/kg	1,360 mg		
PIPERACILLIN & TAZOBACTAM	<40 kg & >9 mo	IV	100 mg/kg	1,700 mg		
PIPERACILLIN & TAZOBACTAM	>40 kg	IV	3.375 Gm per dose			
VANCOMYCIN		IV	15 mg/kg	255 mg		
ANTINAUSEA						
METOCLOPROMIDE		IV	0.2 mg/kg	3.4 mg	5 mg/mL	0.68 mL
DIPHENHYDRAMINE		IV/IM	1.25 mg/kg	21.25 mg	50 mg/mL	0.425 mL
SCOPOLAMINE		IV/IM	6 mcg/kg	102 mcg	400 mcg/mL	0.255 mL
MISCELLANEOUS MEDS						
AMINOCAPROIC ACID		IV	100 mg/kg	1,700 mg	250 mg/mL	6.8 mL
DESMOPRESSIN		IV/SQ	0.3 mcg/kg	5.1 mcg	4 mcg/mL	1.275 mL
DEXAMETHASONE	croup	IV	0.6 mg/kg	10.2 mg	4 mg/mL	2.55 mL
HYDROCORTISONE		IV/IO	3 mg/kg	51 mg	100 mg/mL	0.51 mL

17 KG

1 year ← 13 kg and up

Ventilation: trained rescuer	1 breath q 6-8 sec (8-10 breaths/minute) about 1 second/ breath–visible chest rise; if intubated, continuous compressions without pause for ventilations
Pulse check	carotid or femoral
Compression	heel of 1 hand or both hands one atop the other–lower half of sternum between nipples
Depth	2 inches (5 cm) or at least 1/3 chest depth
Rate	at least 100 compressions per minute
Compress/vent ratio	30:2 single rescuer / 15:2 healthcare providers
Foreign body obstruction	Heimlich maneuver / Never perform a blind finger-sweep. Open the mouth and look for object; if you see it, remove it.

sync cardioversion	0.5 J/kg	8.5 J
repeat	1 J/kg	17 J
defibrillation	2 J/kg	34 J
repeat	4 J/kg	68 J

IV Bolus Drugs		dose	mg to pt	supplied	mL to give
ADENOSINE	IV	0.1 mg/kg	1.7 mg	3 mg/mL	0.57 mL
ADENOSINE repeat dose	IV	0.2 mg/kg	3.4 mg	3 mg/mL	1.13 mL
AMIODARONE	IV/IO	5 mg/kg	85 mg	50 mg/mL	1.70 mL
ATROPINE	IV/IM	0.02 mg/kg	0.34 mg	0.4 mg/mL	0.85 mL
ATROPINE	ETT	0.04 mg/kg	0.68 mg	0.4 mg/mL	1.70 mL
CALCIUM CHLORIDE	IV	20 mg/kg	340 mg	100 mg/mL	3.40 mL
CALCIUM GLUCONATE	IV/IO	60 mg/kg	800 mg	100 mg/mL	8.00 mL
DANTROLENE	IV	2.5 mg/kg	30 mg		
EPHEDRINE	IV	0.15 mg/kg	2.55 mg	10 mg/mL	0.26 mL
EPINEPHRINE (1:10,000)	IV/IO	0.01 mg/kg	0.17 mg	0.1 mg/mL	1.70 mL
EPINEPHRINE (1:1,000)	ETT	0.1 mg/kg	1.7 mg	1 mg/mL	1.70 mL
ESMOLOL	IV	0.5 mg/kg	8.5 mg	10 mg/mL	0.85 mL
LABETALOL	IV	0.2 mg/kg	3.4 mg	5 mg/mL	0.68 mL
LIDOCAINE	IV/IO	1 mg/kg	17 mg	20 mg/mL	0.85 mL
NEOSYNEPHRINE	IV	5 mcg/kg	85 mcg	100 mcg/mL	0.85 mL
ROMAZICON	IV	0.01 mg/kg	0.17 mg	0.1 mg/mL	1.70 mL
VASOPRESSIN	IV/IO	0.4 unit/kg	6.8 units	20 u/mL	0.34 mL

18 KG MAINTENANCE IV FLUIDS: 56 ML/HR

common pediatric drugs		route	dose	mg to pt	supplied	mL to give
ATROPINE	vagolytic	IV	0.02 mg/kg	0.36 mg	0.4 mg/mL	0.9 mL
GLYCOPYRROLATE	vagolytic	IV	0.004 mg/kg	0.072 mg	0.2 mg/mL	0.36 mL
MIDAZOLAM		IV	0.05 mg/kg	0.6 mg	1 mg/mL	0.6 mL
MIDAZOLAM		PO	0.5 mg/kg	9 mg	1 mg/mL	9 mL
MIDAZOLAM		IN	0.2 mg/kg	3.6 mg	1 mg/mL	3.6 mL
SUCCINYLCHOLINE		IV	2 mg/kg	36 mg	20 mg/mL	1.8 mL
SUCCINYLCHOLINE		IM	4 mg/kg	72 mg	20 mg/mL	3.6 mL
PROPOFOL		IV	3 mg/kg	54 mg	10 mg/mL	5.4 mL
ETOMIDATE	>10 y	IV	0.3 mg/kg	5.4 mg	2 mg/mL	2.7 mL
FENTANYL		IV	1 mcg/kg	18 mcg	50 mcg/mL	0.36 mL
FENTANYL		IN	2 mcg/kg	36 mcg	50 mcg/mL	0.72 mL
MORPHINE	<6 mo	IV/IM	0.05 mg/kg	0.9 mg	10 mg/mL	0.09 mL
MORPHINE	>6 mo	IV/IM	0.1 mg/kg	1.8 mg	10 mg/mL	0.18 mL
TORADOL	>2-16 y	IV	0.5 mg/kg	9 mg	30 mg/mL	0.3 mL
TORADOL	>2-16 y	IM	1 mg/kg	18 mg	30 mg/mL	0.6 mL
ACETAMINOPHEN		PR	20 mg/kg	360 mg		
ACETAMINOPHEN	2-12 y	IV	15 mg/kg	270 mg	10 mg/mL	27 mL
CISATRACURIUM		IV	0.1 mg/kg	1.8 mg	2 mg/mL	0.9 mL
PANCURONIUM	<1 mo	IV	0.02 mg/kg	0.36 mg	1 mg/mL	0.36 mL
PANCURONIUM	>1 mo	IV	0.1 mg/kg	1.8 mg	1 mg/mL	1.8 mL
ROCURONIUM		IV	0.6 mg/kg	10.8 mg	10 mg/mL	1.08 mL
ROCURONIUM	RSI	IV	1.2 mg/kg	21.6 mg	10 mg/mL	2.16 mL
VECURONIUM		IV	0.1 mg/kg	1.8 mg	1 mg/mL	1.8 mL
GLYCOPYRROLATE	reversal	IV	0.007 mg/kg	0.126 mg	0.2 mg/mL	0.63 mL
NEOSTIGMINE		IV	0.07 mg/kg	1.26 mg	1 mg/mL	1.26 mL
DEXAMETHASONE		IV	0.25 mg/kg	4.5 mg	10 mg/mL	0.45 mL
ONDANSETRON		IV	0.15 mg/kg	2.7 mg	2 mg/mL	1.35 mL

additional pediatric drugs	route	dose	mg to pt	supplied	mL to give
PREMED/SEDATION; VAGOLYTIC/ANTISIALAGOGUE; GIVE IM 30-60 MIN PREOP					
ATROPINE	IM	0.02 mg/kg	0.36 mg	0.4 mg/mL	0.9 mL
GLYCOPYRROLATE	IM	0.004 mg/kg	0.009 mg	0.2 mg/mL	0.045 mL
MIDAZOLAM	IM	0.1 mg/kg	0.5 mg	1 mg/mL	0.5 mL
DEXMEDETOMIDINE load dose	IV	0.5 mcg/kg	1 mcg	4 mcg/mL	0.25 mL
INDUCTION					
KETAMINE	IV	2 mg/kg	36 mg	10 mg/mL	3.6 mL
KETAMINE	IM/PR	5 mg/kg	90 mg	10 mg/mL	9 mL
OPIOIDS/NONOPIOIDS					
FENTANYL high dose	IV	4 mcg/kg	72 mcg	50 mcg/mL	1.44 mL
FENTANYL cardiac	IV	10 mcg/kg	180 mcg	50 mcg/mL	3.6 mL
HYDROMORPHONE < 6 mo	IV/SQ	0.005 mg/kg	0.09 mg	10 mg/mL	0.009 mL
HYDROMORPHONE > 6 mo	IV/SQ	0.015 mg/kg	0.27 mg	10 mg/mL	0.027 mL
REMIFENTANIL	IV	0.5 mcg/kg	1 mcg	50 mcg/mL	0.02 mL
SUFENTANIL	IV	0.5 mcg/kg	9 mcg	50 mcg/mL	0.18 mL
REVERSALS					
ATROPINE	IV	0.02 mg/kg	0.36 mg	0.4 mg/mL	0.9 mL
EDROPHONIUM neonate	IV	0.1 mg single dose		10	0.01 mL
EDROPHONIUM > 2 mo	IV	0.04 mg/kg	0.72 mg	10	0.072 mL
FLUMAZENIL	IV	0.01 mg/kg	0.18 mg	0.1 mg/mL	1.8 mL
NALOXONE < 5 y; < 20 kg	IV/IM	0.1 mg/kg	1.8 mg	0.4 mg/mL	4.5 mL
NALOXONE > 5 y; > 20 kg	IV/IM	2 mg per dose		0.4 mg/mL	5 mL
NALOXONE	ETT	0.3 mg/kg	5.4 mg	0.4 mg/mL	13.5 mL

additional pediatric drugs		route	dose	mg to pt	supplied	mL to give
ANTIBIOTICS						
AMPICILLIN	<6 y	IV	50 mg/kg	300 mg		
AMPICILLIN	>6 y	IV	50 mg/kg	900 mg		
AMPICILLIN & SULBACTUM	>1 mo	IV	50 mg/kg	900 mg		
CEFAZOLIN		IV	25 mg/kg	450 mg		
CLINDAMYCIN		IV	10 mg/kg	180 mg		
ERTAPENEM	3 mo-12 y	IV	15 mg/kg	270 mg		
ERTAPENEM	>12 y	IV	1 Gm	per dose		
GENTAMICIN		IV	2 mg/kg	36 mg		
LEVOFLOXACIN		IV	10 mg/kg	180 mg		
METRONIDAZOLE		IV	10 mg/kg	180 mg		
PIPERACILLIN & TAZOBACTAM	<40 kg & 2-9 mo	IV	80 mg/kg	1,440 mg		
PIPERACILLIN & TAZOBACTAM	<40 kg & >9 mo	IV	100 mg/kg	1,800 mg		
PIPERACILLIN & TAZOBACTAM	>40 kg	IV	3.375 Gm per dose			
VANCOMYCIN		IV	15 mg/kg	270 mg		
ANTINAUSEA						
METOCLOPROMIDE		IV	0.2 mg/kg	3.6 mg	5 mg/mL	0.72 mL
DIPHENHYDRAMINE		IV/IM	1.25 mg/kg	22.5 mg	50 mg/mL	0.45 mL
SCOPOLAMINE		IV/IM	6 mcg/kg	108 mcg	400 mcg/mL	0.27 mL
MISCELLANEOUS MEDS						
AMINOCAPROIC ACID		IV	100 mg/kg	1,800 mg	250 mg/mL	7.2 mL
DESMOPRESSIN		IV/SQ	0.3 mcg/kg	5.4 mcg	4 mcg/mL	1.35 mL
DEXAMETHASONE	croup	IV	0.6 mg/kg	10.8 mg	4 mg/mL	2.7 mL
HYDROCORTISONE		IV/IO	3 mg/kg	54 mg	100 mg/mL	0.54 mL

18 KG

1 year ← 13 kg and up

Ventilation: trained rescuer	1 breath q 6-8 sec (8-10 breaths/minute) about 1 second/ breath-visible chest rise; if intubated, continuous compressions without pause for ventilations
Pulse check	carotid or femoral
Compression	heel of 1 hand or both hands one atop the other–lower half of sternum between nipples
Depth	2 inches (5 cm) or at least 1/3 chest depth
Rate	at least 100 compressions per minute
Compress/vent ratio	30:2 single rescuer 15:2 healthcare providers
Foreign body obstruction	Heimlich maneuver Never perform a blind finger-sweep. Open the mouth and look for object; if you see it, remove it.

sync cardioversion	0.5 J/kg	9 J
repeat	1 J/kg	18 J
defibrillation	2 J/kg	36 J
repeat	4 J/kg	72 J

IV Bolus Drugs		dose	mg to pt	supplied	mL to give
ADENOSINE	IV	0.1 mg/kg	1.8 mg	3 mg/mL	0.60 mL
ADENOSINE repeat dose	IV	0.2 mg/kg	3.6 mg	3 mg/mL	1.20 mL
AMIODARONE	IV/IO	5 mg/kg	90 mg	50 mg/mL	1.80 mL
ATROPINE	IM/IV	0.02 mg/kg	0.36 mg	0.4 mg/mL	0.90 mL
ATROPINE	ETT	0.04 mg/kg	0.72 mg	0.4 mg/mL	1.80 mL
CALCIUM CHLORIDE	IV	20 mg/kg	360 mg	100 mg/mL	3.60 mL
CALCIUM GLUCONATE	IV/IO	60 mg/kg	800 mg	100 mg/mL	8.00 mL
DANTROLENE	IV	2.5 mg/kg	30 mg		
EPHEDRINE	IV	0.15 mg/kg	2.7 mg	10 mg/mL	0.27 mL
EPINEPHRINE (1:10,000)	IV/IO	0.01 mg/kg	0.18 mg	0.1 mg/mL	1.80 mL
EPINEPHRINE (1:1,000)	ETT	0.1 mg/kg	1.8 mg	1 mg/mL	1.80 mL
ESMOLOL	IV	0.5 mg/kg	9 mg	10 mg/mL	0.90 mL
LABETALOL	IV	0.2 mg/kg	3.6 mg	5 mg/mL	0.72 mL
LIDOCAINE	IV/IO	1 mg/kg	18 mg	20 mg/mL	0.90 mL
NEOSYNEPHRINE	IV	5 mcg/kg	90 mcg	100 mcg/mL	0.90 mL
ROMAZICON	IV	0.01 mg/kg	0.18 mg	0.1 mg/mL	1.80 mL
VASOPRESSIN	IV/IO	0.4 unit/kg	7.2 units	20 u/mL	0.36 mL

19 KG MAINTENANCE IV FLUIDS: 58 ML/HR

common pediatric drugs		route	dose	mg to pt	supplied	mL to give
ATROPINE	vagolytic	IV	0.02 mg/kg	0.38 mg	0.4 mg/mL	0.95 mL
GLYCOPYRROLATE	vagolytic	IV	0.004 mg/kg	0.076 mg	0.2 mg/mL	0.38 mL
MIDAZOLAM		IV	0.05 mg/kg	0.6 mg	1 mg/mL	0.6 mL
MIDAZOLAM		PO	0.5 mg/kg	9.5 mg	1 mg/mL	9.5 mL
MIDAZOLAM		IN	0.2 mg/kg	3.8 mg	1 mg/mL	3.8 mL
SUCCINYLCHOLINE		IV	2 mg/kg	38 mg	20 mg/mL	1.9 mL
SUCCINYLCHOLINE		IM	4 mg/kg	76 mg	20 mg/mL	3.8 mL
PROPOFOL		IV	3 mg/kg	57 mg	10 mg/mL	5.7 mL
ETOMIDATE	>10 y	IV	0.3 mg/kg	5.7 mg	2 mg/mL	2.85 mL
FENTANYL		IV	1 mcg/kg	19 mcg	50 mcg/mL	0.38 mL
FENTANYL		IN	2 mcg/kg	38 mcg	50 mcg/mL	0.76 mL
MORPHINE	<6 mo	IV/IM	0.05 mg/kg	0.95 mg	10 mg/mL	0.095 mL
MORPHINE	>6 mo	IV/IM	0.1 mg/kg	1.9 mg	10 mg/mL	0.19 mL
TORADOL	>2-16 y	IV	0.5 mg/kg	9.5 mg	30 mg/mL	0.317 mL
TORADOL	>2-16 y	IM	1 mg/kg	19 mg	30 mg/mL	0.633 mL
ACETAMINOPHEN		PR	20 mg/kg	380 mg		
ACETAMINOPHEN	2-12 y	IV	15 mg/kg	285 mg	10 mg/mL	28.5 mL
CISATRACURIUM		IV	0.1 mg/kg	1.9 mg	2 mg/mL	0.95 mL
PANCURONIUM	<1 mo	IV	0.02 mg/kg	0.38 mg	1 mg/mL	0.38 mL
PANCURONIUM	>1 mo	IV	0.1 mg/kg	1.9 mg	1 mg/mL	1.9 mL
ROCURONIUM		IV	0.6 mg/kg	11.4 mg	10 mg/mL	1.14 mL
ROCURONIUM	RSI	IV	1.2 mg/kg	22.8 mg	10 mg/mL	2.28 mL
VECURONIUM		IV	0.1 mg/kg	1.9 mg	1 mg/mL	1.9 mL
GLYCOPYRROLATE	reversal	IV	0.007 mg/kg	0.133 mg	0.2 mg/mL	0.665 mL
NEOSTIGMINE		IV	0.07 mg/kg	1.33 mg	1 mg/mL	1.33 mL
DEXAMETHASONE		IV	0.25 mg/kg	4.75 mg	10 mg/mL	0.475 mL
ONDANSETRON		IV	0.15 mg/kg	2.85 mg	2 mg/mL	1.425 mL

additional pediatric drugs	route	dose	mg to pt	supplied	mL to give
PREMED/SEDATION, VAGOLYTIC/ANTISIALAGOGUE: GIVE IM 30-60 MIN PREOP					
ATROPINE	IM	0.02 mg/kg	0.38 mg	0.4 mg/mL	0.95 mL
GLYCOPYRROLATE	IM	0.004 mg/kg	0.009 mg	0.2 mg/mL	0.045 mL
MIDAZOLAM	IM	0.1 mg/kg	0.5 mg	1 mg/mL	0.5 mL
DEXMEDETOMIDINE	IV	load dose 0.5 mcg/kg	1 mcg	4 mcg/mL	0.25 mL
INDUCTION					
KETAMINE	IV	2 mg/kg	38 mg	10 mg/mL	3.8 mL
KETAMINE	IM/PR	5 mg/kg	95 mg	10 mg/mL	9.5 mL
OPIOIDS/NONOPIOIDS					
FENTANYL	IV	high dose 4 mcg/kg	76 mcg	50 mcg/mL	1.52 mL
FENTANYL	IV	cardiac 10 mcg/kg	190 mcg	50 mcg/mL	3.8 mL
HYDROMORPHONE	SQ/IV	< 6 mo 0.005 mg/kg	0.095 mg	10 mg/mL	0.0095 mL
HYDROMORPHONE	SQ/IV	> 6 mo 0.015 mg/kg	0.285 mg	10 mg/mL	0.0285 mL
REMIFENTANIL	IV	0.5 mcg/kg	1 mcg	50 mcg/mL	0.02 mL
SUFENTANIL	IV	0.5 mcg/kg	9.5 mcg	50 mcg/mL	0.19 mL
REVERSALS					
ATROPINE	IV	0.02 mg/kg	0.38 mg	0.4 mg/mL	0.95 mL
EDROPHONIUM	IV	neonate	0.1 mg single dose	10 mg/mL	0.01 mL
EDROPHONIUM	IV	> 2 mo 0.04 mg/kg	0.76 mg	10 mg/mL	0.076 mL
FLUMAZENIL	IV	< 1 y 0.01 mg/kg	0.19 mg	0.1 mg/mL	1.9 mL
NALOXONE	IV/IM	< 5 y; < 20 kg 0.1 mg/kg	1.9 mg	0.4 mg/mL	4.75 mL
NALOXONE	IV/IM	> 5 y; > 20 kg	2 mg per dose	0.4 mg/mL	5 mL
NALOXONE	ETT	0.3 mg/kg	5.7 mg	0.4 mg/mL	14.25 mL

additional pediatric drugs		route	dose	mg to pt	supplied	mL to give
ANTIBIOTICS						
AMPICILLIN	<6 y	IV	50 mg/kg	300 mg		
AMPICILLIN	>6 y	IV	50 mg/kg	950 mg		
AMPICILLIN & SULBACTUM	>1 mo	IV	50 mg/kg	950 mg		
CEFAZOLIN		IV	25 mg/kg	475 mg		
CLINDAMYCIN		IV	10 mg/kg	190 mg		
ERTAPENEM	3 mo-12 y	IV	15 mg/kg	285 mg		
ERTAPENEM	>12 y	IV	1 Gm	per dose		
GENTAMICIN		IV	2 mg/kg	38 mg		
LEVOFLOXACIN		IV	10 mg/kg	190 mg		
METRONIDAZOLE		IV	10 mg/kg	190 mg		
PIPERACILLIN & TAZOBACTAM	<40 kg & 2-9 mo	IV	80 mg/kg	1,520 mg		
PIPERACILLIN & TAZOBACTAM	<40 kg & >9 mo	IV	100 mg/kg	1,900 mg		
PIPERACILLIN & TAZOBACTAM	>40 kg	IV	3.375 Gm per dose			
VANCOMYCIN		IV	15 mg/kg	285 mg		
ANTINAUSEA						
METOCLOPROMIDE		IV	0.2 mg/kg	3.8 mg	5 mg/mL	0.76 mL
DIPHENHYDRAMINE		IV/IM	1.25 mg/kg	23.75 mg	50 mg/mL	0.475 mL
SCOPOLAMINE		IV/IM	6 mcg/kg	114 mcg	400 mcg/mL	0.285 mL
MISCELLANEOUS MEDS						
AMINOCAPROIC ACID		IV	100 mg/kg	1,900 mg	250 mg/mL	7.6 mL
DESMOPRESSIN		IV/SQ	0.3 mcg/kg	5.7 mcg	4 mcg/mL	1.425 mL
DEXAMETHASONE	croup	IV	0.6 mg/kg	11.4 mg	4 mg/mL	2.85 mL
HYDROCORTISONE		IV/IO	3 mg/kg	57 mg	100 mg/mL	0.57 mL

19 KG

1 year → 13 kg and up

Ventilation: trained rescuer	1 breath q 6-8 sec (8-10 breaths/minute) about 1 second/breath-visible chest rise; if intubated, continuous compressions without pause for ventilations
Pulse check	carotid or femoral
Compression	heel of 1 hand or both hands one atop the other—lower half of sternum between nipples
Depth	2 inches (5 cm) or at least 1/3 chest depth
Rate	at least 100 compressions per minute
Compress/vent ratio	30:2 single rescuer 15:2 healthcare providers
Foreign body obstruction	Heimlich maneuver Never perform a blind finger-sweep. Open the mouth and look for object; if you see it, remove it.

sync cardioversion	0.5 J/kg	9.5 J
repeat	1 J/kg	19 J
defibrillation	2 J/kg	38 J
repeat	4 J/kg	76 J

IV Bolus Drugs		dose	mg to pt	supplied	mL to give
ADENOSINE	IV	0.1 mg/kg	1.9 mg	3 mg/mL	0.63 mL
ADENOSINE repeat dose	IV	0.2 mg/kg	3.8 mg	3 mg/mL	1.27 mL
AMIODARONE	IV/IO	5 mg/kg	95 mg	50 mg/mL	1.90 mL
ATROPINE	IM/IV	0.02 mg/kg	0.38 mg	0.4 mg/mL	0.95 mL
ATROPINE	ETT	0.04 mg/kg	0.76 mg	0.4 mg/mL	1.90 mL
CALCIUM CHLORIDE	IV	20 mg/kg	380 mg	100 mg/mL	3.80 mL
CALCIUM GLUCONATE	IV/IO	60 mg/kg	800 mg	100 mg/mL	8.00 mL
DANTROLENE	IV	2.5 mg/kg	30 mg		
EPHEDRINE	IV	0.15 mg/kg	2.85 mg	10 mg/mL	0.29 mL
EPINEPHRINE (1:10,000)	IV/IO	0.01 mg/kg	0.19 mg	0.1 mg/mL	1.90 mL
EPINEPHRINE (1:1,000)	ETT	0.1 mg/kg	1.9 mg	1 mg/mL	1.90 mL
ESMOLOL	IV	0.5 mg/kg	9.5 mg	10 mg/mL	0.95 mL
LABETALOL	IV	0.2 mg/kg	3.8 mg	5 mg/mL	0.76 mL
LIDOCAINE	IV/IO	1 mg/kg	19 mg	20 mg/mL	0.95 mL
NEOSYNEPHRINE	IV	5 mcg/kg	95 mcg	100 mcg/mL	0.95 mL
ROMAZICON	IV	0.01 mg/kg	0.19 mg	0.1 mg/mL	1.90 mL
VASOPRESSIN	IV/IO	0.4 unit/kg	7.6 units	20 u/mL	0.38 mL

20 KG MAINTENANCE IV FLUIDS: 60 ML/HR

common pediatric drugs		route	dose	mg to pt	supplied	mL to give
ATROPINE	vagolytic	IV	0.02 mg/kg	0.4 mg	0.4 mg/mL	1 mL
GLYCOPYRROLATE	vagolytic	IV	0.004 mg/kg	0.08 mg	0.2 mg/mL	0.4 mL
MIDAZOLAM		IV	0.05 mg/kg	0.6 mg	1 mg/mL	0.6 mL
MIDAZOLAM		PO	0.5 mg/kg	10 mg	1 mg/mL	10 mL
MIDAZOLAM		IN	0.2 mg/kg	4 mg	1 mg/mL	4 mL
SUCCINYLCHOLINE		IV	2 mg/kg	40 mg	20 mg/mL	2 mL
SUCCINYLCHOLINE		IM	4 mg/kg	80 mg	20 mg/mL	4 mL
PROPOFOL		IV	3 mg/kg	60 mg	10 mg/mL	6 mL
ETOMIDATE	>10 y	IV	0.3 mg/kg	6 mg	2 mg/mL	3 mL
FENTANYL		IV	1 mcg/kg	20 mcg	50 mcg/mL	0.4 mL
FENTANYL		IN	2 mcg/kg	40 mcg	50 mcg/mL	0.8 mL
MORPHINE	<6 mo	IV/IM	0.05 mg/kg	1 mg	10 mg/mL	0.1 mL
MORPHINE	>6 mo	IV/IM	0.1 mg/kg	2 mg	10 mg/mL	0.2 mL
TORADOL	>2-16 y	IV	0.5 mg/kg	10 mg	30 mg/mL	0.333 mL
TORADOL	>2-16 y	IM	1 mg/kg	20 mg	30 mg/mL	0.667 mL
ACETAMINOPHEN		PR	20 mg/kg	400 mg		
ACETAMINOPHEN	2-12 y	IV	15 mg/kg	300 mg	10 mg/mL	30 mL
CISATRACURIUM		IV	0.1 mg/kg	2 mg	2 mg/mL	1 mL
PANCURONIUM	<1 mo	IV	0.02 mg/kg	0.4 mg	1 mg/mL	0.4 mL
PANCURONIUM	>1 mo	IV	0.1 mg/kg	2 mg	1 mg/mL	2 mL
ROCURONIUM		IV	0.6 mg/kg	12 mg	10 mg/mL	1.2 mL
ROCURONIUM	RSI	IV	1.2 mg/kg	24 mg	10 mg/mL	2.4 mL
VECURONIUM		IV	0.1 mg/kg	2 mg	1 mg/mL	2 mL
GLYCOPYRROLATE	reversal	IV	0.007 mg/kg	0.14 mg	0.2 mg/mL	0.7 mL
NEOSTIGMINE		IV	0.07 mg/kg	1.4 mg	1 mg/mL	1.4 mL
DEXAMETHASONE		IV	0.25 mg/kg	5 mg	10 mg/mL	0.5 mL
ONDANSETRON		IV	0.15 mg/kg	3 mg	2 mg/mL	1.5 mL

additional pediatric drugs	route	dose	mg to pt	supplied	mL to give
PREMED/SEDATION; VAGOLYTIC/ANTISIALAGOGUE; GIVE IM 30-60 MIN PREOP					
ATROPINE	IM	0.02 mg/kg	0.4 mg	0.4 mg/mL	1 mL
GLYCOPYRROLATE	IM	0.004 mg/kg	0.009 mg	0.2 mg/mL	0.045 mL
MIDAZOLAM	IM	0.1 mg/kg	0.5 mg	1 mg/mL	0.5 mL
DEXMEDETOMIDINE load dose	IV	0.5 mcg/kg	1 mcg	4 mcg/mL	0.25 mL
INDUCTION					
KETAMINE	IV	2 mg/kg	40 mg	10 mg/mL	4 mL
KETAMINE	IM/PR	5 mg/kg	100 mg	10 mg/mL	10 mL
OPIOIDS/NONOPIOIDS					
FENTANYL high dose	IV	4 mcg/kg	80 mcg	50 mcg/mL	1.6 mL
FENTANYL cardiac	IV	10 mcg/kg	200 mcg	50 mcg/mL	4 mL
HYDROMORPHONE < 6 mo	IV/SQ	0.005 mg/kg	0.1 mg	10 mg/mL	0.01 mL
HYDROMORPHONE > 6 mo	IV/SQ	0.015 mg/kg	0.3 mg	10 mg/mL	0.03 mL
REMIFENTANIL	IV	0.5 mcg/kg	1 mcg	50 mcg/mL	0.02 mL
SUFENTANIL	IV	0.5 mcg/kg	10 mcg	50 mcg/mL	0.2 mL
REVERSALS					
ATROPINE	IV	0.02 mg/kg	0.4 mg	0.4 mg/mL	1 mL
EDROPHONIUM neonate	IV	0.1 mg single dose		10 mg/mL	0.01 mL
EDROPHONIUM > 2 mo	IV	0.04 mg/kg	0.8 mg	10 mg/mL	0.08 mL
FLUMAZENIL	IV	0.01 mg/kg	0.2 mg	0.1 mg/mL	2 mL
NALOXONE < 5 y; < 20 kg	IV/IM	0.1 mg/kg	2 mg	0.4 mg/mL	5 mL
NALOXONE > 5 y; > 20 kg	IV/IM	2 mg per dose		0.4 mg/mL	5 mL
NALOXONE	ETT	0.3 mg/kg	6 mg	0.4 mg/mL	15 mL

additional pediatric drugs		route	dose	mg to pt	supplied	mL to give
ANTIBIOTICS						
AMPICILLIN	<6 y	IV	50 mg/kg	300 mg		
AMPICILLIN	>6 y	IV	50 mg/kg	1,000 mg		
AMPICILLIN & SULBACTUM	>1 mo	IV	50 mg/kg	1,000 mg		
CEFAZOLIN		IV	25 mg/kg	500 mg		
CLINDAMYCIN		IV	10 mg/kg	200 mg		
ERTAPENEM	3 mo-12 y	IV	15 mg/kg	300 mg		
ERTAPENEM	>12 y	IV	1 Gm	per dose		
GENTAMICIN		IV	2 mg/kg	40 mg		
LEVOFLOXACIN		IV	10 mg/kg	200 mg		
METRONIDAZOLE		IV	10 mg/kg	200 mg		
PIPERACILLIN & TAZOBACTAM	<40 kg & 2-9 mo	IV	80 mg/kg	1,600 mg		
PIPERACILLIN & TAZOBACTAM	<40 kg & >9 mo	IV	100 mg/kg	2,000 mg		
PIPERACILLIN & TAZOBACTAM	>40 kg	IV	3.375 Gm per dose			
VANCOMYCIN		IV	15 mg/kg	300 mg		
ANTINAUSEA						
METOCLOPROMIDE		IV	0.2 mg/kg	4 mg	5 mg/mL	0.8 mL
DIPHENHYDRAMINE		IV/IM	1.25 mg/kg	25 mg	50 mg/mL	0.5 mL
SCOPOLAMINE		IV/IM	6 mcg/kg	120 mcg	400 mcg/mL	0.3 mL
MISCELLANEOUS MEDS						
AMINOCAPROIC ACID		IV	100 mg/kg	2,000 mg	250 mg/mL	8 mL
DESMOPRESSIN		IV/SQ	0.3 mcg/kg	6 mcg	4 mcg/mL	1.5 mL
DEXAMETHASONE	croup	IV	0.6 mg/kg	12 mg	4 mg/mL	3 mL
HYDROCORTISONE		IV/IO	3 mg/kg	60 mg	100 mg/mL	0.6 mL

20 KG

1 year → 13 kg and up

Ventilation: trained rescuer	1 breath q 6-8 sec (8-10 breaths/minute) about 1 second/ breath–visible chest rise; if intubated, continuous compressions without pause for ventilations
Pulse check	carotid or femoral
Compression	heel of 1 hand or both hands one atop the other–lower half of sternum between nipples
Depth	2 inches (5 cm) or at least 1/3 chest depth
Rate	at least 100 compressions per minute
Compress/vent ratio	30:2 single rescuer 15:2 2 healthcare providers
Foreign body obstruction	Heimlich maneuver Never perform a blind finger-sweep. Open the mouth and look for object; if you see it, remove it.

sync cardioversion	0.5 J/kg	10 J
defibrillation	1 J/kg	20 J
repeat	2 J/kg	40 J
repeat	4 J/kg	80 J

IV Bolus Drugs		dose	mg to pt	supplied	mL to give
ADENOSINE	IV	0.1 mg/kg	2 mg	3 mg/mL	0.67 mL
ADENOSINE repeat dose	IV	0.2 mg/kg	4 mg	3 mg/mL	1.33 mL
AMIODARONE	IV/IO	5 mg/kg	100 mg	50 mg/mL	2.00 mL
ATROPINE	IV/IM	0.02 mg/kg	0.4 mg	0.4 mg/mL	1.00 mL
ATROPINE	ETT	0.04 mg/kg	0.8 mg	0.4 mg/mL	2.00 mL
CALCIUM CHLORIDE	IV	20 mg/kg	400 mg	100 mg/mL	4.00 mL
CALCIUM GLUCONATE	IV/IO	60 mg/kg	800 mg	100 mg/mL	8.00 mL
DANTROLENE	IV	2.5 mg/kg	30 mg		
EPHEDRINE	IV	0.15 mg/kg	3 mg	10 mg/mL	0.30 mL
EPINEPHRINE (1:10,000)	IV/IO	0.01 mg/kg	0.2 mg	0.1 mg/mL	2.00 mL
EPINEPHRINE (1:1,000)	ETT	0.1 mg/kg	2 mg	1 mg/mL	2.00 mL
ESMOLOL	IV	0.5 mg/kg	10 mg	10 mg/mL	1.00 mL
LABETALOL	IV	0.2 mg/kg	4 mg	5 mg/mL	0.80 mL
LIDOCAINE	IV/IO	1 mg/kg	20 mg	20 mg/mL	1.00 mL
NEOSYNEPHRINE	IV	5 mcg/kg	100 mcg	100 mcg/mL	1.00 mL
ROMAZICON	IV	0.01 mg/kg	0.2 mg	0.1 mg/mL	2.00 mL
VASOPRESSIN	IV/IO	0.4 unit/kg	8 units	20 u/mL	0.40 mL

21 KG MAINTENANCE IV FLUIDS: 61 ML/HR

common pediatric drugs		route	dose	mg to pt	supplied	mL to give
ATROPINE	vagolytic	IV	0.02 mg/kg	0.42 mg	0.4 mg/mL	1.05 mL
GLYCOPYRROLATE	vagolytic	IV	0.004 mg/kg	0.084 mg	0.2 mg/mL	0.42 mL
MIDAZOLAM		IV	0.05 mg/kg	0.6 mg	1 mg/mL	0.6 mL
MIDAZOLAM		PO	0.5 mg/kg	10.5 mg	1 mg/mL	10.5 mL
MIDAZOLAM		IN	0.2 mg/kg	4.2 mg	1 mg/mL	4.2 mL
SUCCINYLCHOLINE		IV	2 mg/kg	42 mg	20 mg/mL	2.1 mL
SUCCINYLCHOLINE		IM	4 mg/kg	84 mg	20 mg/mL	4.2 mL
PROPOFOL		IV	3 mg/kg	63 mg	10 mg/mL	6.3 mL
ETOMIDATE	>10 y	IV	0.3 mg/kg	6.3 mg	2 mg/mL	3.15 mL
FENTANYL		IV	1 mcg/kg	21 mcg	50 mcg/mL	0.42 mL
FENTANYL		IN	2 mcg/kg	42 mcg	50 mcg/mL	0.84 mL
MORPHINE	<6 mo	IV/IM	0.05 mg/kg	1.05 mg	10 mg/mL	0.105 mL
MORPHINE	>6 mo	IV/IM	0.1 mg/kg	2.1 mg	10 mg/mL	0.21 mL
TORADOL	>2-16 y	IV	0.5 mg/kg	10.5 mg	30 mg/mL	0.35 mL
TORADOL	>2-16 y	IM	1 mg/kg	21 mg	30 mg/mL	0.7 mL
ACETAMINOPHEN		PR	20 mg/kg	420 mg		
ACETAMINOPHEN	2-12 y	IV	15 mg/kg	315 mg	10 mg/mL	31.5 mL
CISATRACURIUM		IV	0.1 mg/kg	2.1 mg	2 mg/mL	1.05 mL
PANCURONIUM	<1 mo	IV	0.02 mg/kg	0.42 mg	1 mg/mL	0.42 mL
PANCURONIUM	>1 mo	IV	0.1 mg/kg	2.1 mg	1 mg/mL	2.1 mL
ROCURONIUM		IV	0.6 mg/kg	12.6 mg	10 mg/mL	1.26 mL
ROCURONIUM	RSI	IV	1.2 mg/kg	25.2 mg	10 mg/mL	2.52 mL
VECURONIUM		IV	0.1 mg/kg	2.1 mg	1 mg/mL	2.1 mL
GLYCOPYRROLATE	reversal	IV	0.007 mg/kg	0.147 mg	0.2 mg/mL	0.735 mL
NEOSTIGMINE		IV	0.07 mg/kg	1.47 mg	1 mg/mL	1.47 mL
DEXAMETHASONE		IV	0.25 mg/kg	5.25 mg	10 mg/mL	0.525 mL
ONDANSETRON		IV	0.15 mg/kg	3.15 mg	2 mg/mL	1.575 mL

additional pediatric drugs	route	dose		mg to pt	supplied	mL to give
PREMED/SEDATION; VAGOLYTIC/ANTISIALAGOGUE; GIVE IM 30-60 MIN PREOP						
ATROPINE	IM		0.02 mg/kg	0.42 mg	0.4 mg/mL	1.05 mL
GLYCOPYRROLATE	IM		0.004 mg/kg	0.000 600 mg	0.2 mg/mL	0.045 mL
MIDAZOLAM	IM		0.1 mg/kg	0.5 mg	1 mg/mL	0.5 mL
DEXMEDETOMIDINE load dose	IV		0.5 mcg/kg	1 mcg	4 mcg/mL	0.25 mL
INDUCTION						
KETAMINE	IV		2 mg/kg	42 mg	10 mg/mL	4.2 mL
KETAMINE	IM/PR		5 mg/kg	105 mg	10 mg/mL	10.5 mL
OPIOIDS/NONOPIOIDS						
FENTANYL	IV	high dose	4 mcg/kg	84 mcg	50 mcg/mL	1.68 mL
FENTANYL	IV	cardiac	10 mcg/kg	210 mcg	50 mcg/mL	4.2 mL
HYDROMORPHONE	IV/SQ	< 6 mo	0.005 mg/kg	0.105 mg	10 mg/mL	0.0105 mL
HYDROMORPHONE	IV/SQ	> 6 mo	0.015 mg/kg	0.315 mg	10 mg/mL	0.0315 mL
REMIFENTANIL	IV		0.5 mcg/kg	1 mcg	50 mcg/mL	0.02 mL
SUFENTANIL	IV		0.5 mcg/kg	10.5 mcg	50 mcg/mL	0.21 mL
REVERSALS						
ATROPINE	IV		0.02 mg/kg	0.42 mg	0.4 mg/mL	1.05 mL
EDROPHONIUM	IV	neonate	0.1 mg single dose		10 mg/mL	0.01 mL
EDROPHONIUM	IV	> 2 mo	0.04 mg/kg	0.84 mg	10 mg/mL	0.084 mL
FLUMAZENIL	IV	< 1 y	0.01 mg/kg	0.2 mg	0.1 mg/mL	2 mL
NALOXONE	IM/IV	< 5 y; < 20 kg	0.1 mg/kg	2 mg	0.4 mg/mL	5 mL
NALOXONE	IM/IV	< 5 y; > 20 kg	2 mg per dose		0.4 mg/mL	5 mL
NALOXONE	ETT		0.3 mg/kg	6.3 mg	0.4 mg/mL	15.75 mL

additional pediatric drugs		route	dose	mg to pt	supplied	mL to give
ANTIBIOTICS						
AMPICILLIN	<6 y	IV	50 mg/kg	300 mg		
AMPICILLIN	>6 y	IV	50 mg/kg	1,050 mg		
AMPICILLIN & SULBACTUM	>1 mo	IV	50 mg/kg	1,050 mg		
CEFAZOLIN		IV	25 mg/kg	525 mg		
CLINDAMYCIN		IV	10 mg/kg	210 mg		
ERTAPENEM	3 mo-12 y	IV	15 mg/kg	315 mg		
ERTAPENEM	>12 y	IV	1 Gm	per dose		
GENTAMICIN		IV	2 mg/kg	42 mg		
LEVOFLOXACIN		IV	10 mg/kg	210 mg		
METRONIDAZOLE		IV	10 mg/kg	210 mg		
PIPERACILLIN & TAZOBACTAM	<40 kg & 2-9 mo	IV	80 mg/kg	1,680 mg		
PIPERACILLIN & TAZOBACTAM	<40 kg & >9 mo	IV	100 mg/kg	2,100 mg		
PIPERACILLIN & TAZOBACTAM	>40 kg	IV	3.375 Gm per dose			
VANCOMYCIN		IV	15 mg/kg	315 mg		
ANTINAUSEA						
METOCLOPROMIDE		IV	0.2 mg/kg	4.2 mg	5 mg/mL	0.84 mL
DIPHENHYDRAMINE		IV/IM	1.25 mg/kg	26.25 mg	50 mg/mL	0.525 mL
SCOPOLAMINE		IV/IM	6 mcg/kg	126 mcg	400 mcg/mL	0.315 mL
MISCELLANEOUS MEDS						
AMINOCAPROIC ACID		IV	100 mg/kg	2,100 mg	250 mg/mL	8.4 mL
DESMOPRESSIN		IV/SQ	0.3 mcg/kg	6.3 mcg	4 mcg/mL	1.575 mL
DEXAMETHASONE	croup	IV	0.6 mg/kg	12.6 mg	4 mg/mL	3.15 mL
HYDROCORTISONE		IV/IO	3 mg/kg	63 mg	100 mg/mL	0.63 mL

6 Pediatric Pharmacology: Perioperative and Emergency Drugs

21 KG

1 year → 13 kg and up

Ventilation: trained rescuer	1 breath q 6-8 sec (8-10 breaths/minute) about 1 second/ breath-visible chest rise; if intubated, continuous compressions without pause for ventilations
Pulse check	carotid or femoral
Compression	heel of 1 hand or both hands one atop the other—lower half of sternum between nipples
Depth	2 inches (5 cm) or at least 1/3 chest depth
Rate	at least 100 compressions per minute
Compress/vent ratio	30:2 single rescuer / 15:2 2 healthcare providers
Foreign body obstruction	Heimlich maneuver / Never perform a blind finger-sweep. Open the mouth and look for object; if you see it, remove it.

sync cardioversion	0.5 J/kg	10.5 J
repeat	1 J/kg	21 J
defibrillation	2 J/kg	42 J
repeat	4 J/kg	84 J

IV Bolus Drugs		dose	mg to pt	supplied	mL to give
ADENOSINE	IV	0.1 mg/kg	2.1 mg	3 mg/mL	0.70 mL
ADENOSINE repeat dose	IV	0.2 mg/kg	4.2 mg	3 mg/mL	1.40 mL
AMIODARONE	IV/IO	5 mg/kg	105 mg	50 mg/mL	2.10 mL
ATROPINE	IV/IM	0.02 mg/kg	0.42 mg	0.4 mg/mL	1.05 mL
ATROPINE	ETT	0.04 mg/kg	0.84 mg	0.4 mg/mL	2.10 mL
CALCIUM CHLORIDE	IV	20 mg/kg	420 mg	100 mg/mL	4.20 mL
CALCIUM GLUCONATE	IV/IO	60 mg/kg	800 mg	100 mg/mL	8.00 mL
DANTROLENE	IV	2.5 mg/kg	30 mg		
EPHEDRINE	IV	0.15 mg/kg	3.15 mg	10 mg/mL	0.32 mL
EPINEPHRINE (1:10,000)	IV/IO	0.01 mg/kg	0.21 mg	0.1 mg/mL	2.10 mL
EPINEPHRINE (1:1,000)	ETT	0.1 mg/kg	2.1 mg	1 mg/mL	2.10 mL
ESMOLOL	IV	0.5 mg/kg	10.5 mg	10 mg/mL	1.05 mL
LABETALOL	IV	0.2 mg/kg	4.2 mg	5 mg/mL	0.84 mL
LIDOCAINE	IV/IO	1 mg/kg	21 mg	20 mg/mL	1.05 mL
NEOSYNEPHRINE	IV	5 mcg/kg	105 mcg	100 mcg/mL	1.05 mL
ROMAZICON	IV	0.01 mg/kg	0.2 mg	0.1 mg/mL	2.00 mL
VASOPRESSIN	IV/IO	0.4 unit/kg	8.4 units	20 u/mL	0.42 mL

22 KG MAINTENANCE IV FLUIDS: 62 ML/HR

common pediatric drugs		route	dose	mg to pt	supplied	mL to give
ATROPINE	vagolytic	IV	0.02 mg/kg	0.44 mg	0.4 mg/mL	1.1 mL
GLYCOPYRROLATE	vagolytic	IV	0.004 mg/kg	0.088 mg	0.2 mg/mL	0.44 mL
MIDAZOLAM		IV	0.05 mg/kg	0.6 mg	1 mg/mL	0.6 mL
MIDAZOLAM		PO	0.5 mg/kg	11 mg	1 mg/mL	11 mL
MIDAZOLAM		IN	0.2 mg/kg	4.4 mg	1 mg/mL	4.4 mL
SUCCINYLCHOLINE		IV	2 mg/kg	44 mg	20 mg/mL	2.2 mL
SUCCINYLCHOLINE		IM	4 mg/kg	88 mg	20 mg/mL	4.4 mL
PROPOFOL		IV	3 mg/kg	66 mg	10 mg/mL	6.6 mL
ETOMIDATE	>10 y	IV	0.3 mg/kg	6.6 mg	2 mg/mL	3.3 mL
FENTANYL		IV	1 mcg/kg	22 mcg	50 mcg/mL	0.44 mL
FENTANYL		IN	2 mcg/kg	44 mcg	50 mcg/mL	0.88 mL
MORPHINE	<6 mo	IV/IM	0.05 mg/kg	1.1 mg	10 mg/mL	0.11 mL
MORPHINE	>6 mo	IV/IM	0.1 mg/kg	2.2 mg	10 mg/mL	0.22 mL
TORADOL	>2-16 y	IV	0.5 mg/kg	11 mg	30 mg/mL	0.367 mL
TORADOL	>2-16 y	IM	1 mg/kg	22 mg	30 mg/mL	0.733 mL
ACETAMINOPHEN		PR	20 mg/kg	440 mg		
ACETAMINOPHEN	2-12 y	IV	15 mg/kg	330 mg	10 mg/mL	33 mL
CISATRACURIUM		IV	0.1 mg/kg	2.2 mg	2 mg/mL	1.1 mL
PANCURONIUM	<1 mo	IV	0.02 mg/kg	0.44 mg	1 mg/mL	0.44 mL
PANCURONIUM	>1 mo	IV	0.1 mg/kg	2.2 mg	1 mg/mL	2.2 mL
ROCURONIUM		IV	0.6 mg/kg	13.2 mg	10 mg/mL	1.32 mL
ROCURONIUM	RSI	IV	1.2 mg/kg	26.4 mg	10 mg/mL	2.64 mL
VECURONIUM		IV	0.1 mg/kg	2.2 mg	1 mg/mL	2.2 mL
GLYCOPYRROLATE	reversal	IV	0.007 mg/kg	0.154 mg	0.2 mg/mL	0.77 mL
NEOSTIGMINE		IV	0.07 mg/kg	1.54 mg	1 mg/mL	1.54 mL
DEXAMETHASONE		IV	0.25 mg/kg	5.5 mg	10 mg/mL	0.55 mL
ONDANSETRON		IV	0.15 mg/kg	3.3 mg	2 mg/mL	1.65 mL

additional pediatric drugs	route	dose	mg to pt	supplied	mL to give
PREMED/SEDATION; VAGOLYTIC/ANTISIALAGOGUE; GIVE IM 30-60 MIN PREOP					
ATROPINE	IM	0.02 mg/kg	0.44 mg	0.4 mg/mL	1.1 mL
GLYCOPYRROLATE	IM	0.004 mg/kg	0.009 mg	0.2 mg/mL	0.045 mL
MIDAZOLAM	IM	0.1 mg/kg	0.5 mg	1 mg/mL	0.5 mL
DEXMEDETOMIDINE load dose	IV	0.5 mcg/kg	1 mcg	4 mcg/mL	0.25 mL
INDUCTION					
KETAMINE	IV	2 mg/kg	44 mg	10 mg/mL	4.4 mL
KETAMINE	IM/PR	5 mg/kg	110 mg	10 mg/mL	11 mL
OPIOIDS/NONOPIOIDS					
FENTANYL	IV	high dose	4 mcg/kg	88 mcg	50 mcg/mL	1.76 mL
FENTANYL	IV	cardiac	10 mcg/kg	220 mcg	50 mcg/mL	4.4 mL
HYDROMORPHONE	IV/SQ	< 6 mo	0.005 mg/kg	0.11 mg	10 mg/mL	0.011 mL
HYDROMORPHONE	IV/SQ	> 6 mo	0.015 mg/kg	0.33 mg	10 mg/mL	0.033 mL
REMIFENTANIL	IV	0.5 mcg/kg	1 mcg	50 mcg/mL	0.02 mL
SUFENTANIL	IV	0.5 mcg/kg	11 mcg	50 mcg/mL	0.22 mL
REVERSALS					
ATROPINE	IV	0.02 mg/kg	0.44 mg	0.4 mg/mL	1.1 mL
EDROPHONIUM	IV	neonate	0.1 mg single dose		10 mg/mL	0.01 mL
EDROPHONIUM	IV	> 2 mo	0.04 mg/kg	0.88 mg	10 mg/mL	0.088 mL
FLUMAZENIL	IV	<1 y	0.01 mg/kg	0.2 mg	0.1 mg/mL	2 mL
NALOXONE	IV/IM	<5 y; <20 kg	0.1 mg/kg	2 mg	0.4 mg/mL	5 mL
NALOXONE	IV/IM	<5 y; >20 kg	2 mg per dose		0.4 mg/mL	5 mL
NALOXONE	ETT	0.3 mg/kg	6.6 mg	0.4 mg/mL	16.5 mL

additional pediatric drugs		route	dose	mg to pt	supplied	mL to give
ANTIBIOTICS						
AMPICILLIN	<6 y	IV	50 mg/kg	300 mg		
AMPICILLIN	>6 y	IV	50 mg/kg	1,100 mg		
AMPICILLIN & SULBACTUM	>1 mo	IV	50 mg/kg	1,100 mg		
CEFAZOLIN		IV	25 mg/kg	550 mg		
CLINDAMYCIN		IV	10 mg/kg	220 mg		
ERTAPENEM	3 mo-12 y	IV	15 mg/kg	330 mg		
ERTAPENEM	>12 y	IV	1 Gm	per dose		
GENTAMICIN		IV	2 mg/kg	44 mg		
LEVOFLOXACIN		IV	10 mg/kg	220 mg		
METRONIDAZOLE		IV	10 mg/kg	220 mg		
PIPERACILLIN & TAZOBACTAM	<40 kg & 2-9 mo	IV	80 mg/kg	1,760 mg		
PIPERACILLIN & TAZOBACTAM	<40 kg & >9 mo	IV	100 mg/kg	2,200 mg		
PIPERACILLIN & TAZOBACTAM	>40 kg	IV	3.375 Gm per dose			
VANCOMYCIN		IV	15 mg/kg	330 mg		
ANTINAUSEA						
METOCLOPROMIDE		IV	0.2 mg/kg	4.4 mg	5 mg/mL	0.88 mL
DIPHENHYDRAMINE		IV/IM	1.25 mg/kg	27.5 mg	50 mg/mL	0.55 mL
SCOPOLAMINE		IV/IM	6 mcg/kg	132 mcg	400 mcg/mL	0.33 mL
MISCELLANEOUS MEDS						
AMINOCAPROIC ACID		IV	100 mg/kg	2,200 mg	250 mg/mL	8.8 mL
DESMOPRESSIN		IV/SQ	0.3 mcg/kg	6.6 mcg	4 mcg/mL	1.65 mL
DEXAMETHASONE	croup	IV	0.6 mg/kg	13.2 mg	4 mg/mL	3.3 mL
HYDROCORTISONE		IV/IO	3 mg/kg	66 mg	100 mg/mL	0.66 mL

22 KG

1 year ← 13 kg and up

Ventilation: trained rescuer	1 breath q 6-8 sec (8-10 breaths/minute) about 1 second/ breath-visible chest rise; if intubated, continuous compressions without pause for ventilations
Pulse check	carotid or femoral
Compression	heel of 1 hand or both hands one atop the other—lower half of sternum between nipples
Depth	2 inches (5 cm) or at least 1/3 chest depth
Rate	at least 100 compressions per minute
Compress/vent ratio	30:2 single rescuer 15:2 healthcare providers
Foreign body obstruction	Heimlich maneuver Never perform a blind finger-sweep. Open the mouth and look for object; if you see it, remove it.

sync cardioversion	0.5 J/kg	11 J
repeat	1 J/kg	22 J
defibrillation	2 J/kg	44 J
repeat	4 J/kg	88 J

IV Bolus Drugs		dose	mg to pt	supplied	mL to give
ADENOSINE	IV	0.1 mg/kg	2.2 mg	3 mg/mL	0.73 mL
ADENOSINE repeat dose	IV	0.2 mg/kg	4.4 mg	3 mg/mL	1.47 mL
AMIODARONE	IV/IO	5 mg/kg	110 mg	50 mg/mL	2.20 mL
ATROPINE	IM/IV	0.02 mg/kg	0.44 mg	0.4 mg/mL	1.10 mL
ATROPINE	ETT	0.04 mg/kg	0.88 mg	0.4 mg/mL	2.20 mL
CALCIUM CHLORIDE	IV	20 mg/kg	440 mg	100 mg/mL	4.40 mL
CALCIUM GLUCONATE	IV/IO	60 mg/kg	800 mg	100 mg/mL	8.00 mL
DANTROLENE	IV	2.5 mg/kg 30 mg			
EPHEDRINE	IV	0.15 mg/kg	3.3 mg	10 mg/mL	0.33 mL
EPINEPHRINE (1:10,000)	IV/IO	0.01 mg/kg	0.22 mg	0.1 mg/mL	2.20 mL
EPINEPHRINE (1:1,000)	ETT	0.1 mg/kg	2.2 mg	1 mg/mL	2.20 mL
ESMOLOL	IV	0.5 mg/kg	11 mg	10 mg/mL	1.10 mL
LABETALOL	IV	0.2 mg/kg	4.4 mg	5 mg/mL	0.88 mL
LIDOCAINE	IV/IO	1 mg/kg	22 mg	20 mg/mL	1.10 mL
NEOSYNEPHRINE	IV	5 mcg/kg	110 mcg	100 mcg/mL	1.10 mL
ROMAZICON	IV	0.01 mg/kg	0.2 mg	0.1 mg/mL	2.00 mL
VASOPRESSIN	IV/IO	0.4 unit/kg	8.8 units	20 u/mL	0.44 mL

23 KG MAINTENANCE IV FLUIDS: 63 ML/HR

common pediatric drugs		route	dose	mg to pt	supplied	mL to give
ATROPINE	vagolytic	IV	0.02 mg/kg	0.46 mg	0.4 mg/mL	1.15 mL
GLYCOPYRROLATE	vagolytic	IV	0.004 mg/kg	0.092 mg	0.2 mg/mL	0.46 mL
MIDAZOLAM		IV	0.05 mg/kg	0.6 mg	1 mg/mL	0.6 mL
MIDAZOLAM		PO	0.5 mg/kg	11.5 mg	1 mg/mL	11.5 mL
MIDAZOLAM		IN	0.2 mg/kg	4.6 mg	1 mg/mL	4.6 mL
SUCCINYLCHOLINE		IV	2 mg/kg	46 mg	20 mg/mL	2.3 mL
SUCCINYLCHOLINE		IM	4 mg/kg	92 mg	20 mg/mL	4.6 mL
PROPOFOL		IV	3 mg/kg	69 mg	10 mg/mL	6.9 mL
ETOMIDATE	>10 y	IV	0.3 mg/kg	6.9 mg	2 mg/mL	3.45 mL
FENTANYL		IV	1 mcg/kg	23 mcg	50 mcg/mL	0.46 mL
FENTANYL		IN	2 mcg/kg	46 mcg	50 mcg/mL	0.92 mL
MORPHINE	<6 mo	IV/IM	0.05 mg/kg	1.15 mg	10 mg/mL	0.115 mL
MORPHINE	>6 mo	IV/IM	0.1 mg/kg	2.3 mg	10 mg/mL	0.23 mL
TORADOL	>2-16 y	IV	0.5 mg/kg	11.5 mg	30 mg/mL	0.383 mL
TORADOL	>2-16 y	IM	1 mg/kg	23 mg	30 mg/mL	0.767 mL
ACETAMINOPHEN		PR	20 mg/kg	460 mg		
ACETAMINOPHEN	2-12 y	IV	15 mg/kg	345 mg	10 mg/mL	34.5 mL
CISATRACURIUM		IV	0.1 mg/kg	2.3 mg	2 mg/mL	1.15 mL
PANCURONIUM	<1 mo	IV	0.02 mg/kg	0.46 mg	1 mg/mL	0.46 mL
PANCURONIUM	>1 mo	IV	0.1 mg/kg	2.3 mg	1 mg/mL	2.3 mL
ROCURONIUM		IV	0.6 mg/kg	13.8 mg	10 mg/mL	1.38 mL
ROCURONIUM	RSI	IV	1.2 mg/kg	27.6 mg	10 mg/mL	2.76 mL
VECURONIUM		IV	0.1 mg/kg	2.3 mg	1 mg/mL	2.3 mL
GLYCOPYRROLATE	reversal	IV	0.007 mg/kg	0.161 mg	0.2 mg/mL	0.805 mL
NEOSTIGMINE		IV	0.07 mg/kg	1.61 mg	1 mg/mL	1.61 mL
DEXAMETHASONE		IV	0.25 mg/kg	5.75 mg	10 mg/mL	0.575 mL
ONDANSETRON		IV	0.15 mg/kg	3.45 mg	2 mg/mL	1.725 mL

additional pediatric drugs	route	dose	mg to pt	supplied	mL to give
PREMED/SEDATION; VAGOLYTIC/ANTISIALAGOGUE; GIVE IM 30-60 MIN PREOP					
ATROPINE	IM	0.02 mg/kg	0.46 mg	0.4 mg/mL	1.15 mL
GLYCOPYRROLATE	IM	0.004 mg/kg	0.009 mg	0.2 mg/mL	0.045 mL
MIDAZOLAM	IM	0.1 mg/kg	0.5 mg	1 mg/mL	0.5 mL
DEXMEDETOMIDINE load dose	IV	0.5 mcg/kg	1 mcg	4 mcg/mL	0.25 mL
INDUCTION					
KETAMINE	IV	2 mg/kg	46 mg	10 mg/mL	4.6 mL
KETAMINE	IM/PR	5 mg/kg	115 mg	10 mg/mL	11.5 mL
OPIOIDS/NONOPIOIDS					
FENTANYL high dose	IV	4 mcg/kg	92 mcg	50 mcg/mL	1.84 mL
FENTANYL cardiac	IV	10 mcg/kg	230 mcg	50 mcg/mL	4.6 mL
HYDROMORPHONE < 6 mo	IV/SQ	0.005 mg/kg	0.115 mg	10 mg/mL	0.0115 mL
HYDROMORPHONE > 6 mo	IV/SQ	0.015 mg/kg	0.345 mg	10 mg/mL	0.0345 mL
REMIFENTANIL	IV	0.5 mcg/kg	1 mcg	50 mcg/mL	0.02 mL
SUFENTANIL	IV	0.5 mcg/kg	11.5 mcg	50 mcg/mL	0.23 mL
REVERSALS					
ATROPINE	IV	0.02 mg/kg	0.46 mg	0.4 mg/mL	1.15 mL
EDROPHONIUM neonate	IV	0.1 mg single dose		10 mg/mL	0.01 mL
EDROPHONIUM > 2 mo	IV	0.04 mg/kg	0.92 mg	10 mg/mL	0.092 mL
FLUMAZENIL > 1 y	IV	0.01 mg/kg	0.2 mg	0.1 mg/mL	2 mL
NALOXONE < 5 y; < 20 kg	IV/IM	0.1 mg/kg	2 mg	0.4 mg/mL	5 mL
NALOXONE > 5 y; > 20 kg	IV/IM	2 mg per dose		0.4 mg/mL	5 mL
NALOXONE	ETT	0.3 mg/kg	6.9 mg	0.4 mg/mL	17.25 mL

additional pediatric drugs		route	dose	mg to pt	supplied	mL to give
ANTIBIOTICS						
AMPICILLIN	<6 y	IV	50 mg/kg	300 mg		
AMPICILLIN	>6 y	IV	50 mg/kg	1,150 mg		
AMPICILLIN & SULBACTUM	>1 mo	IV	50 mg/kg	1,150 mg		
CEFAZOLIN		IV	25 mg/kg	575 mg		
CLINDAMYCIN		IV	10 mg/kg	230 mg		
ERTAPENEM	3 mo-12 y	IV	15 mg/kg	345 mg		
ERTAPENEM	>12 y	IV	1 Gm	per dose		
GENTAMICIN		IV	2 mg/kg	46 mg		
LEVOFLOXACIN		IV	10 mg/kg	230 mg		
METRONIDAZOLE		IV	10 mg/kg	230 mg		
PIPERACILLIN & TAZOBACTAM	<40 kg & 2-9 mo	IV	80 mg/kg	1,840 mg		
PIPERACILLIN & TAZOBACTAM	<40 kg & >9 mo	IV	100 mg/kg	2,300 mg		
PIPERACILLIN & TAZOBACTAM	>40 kg	IV	3.375 Gm per dose			
VANCOMYCIN		IV	15 mg/kg	345 mg		
ANTINAUSEA						
METOCLOPROMIDE		IV	0.2 mg/kg	4.6 mg	5 mg/mL	0.92 mL
DIPHENHYDRAMINE		IV/IM	1.25 mg/kg	28.75 mg	50 mg/mL	0.575 mL
SCOPOLAMINE		IV/IM	6 mcg/kg	138 mcg	400 mcg/mL	0.345 mL
MISCELLANEOUS MEDS						
AMINOCAPROIC ACID		IV	100 mg/kg	2,300 mg	250 mg/mL	9.2 mL
DESMOPRESSIN		IV/SQ	0.3 mcg/kg	6.9 mcg	4 mcg/mL	1.725 mL
DEXAMETHASONE	croup	IV	0.6 mg/kg	13.8 mg	4 mg/mL	3.45 mL
HYDROCORTISONE		IV/IO	3 mg/kg	69 mg	100 mg/mL	0.69 mL

23 KG

1 year ← 13 kg and up

Ventilation:	1 breath q 6-8 sec (8-10 breaths/minute) about 1 second/
trained rescuer	breath-visible chest rise; if intubated, continuous compressions without pause for ventilations
Pulse check	carotid or femoral
Compression	heel of 1 hand or both hands one atop the other-lower half of sternum between nipples
Depth	2 inches (5 cm) or at least 1/3 chest depth
Rate	at least 100 compressions per minute
Compress/vent ratio	30:2 single rescuer
	15:2 healthcare providers
Foreign body obstruction	Heimlich maneuver
	Never perform a blind finger-sweep. Open the mouth and look for object; if you see it, remove it.

sync cardioversion	0.5 J/kg	11.5 J	
	1 J/kg	23 J	repeat
defibrillation	2 J/kg	46 J	
	4 J/kg	92 J	repeat

IV Bolus Drugs		dose	mg to pt	supplied	mL to give
ADENOSINE	IV	0.1 mg/kg	2.3 mg	3 mg/mL	0.77 mL
ADENOSINE	repeat dose	0.2 mg/kg	4.6 mg	3 mg/mL	1.53 mL
AMIODARONE	IV/IO	5 mg/kg	115 mg	50 mg/mL	2.30 mL
ATROPINE	IV/IM	0.02 mg/kg	0.46 mg	0.4 mg/mL	1.15 mL
ATROPINE	ETT	0.04 mg/kg	0.92 mg	0.4 mg/mL	2.30 mL
CALCIUM CHLORIDE	IV	20 mg/kg	460 mg	100 mg/mL	4.60 mL
CALCIUM GLUCONATE	IV/IO	60 mg/kg	800 mg	100 mg/mL	8.00 mL
DANTROLENE	IV	2.5 mg/kg	30 mg		
EPHEDRINE	IV	0.15 mg/kg	3.45 mg	10 mg/mL	0.35 mL
EPINEPHRINE (1:10,000)	IV/IO	0.01 mg/kg	0.23 mg	0.1 mg/mL	2.30 mL
EPINEPHRINE (1:1,000)	ETT	0.1 mg/kg	2.3 mg	1 mg/mL	2.30 mL
ESMOLOL	IV	0.5 mg/kg	11.5 mg	10 mg/mL	1.15 mL
LABETALOL	IV	0.2 mg/kg	4.6 mg	5 mg/mL	0.92 mL
LIDOCAINE	IV/IO	1 mg/kg	23 mg	20 mg/mL	1.15 mL
NEOSYNEPHRINE	IV	5 mcg/kg	115 mcg	100 mcg/mL	1.15 mL
ROMAZICON	IV	0.01 mg/kg	0.2 mg	0.1 mg/mL	2.00 mL
VASOPRESSIN	IV/IO	0.4 unit/kg	9.2 units	20 u/mL	0.46 mL

24 KG MAINTENANCE IV FLUIDS: 64 ML/HR

common pediatric drugs		route	dose	mg to pt	supplied	mL to give
ATROPINE	vagolytic	IV	0.02 mg/kg	0.48 mg	0.4 mg/mL	1.2 mL
GLYCOPYRROLATE	vagolytic	IV	0.004 mg/kg	0.096 mg	0.2 mg/mL	0.48 mL
MIDAZOLAM		IV	0.05 mg/kg	0.6 mg	1 mg/mL	0.6 mL
MIDAZOLAM		PO	0.5 mg/kg	12 mg	1 mg/mL	12 mL
MIDAZOLAM		IN	0.2 mg/kg	4.8 mg	1 mg/mL	4.8 mL
SUCCINYLCHOLINE		IV	2 mg/kg	48 mg	20 mg/mL	2.4 mL
SUCCINYLCHOLINE		IM	4 mg/kg	96 mg	20 mg/mL	4.8 mL
PROPOFOL		IV	3 mg/kg	72 mg	10 mg/mL	7.2 mL
ETOMIDATE	>10 y	IV	0.3 mg/kg	7.2 mg	2 mg/mL	3.6 mL
FENTANYL		IV	1 mcg/kg	24 mcg	50 mcg/mL	0.48 mL
FENTANYL		IN	2 mcg/kg	48 mcg	50 mcg/mL	0.96 mL
MORPHINE	<6 mo	IV/IM	0.05 mg/kg	1.2 mg	10 mg/mL	0.12 mL
MORPHINE	>6 mo	IV/IM	0.1 mg/kg	2.4 mg	10 mg/mL	0.24 mL
TORADOL	>2-16 y	IV	0.5 mg/kg	12 mg	30 mg/mL	0.4 mL
TORADOL	>2-16 y	IM	1 mg/kg	24 mg	30 mg/mL	0.8 mL
ACETAMINOPHEN		PR	20 mg/kg	480 mg		
ACETAMINOPHEN	2-12 y	IV	15 mg/kg	360 mg	10 mg/mL	36 mL
CISATRACURIUM		IV	0.1 mg/kg	2.4 mg	2 mg/mL	1.2 mL
PANCURONIUM	<1 mo	IV	0.02 mg/kg	0.48 mg	1 mg/mL	0.48 mL
PANCURONIUM	>1 mo	IV	0.1 mg/kg	2.4 mg	1 mg/mL	2.4 mL
ROCURONIUM		IV	0.6 mg/kg	14.4 mg	10 mg/mL	1.44 mL
ROCURONIUM	RSI	IV	1.2 mg/kg	28.8 mg	10 mg/mL	2.88 mL
VECURONIUM		IV	0.1 mg/kg	2.4 mg	1 mg/mL	2.4 mL
GLYCOPYRROLATE	reversal	IV	0.007 mg/kg	0.168 mg	0.2 mg/mL	0.84 mL
NEOSTIGMINE		IV	0.07 mg/kg	1.68 mg	1 mg/mL	1.68 mL
DEXAMETHASONE		IV	0.25 mg/kg	6 mg	10 mg/mL	0.6 mL
ONDANSETRON		IV	0.15 mg/kg	3.6 mg	2 mg/mL	1.8 mL

additional pediatric drugs	route	dose	mg to pt	supplied	mL to give
PREMED/SEDATION, VAGOLYTIC/ANTISIALAGOGUE; GIVE IM 30-60 MIN PREOP					
ATROPINE	IM	0.02 mg/kg	0.48 mg	0.4 mg/mL	1.2 mL
GLYCOPYRROLATE	IM	0.004 mg/kg	0.009 mg	0.2 mg/mL	0.045 mL
MIDAZOLAM	IM	0.1 mg/kg	0.5 mg	1 mg/mL	0.5 mL
DEXMEDETOMIDINE load dose	IV	0.5 mcg/kg	1 mcg	4 mcg/mL	0.25 mL
INDUCTION					
KETAMINE	IV	2 mg/kg	48 mg	10 mg/mL	4.8 mL
KETAMINE	IM/PR	5 mg/kg	120 mg	10 mg/mL	12 mL
OPIOIDS/NONOPIOIDS					
FENTANYL	IV	4 mcg/kg	96 mcg	50 mcg/mL	1.92 mL
FENTANYL high dose	IV cardiac	10 mcg/kg	240 mcg	50 mcg/mL	4.8 mL
HYDROMORPHONE < 6 mo	IV/SQ	0.005 mg/kg	0.12 mg	10 mg/mL	0.012 mL
HYDROMORPHONE > 6 mo	IV/SQ	0.015 mg/kg	0.36 mg	10 mg/mL	0.036 mL
REMIFENTANIL	IV	0.5 mcg/kg	1 mcg	50 mcg/mL	0.02 mL
SUFENTANIL	IV	0.5 mcg/kg	12 mcg	50 mcg/mL	0.24 mL
REVERSALS					
ATROPINE	IV	0.02 mg/kg	0.48 mg	0.4 mg/mL	1.2 mL
EDROPHONIUM neonate	IV	0.1 mg single dose		10 mg/mL	0.01 mL
EDROPHONIUM > 2 mo	IV	0.04 mg/kg	0.96 mg	10 mg/mL	0.096 mL
FLUMAZENIL	IV	0.01 mg/kg	0.2 mg	0.1 mg/mL	2 mL
NALOXONE < 5 y; < 20 kg	IV/IM	0.1 mg/kg	6 mg	0.4 mg/mL	5 mL
NALOXONE > 5 y; > 20 kg	IV/IM	2 mg per dose		0.4 mg/mL	5 mL
NALOXONE	ETT	0.3 mg/kg	7.2 mg	0.4 mg/mL	18 mL

additional pediatric drugs		route	dose	mg to pt	supplied	mL to give
ANTIBIOTICS						
AMPICILLIN	<6 y	IV	50 mg/kg	300 mg		
AMPICILLIN	>6 y	IV	50 mg/kg	1,200 mg		
AMPICILLIN & SULBACTUM	>1 mo	IV	50 mg/kg	1,200 mg		
CEFAZOLIN		IV	25 mg/kg	600 mg		
CLINDAMYCIN		IV	10 mg/kg	240 mg		
ERTAPENEM	3 mo-12 y	IV	15 mg/kg	360 mg		
ERTAPENEM	>12 y	IV	1 Gm	per dose		
GENTAMICIN		IV	2 mg/kg	48 mg		
LEVOFLOXACIN		IV	10 mg/kg	240 mg		
METRONIDAZOLE		IV	10 mg/kg	240 mg		
PIPERACILLIN & TAZOBACTAM	<40 kg & 2-9 mo	IV	80 mg/kg	1,920 mg		
PIPERACILLIN & TAZOBACTAM	<40 kg & >9 mo	IV	100 mg/kg	2,400 mg		
PIPERACILLIN & TAZOBACTAM	>40 kg	IV	3.375 Gm per dose			
VANCOMYCIN		IV	15 mg/kg	360 mg		
ANTINAUSEA						
METOCLOPROMIDE		IV	0.2 mg/kg	4.8 mg	5 mg/mL	0.96 mL
DIPHENHYDRAMINE		IV/IM	1.25 mg/kg	30 mg	50 mg/mL	0.6 mL
SCOPOLAMINE		IV/IM	6 mcg/kg	144 mcg	400 mcg/mL	0.36 mL
MISCELLANEOUS MEDS						
AMINOCAPROIC ACID		IV	100 mg/kg	2,400 mg	250 mg/mL	9.6 mL
DESMOPRESSIN		IV/SQ	0.3 mcg/kg	7.2 mcg	4 mcg/mL	1.8 mL
DEXAMETHASONE	croup	IV	0.6 mg/kg	14.4 mg	4 mg/mL	3.6 mL
HYDROCORTISONE		IV/IO	3 mg/kg	72 mg	100 mg/mL	0.72 mL

24 KG

1 year → 13 kg and up

Ventilation: trained rescuer	1 breath q 6-8 sec (8-10 breaths/minute) about 1 second/ breath-visible chest rise; if intubated, continuous compressions without pause for ventilations
Pulse check	carotid or femoral
Compression	heel of 1 hand or both hands one atop the other—lower half of sternum between nipples
Depth	2 inches (5 cm) or at least 1/3 chest depth
Rate	at least 100 compressions per minute
Compress/vent ratio	30:2 single rescuer 15:2 healthcare providers
Foreign body obstruction	Heimlich maneuver Never perform a blind finger-sweep. Open the mouth and look for object; if you see it, remove it.

sync cardioversion	0.5 J/kg	12 J
repeat	1 J/kg	24 J
defibrillation	2 J/kg	48 J
repeat	4 J/kg	96 J

IV Bolus Drugs		dose	mg to pt	supplied	mL to give
ADENOSINE	IV	0.1 mg/kg	2.4 mg	3 mg/mL	0.80 mL
ADENOSINE repeat dose	IV	0.2 mg/kg	4.8 mg	3 mg/mL	1.60 mL
AMIODARONE	IV/IO	5 mg/kg	120 mg	50 mg/mL	2.40 mL
ATROPINE	IM/IV	0.02 mg/kg	0.48 mg	0.4 mg/mL	1.20 mL
ATROPINE	ETT	0.04 mg/kg	0.96 mg	0.4 mg/mL	2.40 mL
CALCIUM CHLORIDE	IV	20 mg/kg	480 mg	100 mg/mL	4.80 mL
CALCIUM GLUCONATE	IV/IO	60 mg/kg	800 mg	100 mg/mL	8.00 mL
DANTROLENE	IV	2.5 mg/kg	60 mg		
EPHEDRINE	IV	0.15 mg/kg	3.6 mg	10 mg/mL	0.36 mL
EPINEPHRINE (1:10,000)	IV/IO	0.01 mg/kg	0.24 mg	0.1 mg/mL	2.40 mL
EPINEPHRINE (1:1,000)	ETT	0.1 mg/kg	2.4 mg	1 mg/mL	2.40 mL
ESMOLOL	IV	0.5 mg/kg	12 mg	10 mg/mL	1.20 mL
LABETALOL	IV	0.2 mg/kg	4.8 mg	5 mg/mL	0.96 mL
LIDOCAINE	IV/IO	1 mg/kg	24 mg	20 mg/mL	1.20 mL
NEOSYNEPHRINE	IV	5 mcg/kg	120 mcg	100 mcg/mL	1.20 mL
ROMAZICON	IV	0.01 mg/kg	0.2 mg	0.1 mg/mL	2.00 mL
VASOPRESSIN	IV/IO	0.4 unit/kg	9.6 units	20 u/mL	0.48 mL

25 KG MAINTENANCE IV FLUIDS: 65 ML/HR

common pediatric drugs		route	dose	mg to pt	supplied	mL to give
ATROPINE	vagolytic	IV	0.02 mg/kg	0.5 mg	0.4 mg/mL	1.25 mL
GLYCOPYRROLATE	vagolytic	IV	0.004 mg/kg	0.1 mg	0.2 mg/mL	0.5 mL
MIDAZOLAM		IV	0.05 mg/kg	0.6 mg	1 mg/mL	0.6 mL
MIDAZOLAM		PO	0.5 mg/kg	12.5 mg	1 mg/mL	12.5 mL
MIDAZOLAM		IN	0.2 mg/kg	5 mg	1 mg/mL	5 mL
SUCCINYLCHOLINE		IV	2 mg/kg	50 mg	20 mg/mL	2.5 mL
SUCCINYLCHOLINE		IM	4 mg/kg	100 mg	20 mg/mL	5 mL
PROPOFOL		IV	3 mg/kg	75 mg	10 mg/mL	7.5 mL
ETOMIDATE	>10 y	IV	0.3 mg/kg	7.5 mg	2 mg/mL	3.75 mL
FENTANYL		IV	1 mcg/kg	25 mcg	50 mcg/mL	0.5 mL
FENTANYL		IN	2 mcg/kg	50 mcg	50 mcg/mL	1 mL
MORPHINE	<6 mo	IV/IM	0.05 mg/kg	1.25 mg	10 mg/mL	0.125 mL
MORPHINE	>6 mo	IV/IM	0.1 mg/kg	2.5 mg	10 mg/mL	0.25 mL
TORADOL	>2-16 y	IV	0.5 mg/kg	12.5 mg	30 mg/mL	0.417 mL
TORADOL	>2-16 y	IM	1 mg/kg	25 mg	30 mg/mL	0.833 mL
ACETAMINOPHEN		PR	20 mg/kg	500 mg		
ACETAMINOPHEN	2-12 y	IV	15 mg/kg	375 mg	10 mg/mL	37.5 mL
CISATRACURIUM		IV	0.1 mg/kg	2.5 mg	2 mg/mL	1.25 mL
PANCURONIUM	<1 mo	IV	0.02 mg/kg	0.5 mg	1 mg/mL	0.5 mL
PANCURONIUM	>1 mo	IV	0.1 mg/kg	2.5 mg	1 mg/mL	2.5 mL
ROCURONIUM		IV	0.6 mg/kg	15 mg	10 mg/mL	1.5 mL
ROCURONIUM	RSI	IV	1.2 mg/kg	30 mg	10 mg/mL	3 mL
VECURONIUM		IV	0.1 mg/kg	2.5 mg	1 mg/mL	2.5 mL
GLYCOPYRROLATE	reversal	IV	0.007 mg/kg	0.175 mg	0.2 mg/mL	0.875 mL
NEOSTIGMINE		IV	0.07 mg/kg	1.75 mg	1 mg/mL	1.75 mL
DEXAMETHASONE		IV	0.25 mg/kg	6.25 mg	10 mg/mL	0.625 mL
ONDANSETRON		IV	0.15 mg/kg	3.75 mg	2 mg/mL	1.875 mL

additional pediatric drugs	route	dose	mg to pt	supplied	mL to give
PREMED/SEDATION; VAGOLYTIC/ANTISIALAGOGUE: GIVE IM 30-60 MIN PREOP					
ATROPINE	IM	0.02 mg/kg	0.5 mg	0.4 mg/mL	1.25 mL
GLYCOPYRROLATE	IM	0.004 mg/kg	0.009 mg	0.2 mg/mL	0.045 mL
MIDAZOLAM	IM	0.1 mg/kg	0.5 mg	1 mg/mL	0.5 mL
DEXMEDETOMIDINE	IV	0.5 mcg/kg load dose	1 mcg	4 mcg/mL	0.25 mL
INDUCTION					
KETAMINE	IV	2 mg/kg	50 mg	10 mg/mL	5 mL
KETAMINE	IM/PR	5 mg/kg	125 mg	10 mg/mL	12.5 mL
OPIOIDS/NONOPIOIDS					
FENTANYL	IV	4 mcg/kg high dose	100 mcg	50 mcg/mL	2 mL
FENTANYL	IV	10 mcg/kg cardiac	250 mcg	50 mcg/mL	5 mL
HYDROMORPHONE	< 6 mo IV/SQ	0.005 mg/kg	0.125 mg	10 mg/mL	0.0125 mL
HYDROMORPHONE	> 6 mo IV/SQ	0.015 mg/kg	0.375 mg	10 mg/mL	0.0375 mL
REMIFENTANIL	IV	0.5 mcg/kg	1 mcg	50 mcg/mL	0.02 mL
SUFENTANIL	IV	0.5 mcg/kg	12.5 mcg	50 mcg/mL	0.25 mL
REVERSALS					
ATROPINE	IV	0.02 mg/kg	0.5 mg	0.4 mg/mL	1.25 mL
EDROPHONIUM	neonate IV	0.1 mg single dose		10 mg/mL	0.01 mL
EDROPHONIUM	> 2 mo IV	0.04 mg/kg	1 mg	10 mg/mL	1.1 mL
FLUMAZENIL	< 1 y IV	0.01 mg/kg	0.2 mg	0.1 mg/mL	2 mL
NALOXONE	< 5 y; < 20 kg IV/IM	0.1 mg/kg	2 mg	0.4 mg/mL	5 mL
NALOXONE	> 5 y; > 20 kg IV/IM	2 mg per dose		0.4 mg/mL	5 mL
NALOXONE	ETT	0.3 mg/kg	7.5 mg	0.4 mg/mL	18.75 mL

additional pediatric drugs		route	dose	mg to pt	supplied	mL to give
ANTIBIOTICS						
AMPICILLIN	<6 y	IV	50 mg/kg	300 mg		
AMPICILLIN	>6 y	IV	50 mg/kg	1,250 mg		
AMPICILLIN & SULBACTUM	>1 mo	IV	50 mg/kg	1,250 mg		
CEFAZOLIN		IV	25 mg/kg	625 mg		
CLINDAMYCIN		IV	10 mg/kg	250 mg		
ERTAPENEM	3 mo-12 y	IV	15 mg/kg	375 mg		
ERTAPENEM	>12 y	IV	1 Gm	per dose		
GENTAMICIN		IV	2 mg/kg	50 mg		
LEVOFLOXACIN		IV	10 mg/kg	250 mg		
METRONIDAZOLE		IV	10 mg/kg	250 mg		
PIPERACILLIN & TAZOBACTAM	<40 kg & 2-9 mo	IV	80 mg/kg	2,000 mg		
PIPERACILLIN & TAZOBACTAM	<40 kg & >9 mo	IV	100 mg/kg	2,500 mg		
PIPERACILLIN & TAZOBACTAM	>40 kg	IV	3.375 Gm per dose			
VANCOMYCIN		IV	15 mg/kg	375 mg		
ANTINAUSEA						
METOCLOPROMIDE		IV	0.2 mg/kg	5 mg	5 mg/mL	1 mL
DIPHENHYDRAMINE		IV/IM	1.25 mg/kg	31.25 mg	50 mg/mL	0.625 mL
SCOPOLAMINE		IV/IM	6 mcg/kg	150 mcg	400 mcg/mL	0.375 mL
MISCELLANEOUS MEDS						
AMINOCAPROIC ACID		IV	100 mg/kg	2,500 mg	250 mg/mL	10 mL
DESMOPRESSIN		IV/SQ	0.3 mcg/kg	7.5 mcg	4 mcg/mL	1.875 mL
DEXAMETHASONE	croup	IV	0.6 mg/kg	15 mg	4 mg/mL	3.75 mL
HYDROCORTISONE		IV/IO	3 mg/kg	75 mg	100 mg/mL	0.75 mL

25 KG

1 year → 13 kg and up

Ventilation: trained rescuer	1 breath q 6-8 sec (8-10 breaths/minute) about 1 second/ breath-visible chest rise; if intubated, continuous compressions without pause for ventilations
Pulse check	carotid or femoral
Compression	heel of 1 hand or both hands one atop the other–lower half of sternum between nipples
Depth	2 inches (5 cm) or at least 1/3 chest depth
Rate	at least 100 compressions per minute
Compress/vent ratio	30:2 single rescuer 15:2 2 healthcare providers
Foreign body obstruction	Heimlich maneuver Never perform a blind finger-sweep. Open the mouth and look for object; if you see it, remove it.

sync cardioversion	0.5 J/kg	12.5 J	
defibrillation	1 J/kg	25 J	repeat
	2 J/kg	50 J	
	4 J/kg	100 J	repeat

IV Bolus Drugs		dose	mg to pt	supplied	mL to give
ADENOSINE		0.1 mg/kg	2.5 mg	3 mg/mL	0.83 mL
ADENOSINE	repeat dose	0.2 mg/kg	5 mg	3 mg/mL	1.67 mL
AMIODARONE		5 mg/kg	125 mg	50 mg/mL	2.50 mL
ATROPINE	IV/IM	0.02 mg/kg	0.5 mg	0.4 mg/mL	1.25 mL
ATROPINE	ETT	0.04 mg/kg	1 mg	0.4 mg/mL	2.50 mL
CALCIUM CHLORIDE	IV	20 mg/kg	500 mg	100 mg/mL	5.00 mL
CALCIUM GLUCONATE	IV/IO	60 mg/kg	800 mg	100 mg/mL	8.00 mL
DANTROLENE		2.5 mg/kg	30 mg		
EPHEDRINE	IV	0.15 mg/kg	3.75 mg	10 mg/mL	0.38 mL
EPINEPHRINE (1:10,000)	IV/IO	0.01 mg/kg	0.25 mg	0.1 mg/mL	2.50 mL
EPINEPHRINE (1:1,000)	ETT	0.1 mg/kg	2.5 mg	1 mg/mL	2.50 mL
ESMOLOL	IV	0.5 mg/kg	12.5 mg	10 mg/mL	1.25 mL
LABETALOL	IV	0.2 mg/kg	5 mg	5 mg/mL	1.00 mL
LIDOCAINE	IV/IO	1 mg/kg	25 mg	100 mcg/mL	1.25 mL
NEOSYNEPHRINE	IV	5 mcg/kg	125 mcg	100 mcg/mL	1.25 mL
ROMAZICON	IV	0.01 mg/kg	0.2 mg	0.1 mg/mL	2.00 mL
VASOPRESSIN	IV/IO	0.4 unit/kg	10 units	20 u/mL	0.50 mL

26 KG MAINTENANCE IV FLUIDS: 66 ML/HR

common pediatric drugs		route	dose	mg to pt	supplied	mL to give
ATROPINE	vagolytic	IV	0.02 mg/kg	0.5 mg	0.4 mg/mL	1.25 mL
GLYCOPYRROLATE	vagolytic	IV	0.004 mg/kg	0.104 mg	0.2 mg/mL	0.52 mL
MIDAZOLAM		IV	0.05 mg/kg	0.6 mg	1 mg/mL	0.6 mL
MIDAZOLAM		PO	0.5 mg/kg	13 mg	1 mg/mL	13 mL
MIDAZOLAM		IN	0.2 mg/kg	5.2 mg	1 mg/mL	5.2 mL
SUCCINYLCHOLINE		IV	2 mg/kg	52 mg	20 mg/mL	2.6 mL
SUCCINYLCHOLINE		IM	4 mg/kg	104 mg	20 mg/mL	5.2 mL
PROPOFOL		IV	3 mg/kg	78 mg	10 mg/mL	7.8 mL
ETOMIDATE	>10 y	IV	0.3 mg/kg	7.8 mg	2 mg/mL	3.9 mL
FENTANYL		IV	1 mcg/kg	26 mcg	50 mcg/mL	0.52 mL
FENTANYL		IN	2 mcg/kg	52 mcg	50 mcg/mL	1.04 mL
MORPHINE	<6 mo	IV/IM	0.05 mg/kg	1.3 mg	10 mg/mL	0.13 mL
MORPHINE	>6 mo	IV/IM	0.1 mg/kg	2.6 mg	10 mg/mL	0.26 mL
TORADOL	>2-16 y	IV	0.5 mg/kg	13 mg	30 mg/mL	0.433 mL
TORADOL	>2-16 y	IM	1 mg/kg	26 mg	30 mg/mL	0.867 mL
ACETAMINOPHEN		PR	20 mg/kg	520 mg		
ACETAMINOPHEN	2-12 y	IV	15 mg/kg	390 mg	10 mg/mL	39 mL
CISATRACURIUM		IV	0.1 mg/kg	2.6 mg	2 mg/mL	1.3 mL
PANCURONIUM	<1 mo	IV	0.02 mg/kg	0.52 mg	1 mg/mL	0.52 mL
PANCURONIUM	>1 mo	IV	0.1 mg/kg	2.6 mg	1 mg/mL	2.6 mL
ROCURONIUM		IV	0.6 mg/kg	15.6 mg	10 mg/mL	1.56 mL
ROCURONIUM	RSI	IV	1.2 mg/kg	31.2 mg	10 mg/mL	3.12 mL
VECURONIUM		IV	0.1 mg/kg	2.6 mg	1 mg/mL	2.6 mL
GLYCOPYRROLATE	reversal	IV	0.007 mg/kg	0.182 mg	0.2 mg/mL	0.91 mL
NEOSTIGMINE		IV	0.07 mg/kg	1.82 mg	1 mg/mL	1.82 mL
DEXAMETHASONE		IV	0.25 mg/kg	6.5 mg	10 mg/mL	0.65 mL
ONDANSETRON		IV	0.15 mg/kg	3.9 mg	2 mg/mL	1.95 mL

additional pediatric drugs	route	dose	mg to pt	supplied	mL to give
PREMED/SEDATION; VAGOLYTIC/ANTISIALAGOGUE; GIVE IM 30–60 MIN PREOP					
ATROPINE	IM	0.02 mg/kg	0.5 mg	0.4 mg/mL	1.25 mL
GLYCOPYRROLATE	IM	0.004 mg/kg	0.009 mg	0.2 mg/mL	0.045 mL
MIDAZOLAM	IM		0.5 mg	1 mg/mL	0.5 mL
DEXMEDETOMIDINE load dose	IV	0.5 mcg/kg	1 mcg	4 mcg/mL	0.25 mL
INDUCTION					
KETAMINE	IV	2 mg/kg	52 mg	10 mg/mL	5.2 mL
KETAMINE	IM/PR	5 mg/kg	130 mg	10 mg/mL	13 mL
OPIOIDS/NONOPIOIDS					
FENTANYL	IV	high dose	4 mcg/kg	104 mcg	50 mcg/mL	2.08 mL
FENTANYL	IV	cardiac	10 mcg/kg	260 mcg	50 mcg/mL	5.2 mL
HYDROMORPHONE	IV/SQ	< 6 mo	0.005 mg/kg	0.13 mg	10 mg/mL	0.013 mL
HYDROMORPHONE	IV/SQ	> 6 mo	0.015 mg/kg	0.39 mg	10 mg/mL	0.039 mL
REMIFENTANIL	IV	0.5 mcg/kg	1 mcg	50 mcg/mL	0.02 mL
SUFENTANIL	IV	0.5 mcg/kg	13 mcg	50 mcg/mL	0.26 mL
REVERSALS					
ATROPINE	IV	0.02 mg/kg	0.5 mg	0.4 mg/mL	1.25 mL
EDROPHONIUM	IV	neonate	0.1 mg single dose		10 mg/mL	0.01 mL
EDROPHONIUM	IV	> 2 mo	1 mg	10 mg/mL	0.104 mL
FLUMAZENIL	IV	> 1 y	0.01 mg/kg	0.2 mg	0.1 mg/mL	2 mL
NALOXONE	IM/IV	< 5 y; < 20 kg	0.1 mg/kg	2 mg	0.4 mg/mL	5 mL
NALOXONE	IM/IV	> 5 y; > 20 kg	2 mg per dose		0.4 mg/mL	5 mL
NALOXONE	ETT	0.3 mg/kg	7.8 mg	0.4 mg/mL	19.5 mL

additional pediatric drugs		route	dose	mg to pt	supplied	mL to give
ANTIBIOTICS						
AMPICILLIN	<6 y	IV	50 mg/kg	300 mg		
AMPICILLIN	>6 y	IV	50 mg/kg	1,300 mg		
AMPICILLIN & SULBACTUM	>1 mo	IV	50 mg/kg	1,300 mg		
CEFAZOLIN		IV	25 mg/kg	650 mg		
CLINDAMYCIN		IV	10 mg/kg	260 mg		
ERTAPENEM	3 mo-12 y	IV	15 mg/kg	390 mg		
ERTAPENEM	>12 y	IV	1 Gm	per dose		
GENTAMICIN		IV	2 mg/kg	52 mg		
LEVOFLOXACIN		IV	10 mg/kg	260 mg		
METRONIDAZOLE		IV	10 mg/kg	260 mg		
PIPERACILLIN & TAZOBACTAM	<40 kg & 2-9 mo	IV	80 mg/kg	2,080 mg		
PIPERACILLIN & TAZOBACTAM	<40 kg & >9 mo	IV	100 mg/kg	2,600 mg		
PIPERACILLIN & TAZOBACTAM	>40 kg	IV	3.375 Gm per dose			
VANCOMYCIN		IV	15 mg/kg	390 mg		
ANTINAUSEA						
METOCLOPROMIDE		IV	0.2 mg/kg	5.2 mg	5 mg/mL	1.04 mL
DIPHENHYDRAMINE		IV/IM	1.25 mg/kg	32.5 mg	50 mg/mL	0.65 mL
SCOPOLAMINE		IV/IM	6 mcg/kg	156 mcg	400 mcg/mL	0.39 mL
MISCELLANEOUS MEDS						
AMINOCAPROIC ACID		IV	100 mg/kg	2,600 mg	250 mg/mL	10.4 mL
DESMOPRESSIN		IV/SQ	0.3 mcg/kg	7.8 mcg	4 mcg/mL	1.95 mL
DEXAMETHASONE	croup	IV	0.6 mg/kg	15.6 mg	4 mg/mL	3.9 mL
HYDROCORTISONE		IV/IO	3 mg/kg	78 mg	100 mg/mL	0.78 mL

26 KG

1 year → 13 kg and up

Ventilation: trained rescuer	1 breath q 6-8 sec (8-10 breaths/minute) about 1 second/ breath-visible chest rise; if intubated, continuous compressions without pause for ventilations
Pulse check	carotid or femoral
Compression	heel of 1 hand or both hands one atop the other—lower half of sternum between nipples
Depth	2 inches (5 cm) or at least 1/3 chest depth
Rate	at least 100 compressions per minute
Compress/vent ratio	30:2 single rescuer 15:2 2 healthcare providers
Foreign body obstruction	Heimlich maneuver Never perform a blind finger-sweep. Open the mouth and look for object; if you see it, remove it.

sync cardioversion	0.5 J/kg	13 J
defibrillation	1 J/kg	26 J
	repeat	
	2 J/kg	52 J
	repeat	
	4 J/kg	104 J

IV Bolus Drugs	dose	mg to pt	supplied	mL to give
ADENOSINE	IV	0.1 mg/kg	2.6 mg	3 mg/mL	0.87 mL
ADENOSINE repeat dose	IV	0.2 mg/kg	5.2 mg	3 mg/mL	1.73 mL
AMIODARONE	IV/IO	5 mg/kg	130 mg	50 mg/mL	2.60 mL
ATROPINE	IV/IM	0.02 mg/kg	0.5 mg	0.4 mg/mL	1.25 mL
ATROPINE	ETT	0.04 mg/kg	1.04 mg	0.4 mg/mL	2.60 mL
CALCIUM CHLORIDE	IV	20 mg/kg	520 mg	100 mg/mL	5.20 mL
CALCIUM GLUCONATE	IV/IO	60 mg/kg	800 mg	100 mg/mL	8.00 mL
DANTROLENE	IV	2.5 mg/kg	30 mg		
EPHEDRINE	IV	0.15 mg/kg	3.9 mg	10 mg/mL	0.39 mL
EPINEPHRINE (1:10,000)	IV/IO	0.01 mg/kg	0.26 mg	0.1 mg/mL	2.60 mL
EPINEPHRINE (1:1,000)	ETT	0.1 mg/kg	2.5 mg	1 mg/mL	2.50 mL
ESMOLOL	IV	0.5 mg/kg	13 mg	10 mg/mL	1.30 mL
LABETALOL	IV	0.2 mg/kg	5.2 mg	5 mg/mL	1.04 mL
LIDOCAINE	IV/IO	1 mg/kg	26 mg	20 mg/mL	1.30 mL
NEOSYNEPHRINE	IV	5 mcg/kg	130 mcg	100 mcg/mL	1.30 mL
ROMAZICON	IV	0.01 mg/kg	0.2 mg	0.1 mg/mL	2.00 mL
VASOPRESSIN	IV/IO	0.4 unit/kg	10.4 units	20 u/mL	0.52 mL

27 KG MAINTENANCE IV FLUIDS: 67 ML/HR

common pediatric drugs		route	dose	mg to pt	supplied	mL to give
ATROPINE	vagolytic	IV	0.02 mg/kg	0.5 mg	0.4 mg/mL	1.25 mL
GLYCOPYRROLATE	vagolytic	IV	0.004 mg/kg	0.108 mg	0.2 mg/mL	0.54 mL
MIDAZOLAM		IV	0.05 mg/kg	0.6 mg	1 mg/mL	0.6 mL
MIDAZOLAM		PO	0.5 mg/kg	13.5 mg	1 mg/mL	13.5 mL
MIDAZOLAM		IN	0.2 mg/kg	5.4 mg	1 mg/mL	5.4 mL
SUCCINYLCHOLINE		IV	2 mg/kg	54 mg	20 mg/mL	2.7 mL
SUCCINYLCHOLINE		IM	4 mg/kg	108 mg	20 mg/mL	5.4 mL
PROPOFOL		IV	3 mg/kg	81 mg	10 mg/mL	8.1 mL
ETOMIDATE	>10 y	IV	0.3 mg/kg	8.1 mg	2 mg/mL	4.05 mL
FENTANYL		IV	1 mcg/kg	27 mcg	50 mcg/mL	0.54 mL
FENTANYL		IN	2 mcg/kg	54 mcg	50 mcg/mL	1.08 mL
MORPHINE	<6 mo	IV/IM	0.05 mg/kg	1.35 mg	10 mg/mL	0.135 mL
MORPHINE	>6 mo	IV/IM	0.1 mg/kg	2.7 mg	10 mg/mL	0.27 mL
TORADOL	>2-16 y	IV	0.5 mg/kg	13.5 mg	30 mg/mL	0.45 mL
TORADOL	>2-16 y	IM	1 mg/kg	27 mg	30 mg/mL	0.9 mL
ACETAMINOPHEN		PR	20 mg/kg	540 mg		
ACETAMINOPHEN	2-12 y	IV	15 mg/kg	405 mg	10 mg/mL	40.5 mL
CISATRACURIUM		IV	0.1 mg/kg	2.7 mg	2 mg/mL	1.35 mL
PANCURONIUM	<1 mo	IV	0.02 mg/kg	0.54 mg	1 mg/mL	0.54 mL
PANCURONIUM	>1 mo	IV	0.1 mg/kg	2.7 mg	1 mg/mL	2.7 mL
ROCURONIUM		IV	0.6 mg/kg	16.2 mg	10 mg/mL	1.62 mL
ROCURONIUM	RSI	IV	1.2 mg/kg	32.4 mg	10 mg/mL	3.24 mL
VECURONIUM		IV	0.1 mg/kg	2.7 mg	1 mg/mL	2.7 mL
GLYCOPYRROLATE	reversal	IV	0.007 mg/kg	0.189 mg	0.2 mg/mL	0.945 mL
NEOSTIGMINE		IV	0.07 mg/kg	1.89 mg	1 mg/mL	1.89 mL
DEXAMETHASONE		IV	0.25 mg/kg	6.75 mg	10 mg/mL	0.675 mL
ONDANSETRON		IV	0.15 mg/kg	4 mg	2 mg/mL	2 mL

additional pediatric drugs	route	dose	mg to pt	supplied	mL to give
PREMED/SEDATION; VAGOLYTIC/ANTISIALAGOGUE; GIVE IM 30-60 MIN PREOP					
ATROPINE	IM	0.02 mg/kg	0.5 mg	0.4 mg/mL	1.25 mL
GLYCOPYRROLATE	IM	0.004 mg/kg	0.009 mg	0.2 mg/mL	0.045 mL
MIDAZOLAM	IM	0.1 mg/kg	0.5 mg	1 mg/mL	0.5 mL
DEXMEDETOMIDINE	IV	load dose 0.5 mcg/kg	1 mcg	4 mcg/mL	0.25 mL
INDUCTION					
KETAMINE	IV	2 mg/kg	54 mg	10 mg/mL	5.4 mL
KETAMINE	IM/PR	5 mg/kg	135 mg	10 mg/mL	13.5 mL
OPIOIDS/NONOPIOIDS					
FENTANYL	IV	high dose 4 mcg/kg	108 mcg	50 mcg/mL	2.16 mL
FENTANYL	IV	cardiac 10 mcg/kg	270 mcg	50 mcg/mL	5.4 mL
HYDROMORPHONE	IV/SO <6 mo	0.005 mg/kg	0.135 mg	10 mg/mL	0.0135 mL
HYDROMORPHONE	IV/SO >6 mo	0.015 mg/kg	0.405 mg	10 mg/mL	0.0405 mL
SUFENTANIL	IV	0.5 mcg/kg	1 mcg	50 mcg/mL	0.02 mL
SUFENTANIL	IV	0.5 mcg/kg	13.5 mcg	50 mcg/mL	0.27 mL
REVERSALS					
ATROPINE	IV	0.02 mg/kg	0.5 mg	0.4 mg/mL	1.25 mL
EDROPHONIUM	IV	neonate	0.1 mg single dose	10 mg/mL	0.01 mL
EDROPHONIUM	IV	>2 y	0.04 mg/kg	1.08 mg	10 mg/mL	0.108 mL
FLUMAZENIL	IV	>1 y	0.01 mg/kg	0.2 mg	0.1 mg/mL	2 mL
NALOXONE	IM/IV	<5 y; <20 kg	0.1 mg/kg	2 mg	0.4 mg/mL	5 mL
NALOXONE	IM/IV	<5 y; <20 kg	2 mg per dose	0.4 mg/mL	5 mL
NALOXONE	ETT	0.3 mg/kg	8.1 mg	0.4 mg/mL	20.25 mL

additional pediatric drugs		route	dose	mg to pt	supplied	mL to give
ANTIBIOTICS						
AMPICILLIN	<6 y	IV	50 mg/kg	300 mg		
AMPICILLIN	>6 y	IV	50 mg/kg	1,350 mg		
AMPICILLIN & SULBACTUM	>1 mo	IV	50 mg/kg	1,350 mg		
CEFAZOLIN		IV	25 mg/kg	675 mg		
CLINDAMYCIN		IV	10 mg/kg	270 mg		
ERTAPENEM	3 mo-12 y	IV	15 mg/kg	405 mg		
ERTAPENEM	>12 y	IV	1 Gm	per dose		
GENTAMICIN		IV	2 mg/kg	54 mg		
LEVOFLOXACIN		IV	10 mg/kg	270 mg		
METRONIDAZOLE		IV	10 mg/kg	270 mg		
PIPERACILLIN & TAZOBACTAM	<40 kg & 2-9 mo	IV	80 mg/kg	2,160 mg		
PIPERACILLIN & TAZOBACTAM	<40 kg & >9 mo	IV	100 mg/kg	2,700 mg		
PIPERACILLIN & TAZOBACTAM	>40 kg	IV	3.375 Gm per dose			
VANCOMYCIN		IV	15 mg/kg	405 mg		
ANTINAUSEA						
METOCLOPROMIDE		IV	0.2 mg/kg	5.4 mg	5 mg/mL	1.08 mL
DIPHENHYDRAMINE		IV/IM	1.25 mg/kg	33.75 mg	50 mg/mL	0.675 mL
SCOPOLAMINE		IV/IM	6 mcg/kg	162 mcg	400 mcg/mL	0.405 mL
MISCELLANEOUS MEDS						
AMINOCAPROIC ACID		IV	100 mg/kg	2,700 mg	250 mg/mL	10.8 mL
DESMOPRESSIN		IV/SQ	0.3 mcg/kg	8.1 mcg	4 mcg/mL	2.025 mL
DEXAMETHASONE	croup	IV	0.6 mg/kg	16 mg	4 mg/mL	4 mL
HYDROCORTISONE		IV/IO	3 mg/kg	81 mg	100 mg/mL	0.81 mL

27 KG

1 year → 13 kg and up

Ventilation: trained rescuer	1 breath q 6-8 sec (8-10 breaths/minute) about 1 second/ breath-visible chest rise; if intubated, continuous compressions without pause for ventilations
Pulse check	carotid or femoral
Compression	heel of 1 hand or both hands one atop the other–lower half of sternum between nipples
Depth	2 inches (5 cm) or at least 1/3 chest depth
Rate	at least 100 compressions per minute
Compress/vent ratio	30:2 single rescuer 15:2 2 healthcare providers
Foreign body obstruction	Heimlich maneuver Never perform a blind finger-sweep. Open the mouth and look for object; if you see it, remove it.

	dose		J
sync cardioversion	0.5 J/kg		13.5 J
defibrillation	1 J/kg	27	27 J
	repeat		54 J
	2 J/kg		54 J
	repeat		108 J
	4 J/kg	108 J	

IV Bolus Drugs		dose	mg to pt	supplied	mL to give
ADENOSINE	IV	0.1 mg/kg	2.7 mg	3 mg	0.90 mL
ADENOSINE repeat dose	IV	0.2 mg/kg	5.4 mg	3 mg/mL	1.80 mL
AMIODARONE	IV/IO	5 mg/kg	135 mg	50 mg	2.70 mL
ATROPINE	IM/IV	0.02 mg/kg	0.5 mg	0.4 mg/mL	1.25 mL
ATROPINE	ETT	0.04 mg/kg	1.08 mg	0.4 mg/mL	2.70 mL
CALCIUM CHLORIDE	IV	20 mg/kg	540 mg	100 mg/mL	5.40 mL
CALCIUM GLUCONATE	IV/IO	60 mg/kg	800 mg	100 mg/mL	8.00 mL
DANTROLENE	IV	2.5 mg/kg	30 mg		
EPHEDRINE	IV	0.15 mg/kg	4.05 mg	10 mg/mL	0.41 mL
EPINEPHRINE (1:10,000)	IV/IO	0.01 mg/kg	0.27 mg	0.1 mg/mL	2.70 mL
EPINEPHRINE (1:1,000)	ETT	0.1 mg/kg	2.5 mg	1 mg/mL	2.50 mL
ESMOLOL	IV	0.5 mg/kg	13.5 mg	10 mg/mL	1.35 mL
LABETALOL	IV	0.2 mg/kg	5.4 mg	5 mg/mL	1.08 mL
LIDOCAINE	IV/IO	1 mg/kg	27 mg	100 mcg/mL	1.35 mL
NEOSYNEPHRINE	IV	5 mcg/kg	135 mcg	100 mcg/mL	1.35 mL
ROMAZICON	IV	0.01 mg/kg	0.2 mg	0.1 mg/mL	2.00 mL
VASOPRESSIN	IV/IO	0.4 unit/kg	10.8 units	20 u/mL	0.54 mL

28 KG MAINTENANCE IV FLUIDS: 68 ML/HR

common pediatric drugs		route	dose	mg to pt	supplied	mL to give
ATROPINE	vagolytic	IV	0.02 mg/kg	0.5 mg	0.4 mg/mL	1.25 mL
GLYCOPYRROLATE	vagolytic	IV	0.004 mg/kg	0.112 mg	0.2 mg/mL	0.56 mL
MIDAZOLAM		IV	0.05 mg/kg	0.6 mg	1 mg/mL	0.6 mL
MIDAZOLAM		PO	0.5 mg/kg	14 mg	1 mg/mL	14 mL
MIDAZOLAM		IN	0.2 mg/kg	5.6 mg	1 mg/mL	5.6 mL
SUCCINYLCHOLINE		IV	2 mg/kg	56 mg	20 mg/mL	2.8 mL
SUCCINYLCHOLINE		IM	4 mg/kg	112 mg	20 mg/mL	5.6 mL
PROPOFOL		IV	3 mg/kg	84 mg	10 mg/mL	8.4 mL
ETOMIDATE	>10 y	IV	0.3 mg/kg	8.4 mg	2 mg/mL	4.2 mL
FENTANYL		IV	1 mcg/kg	28 mcg	50 mcg/mL	0.56 mL
FENTANYL		IN	2 mcg/kg	56 mcg	50 mcg/mL	1.12 mL
MORPHINE	<6 mo	IV/IM	0.05 mg/kg	1.4 mg	10 mg/mL	0.14 mL
MORPHINE	>6 mo	IV/IM	0.1 mg/kg	2.8 mg	10 mg/mL	0.28 mL
TORADOL	>2-16 y	IV	0.5 mg/kg	14 mg	30 mg/mL	0.467 mL
TORADOL	>2-16 y	IM	1 mg/kg	28 mg	30 mg/mL	0.933 mL
ACETAMINOPHEN		PR	20 mg/kg	560 mg		
ACETAMINOPHEN	2-12 y	IV	15 mg/kg	420 mg	10 mg/mL	42 mL
CISATRACURIUM		IV	0.1 mg/kg	2.8 mg	2 mg/mL	1.4 mL
PANCURONIUM	<1 mo	IV	0.02 mg/kg	0.56 mg	1 mg/mL	0.56 mL
PANCURONIUM	>1 mo	IV	0.1 mg/kg	2.8 mg	1 mg/mL	2.8 mL
ROCURONIUM		IV	0.6 mg/kg	16.8 mg	10 mg/mL	1.68 mL
ROCURONIUM	RSI	IV	1.2 mg/kg	33.6 mg	10 mg/mL	3.36 mL
VECURONIUM		IV	0.1 mg/kg	2.8 mg	1 mg/mL	2.8 mL
GLYCOPYRROLATE	reversal	IV	0.007 mg/kg	0.196 mg	0.2 mg/mL	0.98 mL
NEOSTIGMINE		IV	0.07 mg/kg	1.96 mg	1 mg/mL	1.96 mL
DEXAMETHASONE		IV	0.25 mg/kg	7 mg	10 mg/mL	0.7 mL
ONDANSETRON		IV	0.15 mg/kg	4 mg	2 mg/mL	2 mL

additional pediatric drugs	route	dose		mg to pt	supplied	mL to give
PREMED/SEDATION; VAGOLYTIC/ANTISIALAGOGUE; GIVE IM 30-60 MIN PREOP						
ATROPINE	IM	0.02 mg/kg		0.5 mg	0.4 mg/mL	1.25 mL
GLYCOPYRROLATE	IM	0.004 mg/kg		0.009 mg	0.2 mg/mL	0.045 mL
MIDAZOLAM	IM	0.1 mg/kg		0.5 mg	1 mg/mL	0.5 mL
DEXMEDETOMIDINE	IV	load dose	0.5 mcg/kg	1 mcg	4 mcg/mL	0.25 mL
INDUCTION						
KETAMINE	IV	2 mg/kg		56 mg	10 mg/mL	5.6 mL
KETAMINE	IM/PR	5 mg/kg		140 mg	10 mg/mL	14 mL
OPIOIDS/NONOPIOIDS						
FENTANYL	IV	high dose	4 mcg/kg	112 mcg	50 mcg/mL	2.24 mL
FENTANYL	IV	cardiac	10 mcg/kg	280 mcg	50 mcg/mL	5.6 mL
HYDROMORPHONE	IV/SQ	< 6 mo	0.005 mg/kg	0.14 mg	10 mg/mL	0.014 mL
HYDROMORPHONE	IV/SQ	> 6 mo	0.015 mg/kg	0.42 mg	10 mg/mL	0.042 mL
REMIFENTANIL	IV	0.5 mcg/kg		1 mcg	50 mcg/mL	0.02 mL
SUFENTANIL	IV	0.5 mcg/kg		14 mcg	50 mcg/mL	0.28 mL
REVERSALS						
ATROPINE	IV	0.02 mg/kg		0.5 mg	0.4 mg/mL	1.25 mL
EDROPHONIUM	IV	neonate	0.1 mg single dose		10 mg/mL	0.01 mL
EDROPHONIUM	IV	> 2 mo	0.04 mg/kg	1.12 mg	10 mg/mL	0.112 mL
FLUMAZENIL	IV	> 1 y	0.01 mg/kg	0.2 mg	0.1 mg/mL	2 mL
NALOXONE	IV/IM	< 5 y; < 20 kg	0.1 mg/kg	2 mg	0.4 mg/mL	5 mL
NALOXONE	IV/IM	> 5 y; > 20 kg	2 mg per dose		0.4 mg/mL	5 mL
NALOXONE	ETT	0.3 mg/kg		8.4 mg	0.4 mg/mL	21 mL

additional pediatric drugs		route	dose	mg to pt	supplied	mL to give
ANTIBIOTICS						
AMPICILLIN	<6 y	IV	50 mg/kg	300 mg		
AMPICILLIN	>6 y	IV	50 mg/kg	1,400 mg		
AMPICILLIN & SULBACTUM	>1 mo	IV	50 mg/kg	1,400 mg		
CEFAZOLIN		IV	25 mg/kg	700 mg		
CLINDAMYCIN		IV	10 mg/kg	280 mg		
ERTAPENEM	3 mo-12 y	IV	15 mg/kg	420 mg		
ERTAPENEM	>12 y	IV	1 Gm	per dose		
GENTAMICIN		IV	2 mg/kg	56 mg		
LEVOFLOXACIN		IV	10 mg/kg	280 mg		
METRONIDAZOLE		IV	10 mg/kg	280 mg		
PIPERACILLIN & TAZOBACTAM	<40 kg & 2-9 mo	IV	80 mg/kg	2,440 mg		
PIPERACILLIN & TAZOBACTAM	<40 kg & >9 mo	IV	100 mg/kg	2,800 mg		
PIPERACILLIN & TAZOBACTAM	>40 kg	IV	3.375 Gm per dose			
VANCOMYCIN		IV	15 mg/kg	420 mg		
ANTINAUSEA						
METOCLOPROMIDE		IV	0.2 mg/kg	5.6 mg	5 mg/mL	1.12 mL
DIPHENHYDRAMINE		IV/IM	1.25 mg/kg	35 mg	50 mg/mL	0.7 mL
SCOPOLAMINE		IV/IM	6 mcg/kg	168 mcg	400 mcg/mL	0.42 mL
MISCELLANEOUS MEDS						
AMINOCAPROIC ACID		IV	100 mg/kg	2,800 mg	250 mg/mL	11.2 mL
DESMOPRESSIN		IV/SQ	0.3 mcg/kg	8.4 mcg	4 mcg/mL	2.1 mL
DEXAMETHASONE	croup	IV	0.6 mg/kg	16 mg	4 mg/mL	4 mL
HYDROCORTISONE		IV/IO	3 mg/kg	84 mg	100 mg/mL	0.84 mL

28 KG

1 year → 13 kg and up

Ventilation: trained rescuer	1 breath q 6-8 sec (8-10 breaths/minute) about 1 second/ breath-visible chest rise; if intubated, continuous compressions without pause for ventilations
Pulse check	carotid or femoral
Compression	heel of 1 hand or both hands one atop the other–lower half of sternum between nipples
Depth	2 inches (5 cm) or at least 1/3 chest depth
Rate	at least 100 compressions per minute
Compress/vent ratio	30:2 single rescuer 15:2 healthcare providers
Foreign body obstruction	Heimlich maneuver Never perform a blind finger-sweep. Open the mouth and look for object; if you see it, remove it.

sync cardioversion	0.5 J/kg	14 J
repeat	1 J/kg	28 J
defibrillation	2 J/kg	56 J
repeat	4 J/kg	112 J

IV Bolus Drugs		dose	mg to pt	supplied	mL to give
ADENOSINE	IV	0.1 mg/kg	2.8 mg	3 mg/mL	0.93 mL
ADENOSINE repeat dose	IV	0.2 mg/kg	5.6 mg	3 mg/mL	1.87 mL
AMIODARONE	IV/IO	5 mg/kg	140 mg	50 mg/mL	2.80 mL
ATROPINE	IV/IM	0.02 mg/kg	0.5 mg	0.4 mg/mL	1.25 mL
ATROPINE	ETT	0.04 mg/kg	1.12 mg	0.4 mg/mL	2.80 mL
CALCIUM CHLORIDE	IV	20 mg/kg	560 mg	100 mg/mL	5.60 mL
CALCIUM GLUCONATE	IV/IO	60 mg/kg	800 mg	100 mg/mL	8.00 mL
DANTROLENE	IV	2.5 mg/kg	30 mg		
EPHEDRINE	IV	0.15 mg/kg	4.2 mg	10 mg/mL	0.42 mL
EPINEPHRINE (1:10,000)	IV/IO	0.01 mg/kg	0.28 mg	0.1 mg/mL	2.80 mL
EPINEPHRINE (1:1,000)	ETT	0.1 mg/kg	2.5 mg	1 mg/mL	2.50 mL
ESMOLOL	IV	0.5 mg/kg	14 mg	10 mg/mL	1.40 mL
LABETALOL	IV	0.2 mg/kg	5.6 mg	5 mg/mL	1.12 mL
LIDOCAINE	IV/IO	1 mg/kg	28 mg	20 mg/mL	1.40 mL
NEOSYNEPHRINE	IV	5 mcg/kg	140 mcg	100 mcg/mL	1.40 mL
ROMAZICON	IV	0.01 mg/kg	0.2 mg	0.1 mg/mL	2.00 mL
VASOPRESSIN	IV/IO	0.4 unit/kg	11.2 units	20 u/mL	0.56 mL

29 KG MAINTENANCE IV FLUIDS: 69 ML/HR

common pediatric drugs		route	dose	mg to pt	supplied	mL to give
ATROPINE	vagolytic	IV	0.02 mg/kg	0.5 mg	0.4 mg/mL	1.25 mL
GLYCOPYRROLATE	vagolytic	IV	0.004 mg/kg	0.116 mg	0.2 mg/mL	0.58 mL
MIDAZOLAM		IV	0.05 mg/kg	0.6 mg	1 mg/mL	0.6 mL
MIDAZOLAM		PO	0.5 mg/kg	14.5 mg	1 mg/mL	14.5 mL
MIDAZOLAM		IN	0.2 mg/kg	5.8 mg	1 mg/mL	5.8 mL
SUCCINYLCHOLINE		IV	2 mg/kg	58 mg	20 mg/mL	2.9 mL
SUCCINYLCHOLINE		IM	4 mg/kg	116 mg	20 mg/mL	5.8 mL
PROPOFOL		IV	3 mg/kg	87 mg	10 mg/mL	8.7 mL
ETOMIDATE	>10 y	IV	0.3 mg/kg	8.7 mg	2 mg/mL	4.35 mL
FENTANYL		IV	1 mcg/kg	29 mcg	50 mcg/mL	0.58 mL
FENTANYL		IN	2 mcg/kg	58 mcg	50 mcg/mL	1.16 mL
MORPHINE	<6 mo	IV/IM	0.05 mg/kg	1.45 mg	10 mg/mL	0.145 mL
MORPHINE	>6 mo	IV/IM	0.1 mg/kg	2.9 mg	10 mg/mL	0.29 mL
TORADOL	>2-16 y	IV	0.5 mg/kg	14.5 mg	30 mg/mL	0.483 mL
TORADOL	>2-16 y	IM	1 mg/kg	29 mg	30 mg/mL	0.967 mL
ACETAMINOPHEN		PR	20 mg/kg	580 mg		
ACETAMINOPHEN	2-12 y		15 mg/kg	435 mg	10 mg/mL	43.5 mL
CISATRACURIUM		IV	0.1 mg/kg	2.9 mg	2 mg/mL	1.45 mL
PANCURONIUM	<1 mo	IV	0.02 mg/kg	0.58 mg	1 mg/mL	0.58 mL
PANCURONIUM	>1 mo	IV	0.1 mg/kg	2.9 mg	1 mg/mL	2.9 mL
ROCURONIUM		IV	0.6 mg/kg	17.4 mg	10 mg/mL	1.74 mL
ROCURONIUM	RSI	IV	1.2 mg/kg	34.8 mg	10 mg/mL	3.48 mL
VECURONIUM		IV	0.1 mg/kg	2.9 mg	1 mg/mL	2.9 mL
GLYCOPYRROLATE	reversal	IV	0.007 mg/kg	0.203 mg	0.2 mg/mL	1.015 mL
NEOSTIGMINE		IV	0.07 mg/kg	2.03 mg	1 mg/mL	2.03 mL
DEXAMETHASONE		IV	0.25 mg/kg	7.25 mg	10 mg/mL	0.725 mL
ONDANSETRON		IV	0.15 mg/kg	4 mg	2 mg/mL	2 mL

additional pediatric drugs	route	dose	mg to pt	supplied	mL to give
PREMED/SEDATION, VAGOLYTIC/ANTISIALAGOGUE; GIVE IM 30–60 MIN PREOP					
ATROPINE	IM	0.02 mg/kg	0.5 mg	0.4 mg/mL	1.25 mL
GLYCOPYRROLATE	IM	0.004 mg/kg	0.009 mg	0.2 mg/mL	0.045 mL
MIDAZOLAM	IM	0.1 mg/kg	0.5 mg	1 mg/mL	0.5 mL
DEXMEDETOMIDINE load dose	IV	0.5 mcg/kg	1 mcg	4 mcg/mL	0.25 mL
INDUCTION					
KETAMINE	IV	2 mg/kg	55 mg	10 mg/mL	5.8 mL
KETAMINE	IM/PR	5 mg/kg	145 mg	10 mg/mL	14.5 mL
OPIOIDS/NONOPIOIDS					
FENTANYL	IV	4 mcg/kg	116 mcg	50 mcg/mL	2.32 mL
FENTANYL high dose	IV	10 mcg/kg	290 mcg	50 mcg/mL	5.8 mL
HYDROMORPHONE <6 mo	IV/SQ	0.005 mg/kg	0.145 mg	10 mg/mL	0.0145 mL
HYDROMORPHONE >6 mo	IV/SQ	0.015 mg/kg	0.435 mg	10 mg/mL	0.0435 mL
REMIFENTANIL	IV	0.5 mcg/kg	1 mcg	50 mcg/mL	0.02 mL
SUFENTANIL	IV	0.5 mcg/kg	14.5 mcg	50 mcg/mL	0.29 mL
REVERSALS					
ATROPINE	IV	0.02 mg/kg	0.5 mg	0.4 mg/mL	1.25 mL
EDROPHONIUM neonate	IV	0.1 mg single dose		10 mg/mL	0.01 mL
EDROPHONIUM >2 mo	IV	0.04 mg/kg	1.16 mg	10 mg/mL	0.116 mL
FLUMAZENIL >1 y	IV	0.01 mg/kg	0.2 mg	0.1 mg/mL	2 mL
NALOXONE <5 y; <20 kg	IV/IM	0.1 mg/kg	2 mg	0.4 mg/mL	5 mL
NALOXONE >5 y; >20 kg	IV/IM	2 mg per dose		0.4 mg/mL	5 mL
NALOXONE	ETT	0.3 mg/kg	8.7 mg	0.4 mg/mL	21.75 mL

additional pediatric drugs		route	dose	mg to pt	supplied	mL to give
ANTIBIOTICS						
AMPICILLIN	<6 y	IV	50 mg/kg	300 mg		
AMPICILLIN	>6 y	IV	50 mg/kg	1,450 mg		
AMPICILLIN & SULBACTUM	>1 mo	IV	50 mg/kg	1,450 mg		
CEFAZOLIN		IV	25 mg/kg	725 mg		
CLINDAMYCIN		IV	10 mg/kg	290 mg		
ERTAPENEM	3 mo-12 y	IV	15 mg/kg	435 mg		
ERTAPENEM	>12 y	IV	1 Gm	per dose		
GENTAMICIN		IV	2 mg/kg	58 mg		
LEVOFLOXACIN		IV	10 mg/kg	290 mg		
METRONIDAZOLE		IV	10 mg/kg	290 mg		
PIPERACILLIN & TAZOBACTAM	<40 kg & 2-9 mo	IV	80 mg/kg	2,320 mg		
PIPERACILLIN & TAZOBACTAM	<40 kg & >9 mo	IV	100 mg/kg	2,900 mg		
PIPERACILLIN & TAZOBACTAM	>40 kg	IV	3.375 Gm per dose			
VANCOMYCIN		IV	15 mg/kg	435 mg		
ANTINAUSEA						
METOCLOPROMIDE		IV	0.2 mg/kg	5.8 mg	5 mg/mL	1.16 mL
DIPHENHYDRAMINE		IV/IM	1.25 mg/kg	36.25 mg	50 mg/mL	0.725 mL
SCOPOLAMINE		IV/IM	6 mcg/kg	174 mcg	400 mcg/mL	0.435 mL
MISCELLANEOUS MEDS						
AMINOCAPROIC ACID		IV	100 mg/kg	2,900 mg	250 mg/mL	11.6 mL
DESMOPRESSIN		IV/SQ	0.3 mcg/kg	8.7 mcg	4 mcg/mL	2.175 mL
DEXAMETHASONE	croup	IV	0.6 mg/kg	16 mg	4 mg/mL	4 mL
HYDROCORTISONE		IV/IO	3 mg/kg	87 mg	100 mg/mL	0.87 mL

29 KG

1 year → 13 kg and up

Ventilation: trained rescuer:	1 breath q 6-8 sec (8-10 breaths/minute) about 1 second/breath-visible chest rise; if intubated, continuous compressions without pause for ventilations
Pulse check	carotid or femoral
Compression	heel of 1 hand or both hands one atop the other-lower half of sternum between nipples
Depth	2 inches (5 cm) or at least 1/3 chest depth
Rate	at least 100 compressions per minute
Compress/vent ratio	30:2 single rescuer 15:2 healthcare providers
Foreign body obstruction	Heimlich maneuver Never perform a blind finger-sweep. Open the mouth and look for object; if you see it, remove it.

sync cardioversion	0.5 J/kg	14.5 J
defibrillation	1 J/kg	29 J
repeat	2 J/kg	58 J
repeat	4 J/kg	116 J

IV Bolus Drugs		dose	mg to pt	supplied	mL to give
ADENOSINE	IV	0.1 mg/kg	2.9 mg	3 mg/mL	0.97 mL
ADENOSINE	repeat dose	0.2 mg/kg	5.8 mg	3 mg/mL	1.93 mL
AMIODARONE	IV/IO	5 mg/kg	145 mg	50 mg/mL	2.90 mL
ATROPINE	IV/IM	0.02 mg/kg	0.5 mg	0.4 mg/mL	1.25 mL
ATROPINE	ETT	0.04 mg/kg	1.16 mg	0.4 mg/mL	2.90 mL
CALCIUM CHLORIDE	IV	20 mg/kg	580 mg	100 mg/mL	5.80 mL
CALCIUM GLUCONATE	IV/IO	60 mg/kg	800 mg	100 mg/mL	8.00 mL
DANTROLENE	IV	2.5 mg/kg	30 mg		
EPHEDRINE	IV	0.15 mg/kg	4.35 mg	10 mg/mL	0.44 mL
EPINEPHRINE (1:10,000)	IV/IO	0.01 mg/kg	0.29 mg	0.1 mg/mL	2.90 mL
EPINEPHRINE (1:1,000)	ETT	0.1 mg/kg	2.5 mg	1 mg/mL	2.50 mL
ESMOLOL	IV	0.5 mg/kg	14.5 mg	10 mg/mL	1.45 mL
LABETALOL	IV	0.2 mg/kg	5.8 mg	5 mg/mL	1.16 mL
LIDOCAINE	IV/IO	1 mg/kg	29 mg	20 mg/mL	1.45 mL
NEOSYNEPHRINE	IV	5 mcg/kg	145 mcg	100 mcg/mL	1.45 mL
ROMAZICON	IV	0.01 mg/kg	0.2 mg	0.1 mg/mL	2.00 mL
VASOPRESSIN	IV/IO	0.4 unit/kg	11.6 units	20 u/mL	0.58 mL

30 KG MAINTENANCE IV FLUIDS: 70 ML/HR

common pediatric drugs		route	dose	mg to pt	supplied	mL to give
ATROPINE	vagolytic	IV	0.02 mg/kg	0.5 mg	0.4 mg/mL	1.25 mL
GLYCOPYRROLATE	vagolytic	IV	0.004 mg/kg	0.12 mg	0.2 mg/mL	0.6 mL
MIDAZOLAM		IV	0.05 mg/kg	0.6 mg	1 mg/mL	0.6 mL
MIDAZOLAM		PO	0.5 mg/kg	15 mg	1 mg/mL	15 mL
MIDAZOLAM		IN	0.2 mg/kg	6 mg	1 mg/mL	6 mL
SUCCINYLCHOLINE		IV	2 mg/kg	60 mg	20 mg/mL	3 mL
SUCCINYLCHOLINE		IM	4 mg/kg	120 mg	20 mg/mL	6 mL
PROPOFOL		IV	3 mg/kg	90 mg	10 mg/mL	9 mL
ETOMIDATE	>10 y	IV	0.3 mg/kg	9 mg	2 mg/mL	4.5 mL
FENTANYL		IV	1 mcg/kg	30 mcg	50 mcg/mL	0.6 mL
FENTANYL		IN	2 mcg/kg	60 mcg	50 mcg/mL	1.2 mL
MORPHINE	<6 mo	IV/IM	0.05 mg/kg	1.5 mg	10 mg/mL	0.15 mL
MORPHINE	>6 mo	IV/IM	0.1 mg/kg	3 mg	10 mg/mL	0.3 mL
TORADOL	>2-16 y	IV	0.5 mg/kg	15 mg	30 mg/mL	0.5 mL
TORADOL	>2-16 y	IM	1 mg/kg	30 mg	30 mg/mL	1 mL
ACETAMINOPHEN		PR	20 mg/kg	600 mg		
ACETAMINOPHEN	2-12 y	IV	15 mg/kg	450 mg	10 mg/mL	45 mL
CISATRACURIUM		IV	0.1 mg/kg	3 mg	2 mg/mL	1.5 mL
PANCURONIUM	<1 mo	IV	0.02 mg/kg	0.6 mg	1 mg/mL	0.6 mL
PANCURONIUM	>1 mo	IV	0.1 mg/kg	3 mg	1 mg/mL	3 mL
ROCURONIUM		IV	0.6 mg/kg	18 mg	10 mg/mL	1.8 mL
ROCURONIUM	RSI	IV	1.2 mg/kg	36 mg	10 mg/mL	3.6 mL
VECURONIUM		IV	0.1 mg/kg	3 mg	1 mg/mL	3 mL
GLYCOPYRROLATE	reversal	IV	0.007 mg/kg	0.21 mg	0.2 mg/mL	1.05 mL
NEOSTIGMINE		IV	0.07 mg/kg	2.1 mg	1 mg/mL	2.1 mL
DEXAMETHASONE		IV	0.25 mg/kg	7.5 mg	10 mg/mL	0.75 mL
ONDANSETRON		IV	0.15 mg/kg	4 mg	2 mg/mL	2 mL

additional pediatric drugs	route	dose	mg to pt	supplied	mL to give
PREMED/SEDATION, VAGOLYTIC/ANTISIALAGOGUE: GIVE IM 30-60 MIN PREOP					
ATROPINE	IM	0.02 mg/kg	0.5 mg	0.4 mg/mL	1.25 mL
GLYCOPYRROLATE	IM	0.004 mg/kg	0.009 mg	0.2 mg/mL	0.045 mL
MIDAZOLAM	IM	0.1 mg/kg	0.5 mg	1 mg/mL	0.5 mL
DEXMEDETOMIDINE load dose	IV	0.5 mcg/kg	1 mcg	4 mcg/mL	0.25 mL
INDUCTION					
KETAMINE	IV	2 mg/kg	60 mg	10 mg/mL	6 mL
KETAMINE	IM/PR	5 mg/kg	150 mg	10 mg/mL	15 mL
OPIOIDS/NONOPIOIDS					
FENTANYL	IV high dose	4 mcg/kg	120 mcg	50 mcg/mL	2.4 mL
FENTANYL	IV cardiac	10 mcg/kg	300 mcg	50 mcg/mL	6 mL
HYDROMORPHONE <6 mo	IV/SQ	0.005 mg/kg	0.15 mg	10 mg/mL	0.015 mL
HYDROMORPHONE >6 mo	IV/SQ	0.015 mg/kg	0.45 mg	10 mg/mL	0.045 mL
REMIFENTANIL	IV	0.5 mcg/kg	1 mcg	50 mcg/mL	0.02 mL
SUFENTANIL	IV	0.5 mcg/kg	15 mcg	50 mcg/mL	0.3 mL
REVERSALS					
ATROPINE	IV	0.02 mg/kg	0.5 mg	0.4 mg/mL	1.25 mL
EDROPHONIUM	IV neonate	0.1 mg single dose		10 mg/mL	0.01 mL
EDROPHONIUM	IV	0.04 mg/kg	1.2 mg	10 mg/mL	0.12 mL
FLUMAZENIL	IV <1 y	0.01 mg/kg	0.2 mg	0.1 mg/mL	2 mL
NALOXONE	IV/IM <5 y; <20 kg	0.1 mg/kg	2 mg	0.4 mg/mL	5 mL
NALOXONE	IV/IM >5 y; >20 kg	2 mg per dose		0.4 mg/mL	5 mL
NALOXONE	ETT	0.3 mg/kg	9 mg	0.4 mg/mL	22.5 mL

additional pediatric drugs		route	dose	mg to pt	supplied	mL to give
ANTIBIOTICS						
AMPICILLIN	<6 y	IV	50 mg/kg	300 mg		
AMPICILLIN	>6 y	IV	50 mg/kg	1,500 mg		
AMPICILLIN & SULBACTUM	>1 mo	IV	50 mg/kg	1,500 mg		
CEFAZOLIN		IV	25 mg/kg	750 mg		
CLINDAMYCIN		IV	10 mg/kg	300 mg		
ERTAPENEM	3 mo-12 y	IV	15 mg/kg	450 mg		
ERTAPENEM	>12 y	IV	1 Gm	per dose		
GENTAMICIN		IV	2 mg/kg	60 mg		
LEVOFLOXACIN		IV	10 mg/kg	300 mg		
METRONIDAZOLE		IV	10 mg/kg	300 mg		
PIPERACILLIN & TAZOBACTAM	<40 kg & 2-9 mo	IV	80 mg/kg	2,400 mg		
PIPERACILLIN & TAZOBACTAM	<40 kg & >9 mo	IV	100 mg/kg	3,000 mg		
PIPERACILLIN & TAZOBACTAM	>40 kg	IV	3.375 Gm per dose			
VANCOMYCIN		IV	15 mg/kg	450 mg		
ANTINAUSEA						
METOCLOPROMIDE		IV	0.2 mg/kg	6 mg	5 mg/mL	1.2 mL
DIPHENHYDRAMINE		IV/IM	1.25 mg/kg	37.5 mg	50 mg/mL	0.75 mL
SCOPOLAMINE		IV/IM	6 mcg/kg	180 mcg	400 mcg/mL	0.45 mL
MISCELLANEOUS MEDS						
AMINOCAPROIC ACID		IV	100 mg/kg	3,000 mg	250 mg/mL	12 mL
DESMOPRESSIN		IV/SQ	0.3 mcg/kg	9 mcg	4 mcg/mL	2.25 mL
DEXAMETHASONE	croup	IV	0.6 mg/kg	16 mg	4 mg/mL	4 mL
HYDROCORTISONE		IV/IO	3 mg/kg	90 mg	100 mg/mL	0.9 mL

30 KG

1 year → 13 kg and up

Ventilation: trained rescuer	1 breath q 6-8 sec (8-10 breaths/minute) about 1 second/ breath-visible chest rise; if intubated, continuous compressions without pause for ventilations
Pulse check	carotid or femoral
Compression	heel of 1 hand or both hands one atop the other-lower half of sternum between nipples
Depth	2 inches (5 cm) or at least 1/3 chest depth
Rate	at least 100 compressions per minute
Compress/vent ratio	30:2 single rescuer 15:2 2 healthcare providers
Foreign body obstruction	Heimlich maneuver Never perform a blind finger-sweep. Open the mouth and look for object; if you see it, remove it.

sync cardioversion	0.5 J/kg	15 J
	repeat	1 J/kg	30 J
defibrillation	2 J/kg	60 J
	repeat	4 J/kg	120 J

IV Bolus Drugs		dose	mg to pt	supplied	mL to give
ADENOSINE		0.1 mg/kg	3 mg	3 mg/mL	1.00 mL
ADENOSINE repeat dose		0.2 mg/kg	6 mg	3 mg/mL	2.00 mL
AMIODARONE	IV/IO	5 mg/kg	150 mg	50 mg/mL	3.00 mL
ATROPINE	IV/IM	0.02 mg/kg	0.5 mg	0.4 mg/mL	1.25 mL
ATROPINE	ETT	0.04 mg	1.2 mg	0.4 mg	3.00 mL
CALCIUM CHLORIDE	IV	20 mg/kg	600 mg	100 mg/mL	6.00 mL
CALCIUM GLUCONATE	IV/IO	60 mg/kg	800 mg	100 mg/mL	8.00 mL
DANTROLENE	IV	2.5 mg/kg	4.5 mg 30 mg	10 mg/mL	0.45 mL
EPHEDRINE	IV	0.15 mg/kg			
EPINEPHRINE (1:10,000)	IV/IO	0.01 mg/kg	0.3 mg	0.1 mg/mL	3.00 mL
EPINEPHRINE (1:1,000)	ETT	0.1 mg/kg	2.5 mg	1 mg/mL	2.50 mL
ESMOLOL	IV	0.5 mg/kg	15 mg	10 mg/mL	1.50 mL
LABETALOL	IV	0.2 mg/kg	6 mg	5 mg/mL	1.20 mL
LIDOCAINE	IV/IO	1 mg/kg	30 mg	100 mcg/mL	1.50 mL
NEOSYNEPHRINE	IV	5 mcg/kg	150 mcg	100 mcg/mL	1.50 mL
ROMAZICON	IV	0.01 mg/kg	0.2 mg	0.1 mg/mL	2.00 mL
VASOPRESSIN	IV/IO	0.4 unit/kg	12 units	20 u/mL	0.60 mL

31 KG MAINTENANCE IV FLUIDS: 71 ML/HR

common pediatric drugs		route	dose	mg to pt	supplied	mL to give
ATROPINE	vagolytic	IV	0.02 mg/kg	0.5 mg	0.4 mg/mL	1.25 mL
GLYCOPYRROLATE	vagolytic	IV	0.004 mg/kg	0.124 mg	0.2 mg/mL	0.62 mL
MIDAZOLAM		IV	0.05 mg/kg	0.6 mg	1 mg/mL	0.6 mL
MIDAZOLAM		PO	0.5 mg/kg	15.5 mg	1 mg/mL	15.5 mL
MIDAZOLAM		IN	0.2 mg/kg	6.2 mg	1 mg/mL	6.2 mL
SUCCINYLCHOLINE		IV	2 mg/kg	62 mg	20 mg/mL	3.1 mL
SUCCINYLCHOLINE		IM	4 mg/kg	124 mg	20 mg/mL	6.2 mL
PROPOFOL		IV	3 mg/kg	93 mg	10 mg/mL	9.3 mL
ETOMIDATE	>10 y	IV	0.3 mg/kg	9.3 mg	2 mg/mL	4.65 mL
FENTANYL		IV	1 mcg/kg	31 mcg	50 mcg/mL	0.62 mL
FENTANYL		IN	2 mcg/kg	62 mcg	50 mcg/mL	1.24 mL
MORPHINE	<6 mo	IV/IM	0.05 mg/kg	1.55 mg	10 mg/mL	0.155 mL
MORPHINE	>6 mo	IV/IM	0.1 mg/kg	3.1 mg	10 mg/mL	0.31 mL
TORADOL	>2-16 y	IV	0.5 mg/kg	15 mg	30 mg/mL	0.5 mL
TORADOL	>2-16 y	IM	1 mg/kg	30 mg	30 mg/mL	1 mL
ACETAMINOPHEN		PR	20 mg/kg	620 mg		
ACETAMINOPHEN	2-12 y	IV	15 mg/kg	465 mg	10 mg/mL	46.5 mL
CISATRACURIUM		IV	0.1 mg/kg	3.1 mg	2 mg/mL	1.55 mL
PANCURONIUM	<1 mo	IV	0.02 mg/kg	0.62 mg	1 mg/mL	0.62 mL
PANCURONIUM	>1 mo	IV	0.1 mg/kg	3.1 mg	1 mg/mL	3.1 mL
ROCURONIUM		IV	0.6 mg/kg	18.6 mg	10 mg/mL	1.86 mL
ROCURONIUM	RSI	IV	1.2 mg/kg	37.2 mg	10 mg/mL	3.72 mL
VECURONIUM		IV	0.1 mg/kg	3.1 mg	1 mg/mL	3.1 mL
GLYCOPYRROLATE	reversal	IV	0.007 mg/kg	0.217 mg	0.2 mg/mL	1.085 mL
NEOSTIGMINE		IV	0.07 mg/kg	2.17 mg	1 mg/mL	2.17 mL
DEXAMETHASONE		IV	0.25 mg/kg	7.75 mg	10 mg/mL	0.775 mL
ONDANSETRON		IV	0.15 mg/kg	4 mg	2 mg/mL	2 mL

additional pediatric drugs	route	dose		mg to pt	supplied	mL to give
PREMED/SEDATION; VAGOLYTIC/ANTISIALAGOGUE; GIVE IM 30-60 MIN PREOP						
ATROPINE	IM	0.02 mg/kg		0.5 mg	0.4 mg/mL	1.25 mL
GLYCOPYRROLATE	IM	0.004 mg/kg		0.009 mg	0.2 mg/mL	0.045 mL
MIDAZOLAM	IM	0.1 mg/kg		0.5	1 mg/mL	0.5 mL
DEXMEDETOMIDINE load dose	IV	0.5 mcg/kg		1 mcg	4 mcg/mL	0.25 mL
INDUCTION						
KETAMINE	IV	2 mg/kg		62 mg	10 mg/mL	6.2 mL
KETAMINE	IM/PR	5 mg/kg		155 mg	10 mg/mL	15.5 mL
OPIOIDS/NONOPIOIDS						
FENTANYL	IV	high dose	4 mcg/kg	124 mcg	50 mcg/mL	2.48 mL
FENTANYL	IV	cardiac	10 mcg/kg	310 mcg	50 mcg/mL	6.2 mL
HYDROMORPHONE	IV/SQ	< 6 mo	0.005 mg/kg	0.155 mg	10 mg/mL	0.0155 mL
HYDROMORPHONE	IV/SQ	> 6 mo	0.015 mg/kg	0.465 mg	10 mg/mL	0.0465 mL
REMIFENTANIL	IV	0.5 mcg/kg		1 mcg	50 mcg/mL	0.02 mL
SUFENTANIL	IV	0.5 mcg/kg		15.5 mcg	50 mcg/mL	0.31 mL
REVERSALS						
ATROPINE	IV	0.02 mg/kg		0.5 mg	0.4 mg/mL	1.25 mL
EDROPHONIUM	IV	neonate	0.1 mg single dose		10 mg/mL	0.01 mL
EDROPHONIUM	IV	> 2 mo	0.04 mg/kg	1.24 mg	10 mg/mL	0.124 mL
FLUMAZENIL	IV	< 1 y	0.01 mg/kg	0.2 mg	10 mg/mL	2 mL
NALOXONE	IM/IV	< 5 y; < 20 kg	0.1 mg/kg	2 mg	0.4 mg/mL	5 mL
NALOXONE	IM/IV	< 5 y; > 20 kg	2 mg per dose		0.4 mg/mL	5 mL
NALOXONE	ETT	0.3 mg/kg		9.3 mg	0.4 mg/mL	23.25 mL

additional pediatric drugs		route	dose	mg to pt	supplied	mL to give
ANTIBIOTICS						
AMPICILLIN	<6 y	IV	50 mg/kg	300 mg		
AMPICILLIN	>6 y	IV	50 mg/kg	1,550 mg		
AMPICILLIN & SULBACTUM	>1 mo	IV	50 mg/kg	1,550 mg		
CEFAZOLIN		IV	25 mg/kg	775 mg		
CLINDAMYCIN		IV	10 mg/kg	310 mg		
ERTAPENEM	3 mo–12 y	IV	15 mg/kg	465 mg		
ERTAPENEM	>12 y	IV	1 Gm	per dose		
GENTAMICIN		IV	2 mg/kg	62 mg		
LEVOFLOXACIN		IV	10 mg/kg	310 mg		
METRONIDAZOLE		IV	10 mg/kg	310 mg		
PIPERACILLIN & TAZOBACTAM	<40 kg & 2-9 mo	IV	80 mg/kg	2,480 mg		
PIPERACILLIN & TAZOBACTAM	<40 kg & >9 mo	IV	100 mg/kg	3,100 mg		
PIPERACILLIN & TAZOBACTAM	>40 kg	IV	3.375 Gm per dose			
VANCOMYCIN		IV	15 mg/kg	465 mg		
ANTINAUSEA						
METOCLOPROMIDE		IV	0.2 mg/kg	6.2 mg	5 mg/mL	1.24 mL
DIPHENHYDRAMINE		IV/IM	1.25 mg/kg	38.75 mg	50 mg/mL	0.775 mL
SCOPOLAMINE		IV/IM	6 mcg/kg	186 mcg	400 mcg/mL	0.465 mL
MISCELLANEOUS MEDS						
AMINOCAPROIC ACID		IV	100 mg/kg	3,100 mg	250 mg/mL	12.4 mL
DESMOPRESSIN		IV/SQ	0.3 mcg/kg	9.3 mcg	4 mcg/mL	2.325 mL
DEXAMETHASONE	croup	IV	0.6 mg/kg	16 mg	4 mg/mL	4 mL
HYDROCORTISONE		IV/IO	3 mg/kg	93 mg	100 mg/mL	0.93 mL

31 KG

1 year → 13 kg and up

Ventilation: trained rescuer	1 breath q 6-8 sec (8-10 breaths/minute) about 1 second/ breath-visible chest rise; if intubated, continuous compressions without pause for ventilations
Pulse check	carotid or femoral
Compression	heel of 1 hand or both hands one atop the other-lower half of sternum between nipples
Depth	2 inches (5 cm) or at least 1/3 chest depth
Rate	at least 100 compressions per minute
Compress/vent ratio	30:2 single rescuer / 15:2 2 healthcare providers
Foreign body obstruction	Heimlich maneuver / Never perform a blind finger-sweep. Open the mouth and look for object; if you see it, remove it.

sync cardioversion	0.5 J/kg	15.5 J
defibrillation repeat	1 J/kg	31 J
	2 J/kg	62 J
repeat	4 J/kg	124 J

IV Bolus Drugs		dose	mg to pt	supplied	mL to give
ADENOSINE	IV	0.1 mg/kg	3.1 mg	3 mg/mL	1.03 mL
ADENOSINE repeat dose	IV	0.2 mg/kg	6.2 mg	3 mg/mL	2.07 mL
AMIODARONE	IV/IO	5 mg/kg	155 mg	50 mg/mL	3.10 mL
ATROPINE	IV/IM	0.02 mg/kg	0.5 mg	0.4 mg/mL	1.25 mL
ATROPINE	ETT	0.04 mg/kg	1.24 mg	0.4 mg/mL	3.10 mL
CALCIUM CHLORIDE	IV	20 mg/kg	620 mg	100 mg/mL	6.20 mL
CALCIUM GLUCONATE	IV/IO	60 mg/kg	800 mg	100 mg/mL	8.00 mL
DANTROLENE	IV	2.5 mg/kg	30 mg		
EPHEDRINE	IV	0.15 mg/kg	4.65 mg	10 mg/mL	0.47 mL
EPINEPHRINE (1:10,000)	IV/IO	0.01 mg/kg	0.31 mg	0.1 mg/mL	3.10 mL
EPINEPHRINE (1:1,000)	ETT	0.1 mg/kg	2.5 mg	1 mg/mL	2.50 mL
ESMOLOL	IV	0.5 mg/kg	15.5 mg	10 mg/mL	1.55 mL
LABETALOL	IV	0.2 mg/kg	6.2 mg	5 mg/mL	1.24 mL
LIDOCAINE	IV/IO	1 mg/kg	31 mg	20 mg/mL	1.55 mL
NEOSYNEPHRINE	IV	5 mcg/kg	155 mcg	100 mcg/mL	1.55 mL
ROMAZICON	IV	0.01 mg/kg	0.2 mg	0.1 mg/mL	2.00 mL
VASOPRESSIN	IV/IO	0.4 unit/kg	12.4 units	20 u/mL	0.62 mL

32 KG MAINTENANCE IV FLUIDS: 72 ML/HR

common pediatric drugs		route	dose	mg to pt	supplied	mL to give
ATROPINE	vagolytic	IV	0.02 mg/kg	0.5 mg	0.4 mg/mL	1.25 mL
GLYCOPYRROLATE	vagolytic	IV	0.004 mg/kg	0.128 mg	0.2 mg/mL	0.64 mL
MIDAZOLAM		IV	0.05 mg/kg	0.6 mg	1 mg/mL	0.6 mL
MIDAZOLAM		PO	0.5 mg/kg	16 mg	1 mg/mL	16 mL
MIDAZOLAM		IN	0.2 mg/kg	6.4 mg	1 mg/mL	6.4 mL
SUCCINYLCHOLINE		IV	2 mg/kg	64 mg	20 mg/mL	3.2 mL
SUCCINYLCHOLINE		IM	4 mg/kg	128 mg	20 mg/mL	6.4 mL
PROPOFOL		IV	3 mg/kg	96 mg	10 mg/mL	9.6 mL
ETOMIDATE	>10 y	IV	0.3 mg/kg	9.6 mg	2 mg/mL	4.8 mL
FENTANYL		IV	1 mcg/kg	32 mcg	50 mcg/mL	0.64 mL
FENTANYL		IN	2 mcg/kg	64 mcg	50 mcg/mL	1.28 mL
MORPHINE	<6 mo	IV/IM	0.05 mg/kg	1.6 mg	10 mg/mL	0.16 mL
MORPHINE	>6 mo	IV/IM	0.1 mg/kg	3.2 mg	10 mg/mL	0.32 mL
TORADOL	>2-16 y	IV	0.5 mg/kg	15 mg	30 mg/mL	0.5 mL
TORADOL	>2-16 y	IM	1 mg/kg	30 mg	30 mg/mL	1 mL
ACETAMINOPHEN		PR	20 mg/kg	640 mg		
ACETAMINOPHEN	2-12 y	IV	15 mg/kg	480 mg	10 mg/mL	48 mL
CISATRACURIUM		IV	0.1 mg/kg	3.2 mg	2 mg/mL	1.6 mL
PANCURONIUM	<1 mo	IV	0.02 mg/kg	0.64 mg	1 mg/mL	0.64 mL
PANCURONIUM	>1 mo	IV	0.1 mg/kg	3.2 mg	1 mg/mL	3.2 mL
ROCURONIUM		IV	0.6 mg/kg	19.2 mg	10 mg/mL	1.92 mL
ROCURONIUM	RSI	IV	1.2 mg/kg	38.4 mg	10 mg/mL	3.84 mL
VECURONIUM		IV	0.1 mg/kg	3.2 mg	1 mg/mL	3.2 mL
GLYCOPYRROLATE	reversal	IV	0.007 mg/kg	0.224 mg	0.2 mg/mL	1.12 mL
NEOSTIGMINE		IV	0.07 mg/kg	2.24 mg	1 mg/mL	2.24 mL
DEXAMETHASONE		IV	0.25 mg/kg	8 mg	10 mg/mL	0.8 mL
ONDANSETRON		IV	0.15 mg/kg	4 mg	2 mg/mL	2 mL

additional pediatric drugs	route	dose	mg to pt	supplied	mL to give
PREMED/SEDATION; VAGOLYTIC/ANTISIALAGOGUE; GIVE IM 30-60 MIN PREOP					
ATROPINE	IM	0.02 mg/kg	0.5 mg	0.4 mg/mL	1.25 mL
GLYCOPYRROLATE	IM	0.004 mg/kg	0.009 mg	0.2 mg/mL	0.045 mL
MIDAZOLAM	IM	0.1 mg/kg	0.5 mg	1 mg/mL	0.5 mL
DEXMEDETOMIDINE	IV	load dose 0.5 mcg/kg	1 mcg	4 mcg/mL	0.25 mL
INDUCTION					
KETAMINE	IV	2 mg/kg	64 mg	10 mg/mL	6.4 mL
KETAMINE	IM/PR	5 mg/kg	160 mg	10 mg/mL	16 mL
OPIOIDS/NONOPIOIDS					
FENTANYL	IV	high dose 4 mcg/kg	128 mcg	50 mcg/mL	2.56 mL
FENTANYL	IV	cardiac 10 mcg/kg	320 mcg	50 mcg/mL	6.4 mL
HYDROMORPHONE < 6 mo	IV/SQ	0.005 mg/kg	0.16 mg	10 mg/mL	0.016 mL
HYDROMORPHONE > 6 mo	IV/SQ	0.015 mg/kg	0.48 mg	10 mg/mL	0.048 mL
REMIFENTANIL	IV	0.5 mcg/kg	1 mcg	50 mcg/mL	0.02 mL
SUFENTANIL	IV	0.5 mcg/kg	16 mcg	50 mcg/mL	0.32 mL
REVERSALS					
ATROPINE	IV	0.02 mg/kg	0.5 mg	0.4 mg/mL	1.25 mL
EDROPHONIUM neonate	IV	0.1 mg single dose		10 mg/mL	0.01 mL
EDROPHONIUM > 2 mo	IV	0.04 mg/kg	1.28 mg	10 mg/mL	0.128 mL
FLUMAZENIL > 1 y	IV	0.01 mg/kg	0.2 mg	0.1 mg/mL	2 mL
NALOXONE < 5 y; < 20 kg	IM	0.1 mg/kg	2 mg	0.4 mg/mL	5 mL
NALOXONE > 5 y; > 20 kg	IM	2 mg per dose		0.4 mg/mL	5 mL
NALOXONE	ETT	0.3 mg/kg	9.6 mg	0.4 mg/mL	24 mL

additional pediatric drugs		route	dose	mg to pt	supplied	mL to give
ANTIBIOTICS						
AMPICILLIN	<6 y	IV	50 mg/kg	300 mg		
AMPICILLIN	>6 y	IV	50 mg/kg	1,600 mg		
AMPICILLIN & SULBACTUM	>1 mo	IV	50 mg/kg	1,600 mg		
CEFAZOLIN		IV	25 mg/kg	800 mg		
CLINDAMYCIN		IV	10 mg/kg	320 mg		
ERTAPENEM	3 mo-12 y	IV	15 mg/kg	480 mg		
ERTAPENEM	>12 y	IV	1 Gm	per dose		
GENTAMICIN		IV	2 mg/kg	64 mg		
LEVOFLOXACIN		IV	10 mg/kg	320 mg		
METRONIDAZOLE		IV	10 mg/kg	320 mg		
PIPERACILLIN & TAZOBACTAM	<40 kg & 2-9 mo	IV	80 mg/kg	2,560 mg		
PIPERACILLIN & TAZOBACTAM	<40 kg & >9 mo	IV	100 mg/kg	3,200 mg		
PIPERACILLIN & TAZOBACTAM	>40 kg	IV	3.375 Gm per dose			
VANCOMYCIN		IV	15 mg/kg	480 mg		
ANTINAUSEA						
METOCLOPROMIDE		IV	0.2 mg/kg	6.4 mg	5 mg/mL	1.28 mL
DIPHENHYDRAMINE		IV/IM	1.25 mg/kg	40 mg	50 mg/mL	0.8 mL
SCOPOLAMINE		IV/IM	6 mcg/kg	192 mcg	400 mcg/mL	0.48 mL
MISCELLANEOUS MEDS						
AMINOCAPROIC ACID		IV	100 mg/kg	3,200 mg	250 mg/mL	12.8 mL
DESMOPRESSIN		IV/SQ	0.3 mcg/kg	9.6 mcg	4 mcg/mL	2.4 mL
DEXAMETHASONE	croup	IV	0.6 mg/kg	16 mg	4 mg/mL	4 mL
HYDROCORTISONE		IV/IO	3 mg/kg	96 mg	100 mg/mL	0.96 mL

32 KG

1 year ← 13 kg and up

Ventilation: trained rescuer	1 breath q 6-8 sec (8-10 breaths/minute) about 1 second/ breath-visible chest rise; if intubated, continuous compressions without pause for ventilations
Pulse check	carotid or femoral
Compression	heel of 1 hand or both hands one atop the other—lower half of sternum between nipples
Depth	2 inches (5 cm) or at least 1/3 chest depth
Rate	at least 100 compressions per minute
Compress/vent ratio	30:2 single rescuer 15:2 2 healthcare providers
Foreign body obstruction	Heimlich maneuver Never perform a blind finger-sweep. Open the mouth and look for object; if you see it, remove it.

sync cardioversion	0.5 J/kg	16 J	
defibrillation	1 J/kg	32 J	repeat
repeat	2 J/kg	64 J	
repeat	4 J/kg	128 J	

IV Bolus Drugs		dose	mg to pt	supplied	mL to give
ADENOSINE	IV	0.1 mg/kg	3.2 mg	3 mg/mL	1.07 mL
ADENOSINE repeat dose	IV	0.2 mg/kg	6.4 mg	3 mg/mL	2.13 mL
AMIODARONE	IV/IO	5 mg/kg	160 mg	50 mg/mL	3.20 mL
ATROPINE	IM/IV	0.02 mg/kg	0.5 mg	0.4 mg/mL	1.25 mL
ATROPINE	ETT	0.04 mg/kg	1.28 mg	0.4 mg/mL	3.20 mL
CALCIUM CHLORIDE	IV	20 mg/kg	640 mg	100 mg/mL	6.40 mL
CALCIUM GLUCONATE	IV/IO	60 mg/kg	800 mg	100 mg/mL	8.00 mL
DANTROLENE	IV	2.5 mg/kg	30 mg		
EPHEDRINE	IV	0.15 mg/kg	4.8 mg	10 mg/mL	0.48 mL
EPINEPHRINE (1:10,000)	IV/IO	0.01 mg/kg	0.32 mg	0.1 mg/mL	3.20 mL
EPINEPHRINE (1:1,000)	ETT	0.1 mg/kg	2.5 mg	1 mg/mL	2.50 mL
ESMOLOL	IV	0.5 mg/kg	16 mg	10 mg/mL	1.60 mL
LABETALOL	IV	0.2 mg/kg	6.4 mg	5 mg/mL	1.28 mL
LIDOCAINE	IV/IO	1 mg/kg	32 mg	20 mg/mL	1.60 mL
NEOSYNEPHRINE	IV	5 mcg/kg	160 mcg	100 mcg/mL	1.60 mL
ROMAZICON	IV	0.01 mg/kg	0.2 mg	0.1 mg/mL	2.00 mL
VASOPRESSIN	IV/IO	0.4 unit/kg	12.8 units	20 u/mL	0.64 mL

33 KG MAINTENANCE IV FLUIDS: 73 ML/HR

common pediatric drugs		route	dose	mg to pt	supplied	mL to give
ATROPINE	vagolytic	IV	0.02 mg/kg	0.5 mg	0.4 mg/mL	1.25 mL
GLYCOPYRROLATE	vagolytic	IV	0.004 mg/kg	0.132 mg	0.2 mg/mL	0.66 mL
MIDAZOLAM		IV	0.05 mg/kg	0.6 mg	1 mg/mL	0.6 mL
MIDAZOLAM		PO	0.5 mg/kg	16.5 mg	1 mg/mL	16.5 mL
MIDAZOLAM		IN	0.2 mg/kg	6.6 mg	1 mg/mL	6.6 mL
SUCCINYLCHOLINE		IV	2 mg/kg	66 mg	20 mg/mL	3.3 mL
SUCCINYLCHOLINE		IM	4 mg/kg	132 mg	20 mg/mL	6.6 mL
PROPOFOL		IV	3 mg/kg	99 mg	10 mg/mL	9.9 mL
ETOMIDATE	>10 y	IV	0.3 mg/kg	9.9 mg	2 mg/mL	4.95 mL
FENTANYL		IV	1 mcg/kg	33 mcg	50 mcg/mL	0.66 mL
FENTANYL		IN	2 mcg/kg	66 mcg	50 mcg/mL	1.32 mL
MORPHINE	<6 mo	IV/IM	0.05 mg/kg	1.65 mg	10 mg/mL	0.165 mL
MORPHINE	>6 mo	IV/IM	0.1 mg/kg	3.3 mg	10 mg/mL	0.33 mL
TORADOL	>2-16 y	IV	0.5 mg/kg	15 mg	30 mg/mL	0.5 mL
TORADOL	>2-16 y	IM	1 mg/kg	30 mg	30 mg/mL	1 mL
ACETAMINOPHEN		PR	20 mg/kg	660 mg		
ACETAMINOPHEN	2-12 y	IV	15 mg/kg	495 mg	10 mg/mL	49.5 mL
CISATRACURIUM		IV	0.1 mg/kg	3.3 mg	2 mg/mL	1.65 mL
PANCURONIUM	<1 mo	IV	0.02 mg/kg	0.66 mg	1 mg/mL	0.66 mL
PANCURONIUM	>1 mo	IV	0.1 mg/kg	3.3 mg	1 mg/mL	3.3 mL
ROCURONIUM		IV	0.6 mg/kg	19.8 mg	10 mg/mL	1.98 mL
ROCURONIUM	RSI	IV	1.2 mg/kg	39.6 mg	10 mg/mL	3.96 mL
VECURONIUM		IV	0.1 mg/kg	3.3 mg	1 mg/mL	3.3 mL
GLYCOPYRROLATE	reversal	IV	0.007 mg/kg	0.231 mg	0.2 mg/mL	1.155 mL
NEOSTIGMINE		IV	0.07 mg/kg	2.31 mg	1 mg/mL	2.31 mL
DEXAMETHASONE		IV	0.25 mg/kg	8.25 mg	10 mg/mL	0.825 mL
ONDANSETRON		IV	0.15 mg/kg	4 mg	2 mg/mL	2 mL

additional pediatric drugs	route	dose	mg to pt	supplied	mL to give
PREMED/SEDATION; VAGOLYTIC/ANTISIALAGOGUE; GIVE IM 30-60 MIN PREOP					
ATROPINE	IM	0.02 mg/kg	0.5 mg	0.4 mg/mL	1.25 mL
GLYCOPYRROLATE	IM	0.004 mg/kg	0.009 mg	0.2 mg/mL	0.045 mL
MIDAZOLAM	IM	0.1 mg/kg	0.5 mg	1 mg/mL	0.5 mL
DEXMEDETOMIDINE load dose	IV	0.5 mcg/kg	1 mcg	4 mcg/mL	0.25 mL
INDUCTION					
KETAMINE	IV	2 mg/kg	66 mg	10 mg/mL	6.6 mL
KETAMINE	IM/PR	5 mg/kg	165 mg	10 mg/mL	16.5 mL
OPIOIDS/NONOPIOIDS					
FENTANYL	high dose	IV	4 mcg/kg	132 mcg	50 mcg/mL	2.64 mL
FENTANYL	cardiac	IV	10 mcg/kg	330 mcg	50 mcg/mL	6.6 mL
HYDROMORPHONE	< 6 mo	IV/SQ	0.005 mg/kg	0.165 mg	10 mg/mL	0.0165 mL
HYDROMORPHONE	> 6 mo	IV/SQ	0.015 mg/kg	0.495 mg	10 mg/mL	0.0495 mL
SUFENTANIL	IV	0.5 mcg/kg	1 mcg	50 mcg/mL	0.02 mL
SUFENTANIL	IV	0.5 mcg/kg	16.5 mcg	50 mcg/mL	0.33 mL
REVERSALS					
ATROPINE	IV	0.02 mg/kg	0.5 mg	0.4 mg/mL	1.25 mL
EDROPHONIUM	neonate	IV	0.1 mg single dose		10 mg/mL	0.01 mL
EDROPHONIUM	> 2 mo	IV	0.04 mg/kg	1.32 mg	10 mg/mL	0.132 mL
FLUMAZENIL	> 1 y	IV	0.01 mg/kg	0.2 mg	0.1 mg/mL	2 mL
NALOXONE	< 5 y; < 20 kg	IM/IV	0.1 mg/kg	2 mg	0.4 mg/mL	5 mL
NALOXONE	< 5 y; > 20 kg	IM	2 mg per dose		0.4 mg/mL	5 mL
NALOXONE	ETT	0.3 mg/kg	9.9 mg	0.4 mg/mL	24.75 mL

additional pediatric drugs		route	dose	mg to pt	supplied	mL to give
ANTIBIOTICS						
AMPICILLIN	<6 y	IV	50 mg/kg	300 mg		
AMPICILLIN	>6 y	IV	50 mg/kg	1,650 mg		
AMPICILLIN & SULBACTUM	>1 mo	IV	50 mg/kg	1,650 mg		
CEFAZOLIN		IV	25 mg/kg	825 mg		
CLINDAMYCIN		IV	10 mg/kg	330 mg		
ERTAPENEM	3 mo–12 y	IV	15 mg/kg	495 mg		
ERTAPENEM	>12 y	IV	1 Gm	per dose		
GENTAMICIN		IV	2 mg/kg	66 mg		
LEVOFLOXACIN		IV	10 mg/kg	330 mg		
METRONIDAZOLE		IV	10 mg/kg	330 mg		
PIPERACILLIN & TAZOBACTAM	<40 kg & 2-9 mo	IV	80 mg/kg	2,640 mg		
PIPERACILLIN & TAZOBACTAM	<40 kg & >9 mo	IV	100 mg/kg	3,300 mg		
PIPERACILLIN & TAZOBACTAM	>40 kg	IV	3.375 Gm per dose			
VANCOMYCIN		IV	15 mg/kg	495 mg		
ANTINAUSEA						
METOCLOPROMIDE		IV	0.2 mg/kg	6.6 mg	5 mg/mL	1.32 mL
DIPHENHYDRAMINE		IV/IM	1.25 mg/kg	41.25 mg	50 mg/mL	0.825 mL
SCOPOLAMINE		IV/IM	6 mcg/kg	198 mcg	400 mcg/mL	0.495 mL
MISCELLANEOUS MEDS						
AMINOCAPROIC ACID		IV	100 mg/kg	3,300 mg	250 mg/mL	13.2 mL
DESMOPRESSIN		IV/SQ	0.3 mcg/kg	9.9 mcg	4 mcg/mL	2.475 mL
DEXAMETHASONE	croup	IV	0.6 mg/kg	16 mg	4 mg/mL	4 mL
HYDROCORTISONE		IV/IO	3 mg/kg	99 mg	100 mg/mL	0.99 mL

33 KG

1 year ← 13 kg and up

Ventilation: trained rescuer	1 breath q 6-8 sec (8-10 breaths/minute) about 1 second/breath-visible chest rise; if intubated, continuous compressions without pause for ventilations
Pulse check	carotid or femoral
Compression	heel of 1 hand or both hands one atop the other-lower half of sternum between nipples
Depth	2 inches (5 cm) or at least 1/3 chest depth
Rate	at least 100 compressions per minute
Compress/vent ratio	30:2 single rescuer; 15:2 2 healthcare providers
Foreign body obstruction	Heimlich maneuver; Never perform a blind finger-sweep. Open the mouth and look for object; if you see it, remove it.

sync cardioversion	0.5 J/kg	16.5 J
defibrillation	1 J/kg	33 J
repeat	2 J/kg	66 J
repeat	4 J/kg	132 J

IV Bolus Drugs		dose	mg to pt	supplied	mL to give
ADENOSINE	IV	0.1 mg/kg	3.3 mg	3 mg/mL	1.10 mL
ADENOSINE repeat dose	IV	0.2 mg/kg	6.6 mg	3 mg/mL	2.20 mL
AMIODARONE	IV/IO	5 mg/kg	165 mg	50 mg/mL	3.30 mL
ATROPINE	IM/IV	0.02 mg/kg	0.5 mg	0.4 mg/mL	1.25 mL
ATROPINE	ETT	0.04 mg/kg	1.32 mg	0.4 mg/mL	3.30 mL
CALCIUM CHLORIDE	IV	20 mg/kg	660 mg	100 mg/mL	6.60 mL
CALCIUM GLUCONATE	IV/IO	60 mg/kg	800 mg	100 mg/mL	8.00 mL
DANTROLENE		2.5 mg/kg	30 mg		
EPHEDRINE	IV	0.15 mg/kg	4.95 mg	10 mg/mL	0.50 mL
EPINEPHRINE (1:10,000)	IV/IO	0.01 mg/kg	0.33 mg	0.1 mg/mL	3.30 mL
EPINEPHRINE (1:1,000)	ETT	0.1 mg/kg	2.5 mg	1 mg/mL	2.50 mL
ESMOLOL	IV	0.5 mg/kg	16.5 mg	10 mg/mL	1.65 mL
LABETALOL	IV	0.2 mg/kg	6.6 mg	5 mg/mL	1.32 mL
LIDOCAINE	IV/IO	1 mg/kg	33 mg	20 mg/mL	1.65 mL
NEOSYNEPHRINE	IV	5 mcg/kg	165 mcg	100 mcg/mL	1.65 mL
ROMAZICON	IV	0.01 mg/kg	0.2 mg	0.1 mg/mL	2.00 mL
VASOPRESSIN	IV/IO	0.4 unit/kg	13.2 units	20 u/mL	0.66 mL

34 KG MAINTENANCE IV FLUIDS: 74 ML/HR

common pediatric drugs		route	dose	mg to pt	supplied	mL to give
ATROPINE	vagolytic	IV	0.02 mg/kg	0.5 mg	0.4 mg/mL	1.25 mL
GLYCOPYRROLATE	vagolytic	IV	0.004 mg/kg	0.136 mg	0.2 mg/mL	0.68 mL
MIDAZOLAM		IV	0.05 mg/kg	0.6 mg	1 mg/mL	0.6 mL
MIDAZOLAM		PO	0.5 mg/kg	17 mg	1 mg/mL	17 mL
MIDAZOLAM		IN	0.2 mg/kg	6.8 mg	1 mg/mL	6.8 mL
SUCCINYLCHOLINE		IV	2 mg/kg	68 mg	20 mg/mL	3.4 mL
SUCCINYLCHOLINE		IM	4 mg/kg	136 mg	20 mg/mL	6.8 mL
PROPOFOL		IV	3 mg/kg	102 mg	10 mg/mL	10.2 mL
ETOMIDATE	>10 y	IV	0.3 mg/kg	10.2 mg	2 mg/mL	5.1 mL
FENTANYL		IV	1 mcg/kg	34 mcg	50 mcg/mL	0.68 mL
FENTANYL		IN	2 mcg/kg	68 mcg	50 mcg/mL	1.36 mL
MORPHINE	<6 mo	IV/IM	0.05 mg/kg	1.7 mg	10 mg/mL	0.17 mL
MORPHINE	>6 mo	IV/IM	0.1 mg/kg	3.4 mg	10 mg/mL	0.34 mL
TORADOL	>2-16 y	IV	0.5 mg/kg	15 mg	30 mg/mL	0.5 mL
TORADOL	>2-16 y	IM	1 mg/kg	30 mg	30 mg/mL	1 mL
ACETAMINOPHEN		PR	20 mg/kg	680 mg		
ACETAMINOPHEN	2-12 y	IV	15 mg/kg	510 mg	10 mg/mL	51 mL
CISATRACURIUM		IV	0.1 mg/kg	3.4 mg	2 mg/mL	1.7 mL
PANCURONIUM	<1 mo	IV	0.02 mg/kg	0.68 mg	1 mg/mL	0.68 mL
PANCURONIUM	>1 mo	IV	0.1 mg/kg	3.4 mg	1 mg/mL	3.4 mL
ROCURONIUM		IV	0.6 mg/kg	20.4 mg	10 mg/mL	2.04 mL
ROCURONIUM	RSI	IV	1.2 mg/kg	40.8 mg	10 mg/mL	4.08 mL
VECURONIUM		IV	0.1 mg/kg	3.4 mg	1 mg/mL	3.4 mL
GLYCOPYRROLATE	reversal	IV	0.007 mg/kg	0.238 mg	0.2 mg/mL	1.19 mL
NEOSTIGMINE		IV	0.07 mg/kg	2.38 mg	1 mg/mL	2.38 mL
DEXAMETHASONE		IV	0.25 mg/kg	8.5 mg	10 mg/mL	0.85 mL
ONDANSETRON		IV	0.15 mg/kg	4 mg	2 mg/mL	2 mL

additional pediatric drugs	route	dose	mg to pt	supplied	mL to give
PREMED/SEDATION; VAGOLYTIC/ANTISIALAGOGUE; GIVE IM 30–60 MIN PREOP					
ATROPINE	IM	0.02 mg/kg	0.5 mg	0.4 mg/mL	1.25 mL
GLYCOPYRROLATE	IM	0.004 mg/kg	0.009 mg	0.2 mg/mL	0.045 mL
MIDAZOLAM	IM	0.1 mg/kg	0.5 mg	1 mg/mL	0.5 mL
DEXMEDETOMIDINE load dose	IV	0.5 mcg/kg	1 mcg	4 mcg/mL	0.25 mL
INDUCTION					
KETAMINE	IV	2 mg/kg	68 mg	10 mg/mL	6.8 mL
KETAMINE	IM/PR	5 mg/kg	170 mg	10 mg/mL	17 mL
OPIOIDS/NONOPIOIDS					
FENTANYL high dose	IV	4 mcg/kg	136 mcg	50 mcg/mL	2.72 mL
FENTANYL cardiac	IV	10 mcg/kg	340 mcg	50 mcg/mL	6.8 mL
HYDROMORPHONE <6 mo	IV/SQ	0.005 mg/kg	0.17 mg	10 mg/mL	0.017 mL
HYDROMORPHONE >6 mo	IV/SQ	0.015 mg/kg	0.51 mg	10 mg/mL	0.051 mL
REMIFENTANIL	IV	0.5 mcg/kg	1 mcg	50 mcg/mL	0.02 mL
SUFENTANIL	IV	0.5 mcg/kg	17 mcg	50 mcg/mL	0.34 mL
REVERSALS					
ATROPINE	IV	0.02 mg/kg	0.5 mg	0.4 mg/mL	1.25 mL
EDROPHONIUM	IV	neonate	0.1 mg single dose	10 mg/mL	0.01 mL
EDROPHONIUM	IV	0.04 mg/kg	1.36 mg	10 mg/mL	0.136 mL
FLUMAZENIL	IV	>1 y	0.1 mg	0.2 mg	0.1 mg/mL / 2 mL
NALOXONE <5 y; <20 kg	IM	0.1 mg/kg	2 mg	0.4 mg/mL	5 mL
NALOXONE >5 y; >20 kg	IV/IM	2 mg per dose		0.4 mg/mL	5 mL
NALOXONE	ETT	0.3 mg/kg	10.2 mg	0.4 mg/mL	25.5 mL

additional pediatric drugs		route	dose	mg to pt	supplied	mL to give
ANTIBIOTICS						
AMPICILLIN	<6 y	IV	50 mg/kg	300 mg		
AMPICILLIN	>6 y	IV	50 mg/kg	1,700 mg		
AMPICILLIN & SULBACTUM	>1 mo	IV	50 mg/kg	1,700 mg		
CEFAZOLIN		IV	25 mg/kg	850 mg		
CLINDAMYCIN		IV	10 mg/kg	340 mg		
ERTAPENEM	3 mo-12 y	IV	15 mg/kg	510 mg		
ERTAPENEM	>12 y	IV	1 Gm	per dose		
GENTAMICIN		IV	2 mg/kg	68 mg		
LEVOFLOXACIN		IV	10 mg/kg	340 mg		
METRONIDAZOLE		IV	10 mg/kg	340 mg		
PIPERACILLIN & TAZOBACTAM	<40 kg & 2-9 mo	IV	80 mg/kg	2,720 mg		
PIPERACILLIN & TAZOBACTAM	<40 kg & >9 mo	IV	100 mg/kg	3,375 mg		
PIPERACILLIN & TAZOBACTAM	>40 kg	IV	3.375 Gm per dose			
VANCOMYCIN		IV	15 mg/kg	510 mg		
ANTINAUSEA						
METOCLOPROMIDE		IV	0.2 mg/kg	6.8 mg	5 mg/mL	1.36 mL
DIPHENHYDRAMINE		IV/IM	1.25 mg/kg	42.5 mg	50 mg/mL	0.85 mL
SCOPOLAMINE		IV/IM	6 mcg/kg	204 mcg	400 mcg/mL	0.51 mL
MISCELLANEOUS MEDS						
AMINOCAPROIC ACID		IV	100 mg/kg	3,400 mg	250 mg/mL	13.6 mL
DESMOPRESSIN		IV/SQ	0.3 mcg/kg	10.2 mcg	4 mcg/mL	2.55 mL
DEXAMETHASONE	croup	IV	0.6 mg/kg	16 mg	4 mg/mL	4 mL
HYDROCORTISONE		IV/IO	3 mg/kg	100 mg	100 mg/mL	1 mL

34 KG

1 year ← 13 kg and up

Ventilation: trained rescuer	1 breath q 6-8 sec (8-10 breaths/minute) about 1 second/ breath-visible chest rise; if intubated, continuous compressions without pause for ventilations
Pulse check	carotid or femoral
Compression	heel of 1 hand or both hands one atop the other-lower half of sternum between nipples
Depth	2 inches (5 cm) or at least 1/3 chest depth
Rate	at least 100 compressions per minute
Compress/vent ratio	30:2 single rescuer 15:2 2 healthcare providers
Foreign body obstruction	Heimlich maneuver Never perform a blind finger-sweep. Open the mouth and look for object; if you see it, remove it.

sync cardioversion	0.5 J/kg	17 J	
defibrillation	1 J/kg	34 J	repeat
	2 J/kg	68 J	repeat
	4 J/kg	136 J	

IV Bolus Drugs	dose	mg to pt	supplied	mL to give
ADENOSINE	0.1 mg/kg	3.4 mg	3 mg/mL	1.13 mL
ADENOSINE repeat dose	0.2 mg/kg	6.8 mg	3 mg/mL	2.27 mL
AMIODARONE	5 mg/kg	170 mg	50 mg/mL	3.40 mL
ATROPINE	0.02 mg/kg	0.5 mg	0.4 mg/mL	1.25 mL
ATROPINE	0.04 mg/kg	1.36 mg	0.4 mg/mL	3.40 mL
CALCIUM CHLORIDE	20 mg/kg	680 mg	100 mg/mL	6.80 mL
CALCIUM GLUCONATE	60 mg/kg	800 mg	100 mg/mL	8.00 mL
DANTROLENE	2.5 mg/kg	30 mg		
EPHEDRINE	0.15 mg/kg	5.1 mg	10 mg/mL	0.51 mL
EPINEPHRINE (1:10,000)	0.01 mg/kg	0.34 mg	0.1 mg/mL	3.40 mL
EPINEPHRINE (1:1,000)	0.1 mg/kg	2.5 mg	1 mg/mL	2.50 mL
ESMOLOL	0.5 mg/kg	17 mg	10 mg/mL	1.70 mL
LABETALOL	0.2 mg/kg	6.8 mg	5 mg/mL	1.36 mL
LIDOCAINE	1 mg/kg	34 mg	100 mcg/mL	1.70 mL
NEOSYNEPHRINE	5 mcg/kg	170 mcg	100 mcg/mL	1.70 mL
ROMAZICON	0.01 mg/kg	0.2 mg	0.1 mg/mL	2.00 mL
VASOPRESSIN	0.4 unit/kg	13.6 units	20 u/mL	0.68 mL

ATROPINE, EPINEPHRINE (1:10,000), LIDOCAINE, VASOPRESSIN routes include ETT and IO markings per original.

35 KG MAINTENANCE IV FLUIDS: 75 ML/HR

common pediatric drugs	route	dose	mg to pt	supplied	mL to give
ATROPINE	vagolytic IV	0.02 mg/kg	0.5 mg	0.4 mg/mL	1.25 mL
GLYCOPYRROLATE	vagolytic IV	0.004 mg/kg	0.14 mg	0.2 mg/mL	0.7 mL
MIDAZOLAM	IV	0.05 mg/kg	0.6 mg	1 mg/mL	0.6 mL
MIDAZOLAM	PO	0.5 mg/kg	17.5 mg	1 mg/mL	17.5 mL
MIDAZOLAM	IN	0.2 mg/kg	7 mg	1 mg/mL	7 mL
SUCCINYLCHOLINE	IV	2 mg/kg	70 mg	20 mg/mL	3.5 mL
SUCCINYLCHOLINE	IM	4 mg/kg	140 mg	20 mg/mL	7 mL
PROPOFOL	IV	3 mg/kg	105 mg	10 mg/mL	10.5 mL
ETOMIDATE	>10 y IV	0.3 mg/kg	10.5 mg	2 mg/mL	5.25 mL
FENTANYL	IV	1 mcg/kg	35 mcg	50 mcg/mL	0.7 mL
FENTANYL	IN	2 mcg/kg	70 mcg	50 mcg/mL	1.4 mL
MORPHINE	<6 mo IV/IM	0.05 mg/kg	1.75 mg	10 mg/mL	0.175 mL
MORPHINE	>6 mo IV/IM	0.1 mg/kg	3.5 mg	10 mg/mL	0.35 mL
TORADOL	>2-16 y IV	0.5 mg/kg	15 mg	30 mg/mL	0.5 mL
TORADOL	>2-16 y IM	1 mg/kg	30 mg	30 mg/mL	1 mL
ACETAMINOPHEN	PR	20 mg/kg	700 mg		
ACETAMINOPHEN	2-12 y IV	15 mg/kg	525 mg	10 mg/mL	52.5 mL
CISATRACURIUM	IV	0.1 mg/kg	3.5 mg	2 mg/mL	1.75 mL
PANCURONIUM	<1 mo IV	0.02 mg/kg	0.7 mg	1 mg/mL	0.7 mL
PANCURONIUM	>1 mo IV	0.1 mg/kg	3.5 mg	1 mg/mL	3.5 mL
ROCURONIUM	IV	0.6 mg/kg	21 mg	10 mg/mL	2.1 mL
ROCURONIUM	RSI IV	1.2 mg/kg	42 mg	10 mg/mL	4.2 mL
VECURONIUM	IV	0.1 mg/kg	3.5 mg	1 mg/mL	3.5 mL
GLYCOPYRROLATE	reversal IV	0.007 mg/kg	0.245 mg	0.2 mg/mL	1.225 mL
NEOSTIGMINE	IV	0.07 mg/kg	2.45 mg	1 mg/mL	2.45 mL
DEXAMETHASONE	IV	0.25 mg/kg	8.75 mg	10 mg/mL	0.875 mL
ONDANSETRON	IV	0.15 mg/kg	4 mg	2 mg/mL	2 mL

additional pediatric drugs		route	dose	mg to pt	supplied	mL to give
PREMED/SEDATION; VAGOLYTIC/ANTISIAL/AGOGUE; GIVE IM 30–60 MIN PREOP						
ATROPINE		IM	0.02 mg/kg	0.5 mg	0.4 mg/mL	1.25 mL
GLYCOPYRROLATE		IM	0.004 mg/kg	0.009 mg	0.2 mg/mL	0.045 mL
MIDAZOLAM		IM	0.1 mg/kg	0.5 mg	1 mg/mL	0.5 mL
DEXMEDETOMIDINE	load dose	IV	0.5 mcg/kg	1 mcg	4 mcg/mL	0.25 mL
INDUCTION						
KETAMINE		IV	2 mg/kg	70 mg	10 mg/mL	7 mL
KETAMINE		IM/PR	5 mg/kg	175 mg	10 mg/mL	17.5 mL
OPIOIDS/NONOPIOIDS						
FENTANYL	high dose	IV	4 mcg/kg	140 mcg	50 mcg/mL	2.8 mL
FENTANYL	cardiac	IV	10 mcg/kg	350 mcg	50 mcg/mL	7 mL
HYDROMORPHONE	< 6 mo	IV/SQ	0.005 mg/kg	0.175 mg	10 mg/mL	0.0175 mL
HYDROMORPHONE	> 6 mo	IV/SQ	0.015 mg/kg	0.525 mg	10 mg/mL	0.0525 mL
REMIFENTANIL		IV	0.5 mcg/kg	1 mcg	50 mcg/mL	0.02 mL
SUFENTANIL		IV	0.5 mcg/kg	17.5 mcg	50 mcg/mL	0.35 mL
REVERSALS						
ATROPINE		IV	0.02 mg/kg	0.5 mg	0.4 mg/mL	1.25 mL
EDROPHONIUM	neonate	IV	0.1 mg single dose		10 mg/mL	0.01 mL
EDROPHONIUM	> 2 mo	IV	0.04 mg/kg	1.4 mg	10 mg/mL	0.14 mL
FLUMAZENIL	> 1 y	IV	0.01 mg/kg	0.2 mg	0.1 mg/mL	2 mL
NALOXONE	< 5 y; < 20 kg	IM/IV	0.1 mg/kg	2 mg	0.4 mg/mL	5 mL
NALOXONE	> 5 y; > 20 kg	IM/IV	2 mg per dose		0.4 mg/mL	5 mL
NALOXONE		ETT	0.3 mg/kg	10.5 mg	0.4 mg/mL	26.25 mL

additional pediatric drugs		route	dose	mg to pt	supplied	mL to give
ANTIBIOTICS						
AMPICILLIN	<6 y	IV	50 mg/kg	300 mg		
AMPICILLIN	>6 y	IV	50 mg/kg	1,750 mg		
AMPICILLIN & SULBACTUM	>1 mo	IV	50 mg/kg	1,750 mg		
CEFAZOLIN		IV	25 mg/kg	875 mg		
CLINDAMYCIN		IV	10 mg/kg	350 mg		
ERTAPENEM	3 mo-12 y	IV	15 mg/kg	525 mg		
ERTAPENEM	>12 y	IV	1 Gm	per dose		
GENTAMICIN		IV	2 mg/kg	70 mg		
LEVOFLOXACIN		IV	10 mg/kg	350 mg		
METRONIDAZOLE		IV	10 mg/kg	350 mg		
PIPERACILLIN & TAZOBACTAM	<40 kg & 2-9 mo	IV	80 mg/kg	2,800 mg		
PIPERACILLIN & TAZOBACTAM	<40 kg & >9 mo	IV	100 mg/kg	3,375 mg		
PIPERACILLIN & TAZOBACTAM	>40 kg	IV	3.375 Gm per dose			
VANCOMYCIN		IV	15 mg/kg	525 mg		
ANTINAUSEA						
METOCLOPROMIDE		IV	0.2 mg/kg	7 mg	5 mg/mL	1.4 mL
DIPHENHYDRAMINE		IV/IM	1.25 mg/kg	43.75 mg	50 mg/mL	0.875 mL
SCOPOLAMINE		IV/IM	6 mcg/kg	210 mcg	400 mcg/mL	0.525 mL
MISCELLANEOUS MEDS						
AMINOCAPROIC ACID		IV	100 mg/kg	3,500 mg	250 mg/mL	14 mL
DESMOPRESSIN		IV/SQ	0.3 mcg/kg	10.5 mcg	4 mcg/mL	2.625 mL
DEXAMETHASONE	croup	IV	0.6 mg/kg	16 mg	4 mg/mL	4 mL
HYDROCORTISONE		IV/IO	3 mg/kg	100 mg	100 mg/mL	1 mL

35 KG
1 year → 13 kg and up

Ventilation: trained rescuer	1 breath q 6-8 sec (8-10 breaths/minute) about 1 second/ breath-visible chest rise; if intubated, continuous compressions without pause for ventilations
Pulse check	carotid or femoral
Compression	heel of 1 hand or both hands one atop the other–lower half of sternum between nipples
Depth	2 inches (5 cm) or at least 1/3 chest depth
Rate	at least 100 compressions per minute
Compress/vent ratio	30:2 single rescuer
	15:2 2 healthcare providers
Foreign body obstruction	Heimlich maneuver
	Never perform a blind finger-sweep. Open the mouth and look for object; if you see it, remove it.

sync cardioversion		0.5 J/kg	17.5 J
	repeat	1 J/kg	35 J
defibrillation		2 J/kg	70 J
	repeat	4 J/kg	140 J

IV Bolus Drugs		dose	mg to pt	supplied	mL to give
ADENOSINE	IV	0.1 mg/kg	3.5 mg	3 mg/mL	1.17 mL
ADENOSINE repeat dose	IV	0.2 mg/kg	7 mg	3 mg/mL	2.33 mL
AMIODARONE	IV/IO	5 mg/kg	175 mg	50 mg/mL	3.50 mL
ATROPINE	IV/IM	0.02 mg/kg	0.5 mg	0.4 mg/mL	1.25 mL
ATROPINE	ETT	0.04 mg/kg	1.4 mg	0.4 mg/mL	3.50 mL
CALCIUM CHLORIDE	IV	20 mg/kg	700 mg	100 mg/mL	7.00 mL
CALCIUM GLUCONATE	IV/IO	60 mg/kg	800 mg	100 mg/mL	8.00 mL
DANTROLENE	IV	2.5 mg/kg	30 mg		
EPHEDRINE	IV	0.15 mg/kg	5.25 mg	10 mg/mL	0.53 mL
EPINEPHRINE (1:10,000)	IV/IO	0.01 mg/kg	0.35 mg	0.1 mg/mL	3.50 mL
EPINEPHRINE (1:1,000)	ETT	0.1 mg/kg	2.5 mg	1 mg/mL	2.50 mL
ESMOLOL	IV	0.5 mg/kg	17.5 mg	10 mg/mL	1.75 mL
LABETALOL	IV	0.2 mg/kg	7 mg	5 mg/mL	1.40 mL
LIDOCAINE	IV/IO	1 mg/kg	35 mg	20 mg/mL	1.75 mL
NEOSYNEPHRINE	IV	5 mcg/kg	175 mcg	100 mcg/mL	1.75 mL
ROMAZICON	IV	0.01 mg/kg	0.2 mg	0.1 mg/mL	2.00 mL
VASOPRESSIN	IV/IO	0.4 unit/kg	14 units	20 u/mL	0.70 mL

36 KG MAINTENANCE IV FLUIDS: 76 ML/HR

common pediatric drugs		route	dose	mg to pt	supplied	mL to give
ATROPINE	vagolytic	IV	0.02 mg/kg	0.5 mg	0.4 mg/mL	1.25 mL
GLYCOPYRROLATE	vagolytic	IV	0.004 mg/kg	0.144 mg	0.2 mg/mL	0.72 mL
MIDAZOLAM		IV	0.05 mg/kg	0.6 mg	1 mg/mL	0.6 mL
MIDAZOLAM		PO	0.5 mg/kg	18 mg	1 mg/mL	18 mL
MIDAZOLAM		IN	0.2 mg/kg	7.2 mg	1 mg/mL	7.2 mL
SUCCINYLCHOLINE		IV	2 mg/kg	72 mg	20 mg/mL	3.6 mL
SUCCINYLCHOLINE		IM	4 mg/kg	144 mg	20 mg/mL	7.2 mL
PROPOFOL		IV	3 mg/kg	108 mg	10 mg/mL	10.8 mL
ETOMIDATE	>10 y	IV	0.3 mg/kg	10.8 mg	2 mg/mL	5.4 mL
FENTANYL		IV	1 mcg/kg	36 mcg	50 mcg/mL	0.72 mL
FENTANYL		IN	2 mcg/kg	72 mcg	50 mcg/mL	1.44 mL
MORPHINE	<6 mo	IV/IM	0.05 mg/kg	1.8 mg	10 mg/mL	0.18 mL
MORPHINE	>6 mo	IV/IM	0.1 mg/kg	3.6 mg	10 mg/mL	0.36 mL
TORADOL	>2-16 y	IV	0.5 mg/kg	15 mg	30 mg/mL	0.5 mL
TORADOL	>2-16 y	IM	1 mg/kg	30 mg	30 mg/mL	1 mL
ACETAMINOPHEN		PR	20 mg/kg	720 mg		
ACETAMINOPHEN	2-12 y	IV	15 mg/kg	540 mg	10 mg/mL	54 mL
CISATRACURIUM		IV	0.1 mg/kg	3.6 mg	2 mg/mL	1.8 mL
PANCURONIUM	<1 mo	IV	0.02 mg/kg	0.72 mg	1 mg/mL	0.72 mL
PANCURONIUM	>1 mo	IV	0.1 mg/kg	3.6 mg	1 mg/mL	3.6 mL
ROCURONIUM		IV	0.6 mg/kg	21.6 mg	10 mg/mL	2.16 mL
ROCURONIUM	RSI	IV	1.2 mg/kg	43.2 mg	10 mg/mL	4.32 mL
VECURONIUM		IV	0.1 mg/kg	3.6 mg	1 mg/mL	3.6 mL
GLYCOPYRROLATE	reversal	IV	0.007 mg/kg	0.252 mg	0.2 mg/mL	1.26 mL
NEOSTIGMINE		IV	0.07 mg/kg	2.52 mg	1 mg/mL	2.52 mL
DEXAMETHASONE		IV	0.25 mg/kg	9 mg	10 mg/mL	0.9 mL
ONDANSETRON		IV	0.15 mg/kg	4 mg	2 mg/mL	2 mL

additional pediatric drugs	route	dose	mg to pt	supplied	mL to give
PREMED/SEDATION; VAGOLYTIC/ANTISIALAGOGUE; GIVE IM 30-60 MIN PREOP					
ATROPINE	IM	0.02 mg/kg	0.5 mg	0.4 mg/mL	1.25 mL
GLYCOPYRROLATE	IM	0.004 mg/kg	0.009 mg	0.2 mg/mL	0.045 mL
MIDAZOLAM	IM	0.1 mg/kg	0.5 mg	1 mg/mL	0.5 mL
DEXMEDETOMIDINE load dose	IV	0.5 mcg/kg	1 mcg	4 mcg/mL	0.25 mL
INDUCTION					
KETAMINE	IV	2 mg/kg	72 mg	10 mg/mL	7.2 mL
KETAMINE	IM/PR	5 mg/kg	180 mg	10 mg/mL	18 mL
OPIOIDS/NONOPIOIDS					
FENTANYL high dose	IV	4 mcg/kg	144 mcg	50 mcg/mL	2.88 mL
FENTANYL cardiac	IV	10 mcg/kg	360 mcg	50 mcg/mL	7.2 mL
HYDROMORPHONE < 6 mo	IV/SQ	0.005 mg/kg	0.18 mg	10 mg/mL	0.018 mL
HYDROMORPHONE > 6 mo	IV/SQ	0.015 mg/kg	0.54 mg	10 mg/mL	0.054 mL
REMIFENTANIL	IV	0.5 mcg/kg	1 mcg	50 mcg/mL	0.02 mL
SUFENTANIL	IV	0.5 mcg/kg	18 mcg	50 mcg/mL	0.36 mL
REVERSALS					
ATROPINE	IV	0.02 mg/kg	0.5 mg	0.4 mg/mL	1.25 mL
EDROPHONIUM neonate	IV	0.1 mg single dose		10 mg/mL	0.01 mL
EDROPHONIUM > 2 mo	IV	0.04 mg/kg	1.44 mg	10 mg/mL	0.144 mL
FLUMAZENIL > 1 y	IV	0.01 mg/kg	0.2 mg	0.1 mg/mL	2 mL
NALOXONE < 5 y; < 20 kg	IV/IM	0.1 mg/kg	2 mg	0.4 mg/mL	5 mL
NALOXONE > 5 y; > 20 kg	IM	2 mg per dose		0.4 mg/mL	5 mL
NALOXONE	ETT	0.3 mg/kg	10.8 mg	0.4 mg/mL	27 mL

additional pediatric drugs	route	dose	mg to pt	supplied	mL to give
ANTIBIOTICS					
AMPICILLIN <6 y	IV	50 mg/kg	300 mg		
AMPICILLIN >6 y	IV	50 mg/kg	1,800 mg		
AMPICILLIN & SULBACTUM >1 mo	IV	50 mg/kg	1,800 mg		
CEFAZOLIN	IV	25 mg/kg	900 mg		
CLINDAMYCIN	IV	10 mg/kg	360 mg		
ERTAPENEM 3 mo-12 y	IV	15 mg/kg	540 mg		
ERTAPENEM >12 y	IV	1 Gm	per dose		
GENTAMICIN	IV	2 mg/kg	72 mg		
LEVOFLOXACIN	IV	10 mg/kg	360 mg		
METRONIDAZOLE	IV	10 mg/kg	360 mg		
PIPERACILLIN & TAZOBACTAM <40 kg & 2-9 mo	IV	80 mg/kg	2,880 mg		
PIPERACILLIN & TAZOBACTAM <40 kg & >9 mo	IV	100 mg/kg	3,375 mg		
PIPERACILLIN & TAZOBACTAM >40 kg	IV	3.375 Gm per dose			
VANCOMYCIN	IV	15 mg/kg	540 mg		
ANTINAUSEA					
METOCLOPROMIDE	IV	0.2 mg/kg	7.2 mg	5 mg/mL	1.44 mL
DIPHENHYDRAMINE	IV/IM	1.25 mg/kg	45 mg	50 mg/mL	0.9 mL
SCOPOLAMINE	IV/IM	6 mcg/kg	216 mcg	400 mcg/mL	0.54 mL
MISCELLANEOUS MEDS					
AMINOCAPROIC ACID	IV	100 mg/kg	3,600 mg	250 mg/mL	14.4 mL
DESMOPRESSIN	IV/SQ	0.3 mcg/kg	10.8 mcg	4 mcg/mL	2.7 mL
DEXAMETHASONE croup	IV	0.6 mg/kg	16 mg	4 mg/mL	4 mL
HYDROCORTISONE	IV/IO	3 mg/kg	100 mg	100 mg/mL	1 mL

36 KG

1 year → 13 kg and up

Ventilation: trained rescuer	1 breath q 6-8 sec (8-10 breaths/minute) about 1 second/ breath-visible chest rise; if intubated, continuous compressions without pause for ventilations
Pulse check	carotid or femoral
Compression	heel of 1 hand or both hands one atop the other-lower half of sternum between nipples
Depth	2 inches (5 cm) or at least 1/3 chest depth
Rate	at least 100 compressions per minute
Compress/vent ratio	30:2 single rescuer 15:2 2 healthcare providers
Foreign body obstruction	Heimlich maneuver Never perform a blind finger-sweep. Open the mouth and look for object; if you see it, remove it.

sync cardioversion	0.5 J/kg	18 J
repeat	1 J/kg	36 J
defibrillation	2 J/kg	72 J
repeat	4 J/kg	144 J

IV Bolus Drugs	IV	dose	mg to pt	supplied	mL to give
ADENOSINE	IV	0.1 mg/kg	3.6 mg	3 mg/mL	1.20 mL
ADENOSINE repeat dose	IV	0.2 mg/kg	7.2 mg	3 mg/mL	2.40 mL
AMIODARONE	IV/IO	5 mg/kg	180 mg	50 mg/mL	3.60 mL
ATROPINE	IM/IV	0.02 mg/kg	0.5 mg	0.4 mg/mL	1.25 mL
ATROPINE	ETT	0.04 mg/kg	1.44 mg	0.4 mg/mL	3.60 mL
CALCIUM CHLORIDE	IV	20 mg/kg	720 mg	100 mg/mL	7.20 mL
CALCIUM GLUCONATE	IV/IO	60 mg/kg	800 mg	100 mg/mL	8.00 mL
DANTROLENE	IV	2.5 mg/kg	30 mg		
EPHEDRINE	IV	0.15 mg/kg	5.4 mg	10 mg/mL	0.54 mL
EPINEPHRINE (1:10,000)	IV/IO	0.01 mg/kg	0.36 mg	0.1 mg/mL	3.60 mL
EPINEPHRINE (1:1,000)	ETT	0.1 mg/kg	2.5 mg	1 mg/mL	2.50 mL
ESMOLOL	IV	0.5 mg/kg	18 mg	10 mg/mL	1.80 mL
LABETALOL	IV	0.2 mg/kg	7.2 mg	5 mg/mL	1.44 mL
LIDOCAINE	IV/IO	1 mg/kg	36 mg	20 mg/mL	1.80 mL
NEOSYNEPHRINE	IV	5 mcg/kg	180 mcg	100 mcg/mL	1.80 mL
ROMAZICON	IV	0.01 mg/kg	0.2 mg	0.1 mg/mL	2.00 mL
VASOPRESSIN	IV/IO	0.4 unit/kg	14.4 units	20 u/mL	0.72 mL

37 KG MAINTENANCE IV FLUIDS: 77 ML/HR

common pediatric drugs		route	dose	mg to pt	supplied	mL to give
ATROPINE	vagolytic	IV	0.02 mg/kg	0.5 mg	0.4 mg/mL	1.25 mL
GLYCOPYRROLATE	vagolytic	IV	0.004 mg/kg	0.148 mg	0.2 mg/mL	0.74 mL
MIDAZOLAM		IV	0.05 mg/kg	0.6 mg	1 mg/mL	0.6 mL
MIDAZOLAM		PO	0.5 mg/kg	18.5 mg	1 mg/mL	18.5 mL
MIDAZOLAM		IN	0.2 mg/kg	7.4 mg	1 mg/mL	7.4 mL
SUCCINYLCHOLINE		IV	2 mg/kg	74 mg	20 mg/mL	3.7 mL
SUCCINYLCHOLINE		IM	4 mg/kg	148 mg	20 mg/mL	7.4 mL
PROPOFOL		IV	3 mg/kg	111 mg	10 mg/mL	11.1 mL
ETOMIDATE	>10 y	IV	0.3 mg/kg	11.1 mg	2 mg/mL	5.55 mL
FENTANYL		IV	1 mcg/kg	37 mcg	50 mcg/mL	0.74 mL
FENTANYL		IN	2 mcg/kg	74 mcg	50 mcg/mL	1.48 mL
MORPHINE	<6 mo	IV/IM	0.05 mg/kg	1.85 mg	10 mg/mL	0.185 mL
MORPHINE	>6 mo	IV/IM	0.1 mg/kg	3.7 mg	10 mg/mL	0.37 mL
TORADOL	>2-16 y	IV	0.5 mg/kg	15 mg	30 mg/mL	0.5 mL
TORADOL	>2-16 y	IM	1 mg/kg	30 mg	30 mg/mL	1 mL
ACETAMINOPHEN		PR	20 mg/kg	740 mg		
ACETAMINOPHEN	2-12 y	IV	15 mg/kg	555 mg	10 mg/mL	55.5 mL
CISATRACURIUM		IV	0.1 mg/kg	3.7 mg	2 mg/mL	1.85 mL
PANCURONIUM	<1 mo	IV	0.02 mg/kg	0.74 mg	1 mg/mL	0.74 mL
PANCURONIUM	>1 mo	IV	0.1 mg/kg	3.7 mg	1 mg/mL	3.7 mL
ROCURONIUM		IV	0.6 mg/kg	22.2 mg	10 mg/mL	2.22 mL
ROCURONIUM	RSI	IV	1.2 mg/kg	44.4 mg	10 mg/mL	4.44 mL
VECURONIUM		IV	0.1 mg/kg	3.7 mg	1 mg/mL	3.7 mL
GLYCOPYRROLATE	reversal	IV	0.007 mg/kg	0.259 mg	0.2 mg/mL	1.295 mL
NEOSTIGMINE		IV	0.07 mg/kg	2.59 mg	1 mg/mL	2.59 mL
DEXAMETHASONE		IV	0.25 mg/kg	9.25 mg	10 mg/mL	0.925 mL
ONDANSETRON		IV	0.15 mg/kg	4 mg	2 mg/mL	2 mL

additional pediatric drugs	route	dose	mg to pt	supplied	mL to give
PREMED/SEDATION; VAGOLYTIC/ANTISIALAGOGUE; GIVE IM 30-60 MIN PREOP					
ATROPINE	IM	0.02 mg/kg	0.5 mg	0.4 mg/mL	1.25 mL
GLYCOPYRROLATE	IM	0.004 mg/kg	0.009 mg	0.2 mg/mL	0.045 mL
MIDAZOLAM	IM	0.1 mg/kg	0.5 mg	1 mg/mL	0.5
DEXMEDETOMIDINE load dose	IV	0.5 mcg/kg	1 mcg	4 mcg/mL	0.25 mL
INDUCTION					
KETAMINE	IV	2 mg/kg	74 mg	10 mg/mL	7.4 mL
KETAMINE	IM/PR	5 mg/kg	185 mg	10 mg/mL	18.5 mL
OPIOIDS/NONOPIOIDS					
FENTANYL high dose	IV	4 mcg/kg	148 mcg	50 mcg/mL	2.96 mL
FENTANYL cardiac	IV	10 mcg/kg	370 mcg	50 mcg/mL	7.4 mL
HYDROMORPHONE <6 mo	IV/SQ	0.005 mg/kg	0.185 mg	10 mg/mL	0.0185 mL
HYDROMORPHONE >6 mo	IV/SQ	0.015 mg/kg	0.555 mg	10 mg/mL	0.0555 mL
REMIFENTANIL	IV	0.5 mcg/kg	1 mcg	50 mcg/mL	0.02 mL
SUFENTANIL	IV	0.5 mcg/kg	18.5 mcg	50 mcg/mL	0.37 mL
REVERSALS					
ATROPINE	IV	0.02 mg/kg	0.5 mg	0.4 mg/mL	1.25 mL
EDROPHONIUM	neonate	0.1 mg single dose		10 mg/mL	0.01 mL
EDROPHONIUM	>2 mo	0.04 mg/kg	1.48 mg	10 mg/mL	0.148 mL
FLUMAZENIL	>1 y	0.01 mg/kg	0.2 mg	0.1 mg/mL	2 mL
NALOXONE	<5 y; <20 kg	0.1 mg/kg	2 mg	0.4 mg/mL	5 mL
NALOXONE	<5 y; >20 kg	2 mg per dose		0.4 mg/mL	5 mL
NALOXONE	ETT	0.3 mg/kg	11.1 mg	0.4 mg/mL	27.75 mL

additional pediatric drugs		route	dose	mg to pt	supplied	mL to give
ANTIBIOTICS						
AMPICILLIN	<6 y	IV	50 mg/kg	300 mg		
AMPICILLIN	>6 y	IV	50 mg/kg	1,850 mg		
AMPICILLIN & SULBACTUM	>1 mo	IV	50 mg/kg	1,850 mg		
CEFAZOLIN		IV	25 mg/kg	925 mg		
CLINDAMYCIN		IV	10 mg/kg	370 mg		
ERTAPENEM	3 mo-12 y	IV	15 mg/kg	555 mg		
ERTAPENEM	>12 y	IV	1 Gm	per dose		
GENTAMICIN		IV	2 mg/kg	74 mg		
LEVOFLOXACIN		IV	10 mg/kg	370 mg		
METRONIDAZOLE		IV	10 mg/kg	370 mg		
PIPERACILLIN & TAZOBACTAM	<40 kg & 2-9 mo	IV	80 mg/kg	2,960 mg		
PIPERACILLIN & TAZOBACTAM	<40 kg & >9 mo	IV	100 mg/kg	3,375 mg		
PIPERACILLIN & TAZOBACTAM	>40 kg	IV	3.375 Gm per dose			
VANCOMYCIN		IV	15 mg/kg	555 mg		
ANTINAUSEA						
METOCLOPROMIDE		IV	0.2 mg/kg	7.4 mg	5 mg/mL	1.48 mL
DIPHENHYDRAMINE		IV/IM	1.25 mg/kg	46.25 mg	50 mg/mL	0.925 mL
SCOPOLAMINE		IV/IM	6 mcg/kg	222 mcg	400 mcg/mL	0.555 mL
MISCELLANEOUS MEDS						
AMINOCAPROIC ACID		IV	100 mg/kg	3,700 mg	250 mg/mL	14.8 mL
DESMOPRESSIN		IV/SQ	0.3 mcg/kg	11.1 mcg	4 mcg/mL	2.775 mL
DEXAMETHASONE	croup	IV	0.6 mg/kg	16 mg	4 mg/mL	4 mL
HYDROCORTISONE		IV/IO	3 mg/kg	100 mg	100 mg/mL	1 mL

37 KG

1 year ← 13 kg and up

Ventilation: trained rescuer	1 breath q 6-8 sec (8-10 breaths/minute) about 1 second/ breath-visible chest rise; if intubated, continuous compressions without pause for ventilations
Pulse check	carotid or femoral
Compression	heel of 1 hand or both hands one atop the other—lower half of sternum between nipples
Depth	2 inches (5 cm) or at least 1/3 chest depth
Rate	at least 100 compressions per minute
Compress/vent ratio	30:2 single rescuer 15:2 2 healthcare providers
Foreign body obstruction	Heimlich maneuver Never perform a blind finger-sweep. Open the mouth and look for object; if you see it, remove it.

sync cardioversion	0.5 J/kg	18.5 J
repeat	1 J/kg	37 J
defibrillation	2 J/kg	74 J
repeat	4 J/kg	148 J

IV Bolus Drugs		dose	mg to pt	supplied	mL to give
ADENOSINE	IV	0.1 mg/kg	3.7 mg	3 mg/mL	1.23 mL
ADENOSINE repeat dose	IV	0.2 mg/kg	7.4 mg	3 mg/mL	2.47 mL
AMIODARONE	IV/IO	5 mg/kg	185 mg	50 mg/mL	3.70 mL
ATROPINE	IM/IV	0.02 mg/kg	0.5 mg	0.4 mg/mL	1.25 mL
ATROPINE	ETT	0.04 mg/kg	1.48 mg	0.4 mg/mL	3.70 mL
CALCIUM CHLORIDE	IV	20 mg/kg	740 mg	100 mg/mL	7.40 mL
CALCIUM GLUCONATE	IV/IO	60 mg/kg	800 mg	100 mg/mL	8.00 mL
DANTROLENE	IV	2.5 mg/kg	30 mg		
EPHEDRINE	IV	0.15 mg/kg	5.55 mg	10 mg/mL	0.56 mL
EPINEPHRINE (1:10,000)	IV/IO	0.01 mg/kg	0.37 mg	0.1 mg/mL	3.70 mL
EPINEPHRINE (1:1,000)	ETT	0.1 mg/kg	2.5 mg	1 mg/mL	2.50 mL
ESMOLOL	IV	0.5 mg/kg	18.5 mg	10 mg/mL	1.85 mL
LABETALOL	IV	0.2 mg/kg	7.4 mg	5 mg/mL	1.48 mL
LIDOCAINE	IV/IO	1 mg/kg	37 mg	20 mg/mL	1.85 mL
NEOSYNEPHRINE	IV	5 mcg/kg	185 mcg	100 mcg/mL	1.85 mL
ROMAZICON	IV	0.01 mg/kg	0.2 mg	0.1 mg/mL	2.00 mL
VASOPRESSIN	IV/IO	0.4 unit/kg	14.8 units	20 u/mL	0.74 mL

38 KG MAINTENANCE IV FLUIDS: 78 ML/HR

common pediatric drugs		route	dose	mg to pt	supplied	mL to give
ATROPINE	vagolytic	IV	0.02 mg/kg	0.5 mg	0.4 mg/mL	1.25 mL
GLYCOPYRROLATE	vagolytic	IV	0.004 mg/kg	0.152 mg	0.2 mg/mL	0.76 mL
MIDAZOLAM		IV	0.05 mg/kg	0.6 mg	1 mg/mL	0.6 mL
MIDAZOLAM		PO	0.5 mg/kg	19 mg	1 mg/mL	19 mL
MIDAZOLAM		IN	0.2 mg/kg	7.6 mg	1 mg/mL	7.6 mL
SUCCINYLCHOLINE		IV	2 mg/kg	76 mg	20 mg/mL	3.8 mL
SUCCINYLCHOLINE		IM	4 mg/kg	152 mg	20 mg/mL	7.6 mL
PROPOFOL		IV	3 mg/kg	114 mg	10 mg/mL	11.4 mL
ETOMIDATE	>10 y	IV	0.3 mg/kg	11.4 mg	2 mg/mL	5.7 mL
FENTANYL		IV	1 mcg/kg	38 mcg	50 mcg/mL	0.76 mL
FENTANYL		IN	2 mcg/kg	76 mcg	50 mcg/mL	1.52 mL
MORPHINE	<6 mo	IV/IM	0.05 mg/kg	1.9 mg	10 mg/mL	0.19 mL
MORPHINE	>6 mo	IV/IM	0.1 mg/kg	3.8 mg	10 mg/mL	0.38 mL
TORADOL	>2-16 y	IV	0.5 mg/kg	15 mg	30 mg/mL	0.5 mL
TORADOL	>2-16 y	IM	1 mg/kg	30 mg	30 mg/mL	1 mL
ACETAMINOPHEN		PR	20 mg/kg	760 mg		
ACETAMINOPHEN	2-12 y	IV	15 mg/kg	570 mg	10 mg/mL	57 mL
CISATRACURIUM		IV	0.1 mg/kg	3.8 mg	2 mg/mL	1.9 mL
PANCURONIUM	<1 mo	IV	0.02 mg/kg	0.76 mg	1 mg/mL	0.76 mL
PANCURONIUM	>1 mo	IV	0.1 mg/kg	3.8 mg	1 mg/mL	3.8 mL
ROCURONIUM		IV	0.6 mg/kg	22.8 mg	10 mg/mL	2.28 mL
ROCURONIUM	RSI	IV	1.2 mg/kg	45.6 mg	10 mg/mL	4.56 mL
VECURONIUM		IV	0.1 mg/kg	3.8 mg	1 mg/mL	3.8 mL
GLYCOPYRROLATE	reversal	IV	0.007 mg/kg	0.266 mg	0.2 mg/mL	1.33 mL
NEOSTIGMINE		IV	0.07 mg/kg	2.66 mg	1 mg/mL	2.66 mL
DEXAMETHASONE		IV	0.25 mg/kg	9.5 mg	10 mg/mL	0.95 mL
ONDANSETRON		IV	0.15 mg/kg	4 mg	2 mg/mL	2 mL

additional pediatric drugs	route	dose		mg to pt	supplied	mL to give
PREMED/SEDATION; VAGOLYTIC/ANTISIALAGOGUE; GIVE IM 30-60 MIN PREOP						
ATROPINE	IM	0.02 mg/kg		0.5 mg	0.4 mg/mL	1.25 mL
GLYCOPYRROLATE	IM	0.004 mg/kg		0.009 mg	0.2 mg/mL	0.045 mL
MIDAZOLAM	IM	0.1 mg/kg		0.5 mg	1 mg/mL	0.5 mL
DEXMEDETOMIDINE load dose	IV	0.5 mcg/kg		1 mcg	4 mcg/mL	0.25 mL
INDUCTION						
KETAMINE	IV	2 mg/kg		76 mg	10 mg/mL	7.6 mL
KETAMINE	IM/PR	5 mg/kg		190 mg	10 mg/mL	19 mL
OPIOIDS/NONOPIOIDS						
FENTANYL	IV	high dose	4 mcg/kg	152 mcg	50 mcg/mL	3.04 mL
FENTANYL	IV	cardiac	10 mcg/kg	380 mcg	50 mcg/mL	7.6 mL
HYDROMORPHONE	IV/SQ	< 6 mo	0.005 mg/kg	0.19 mg	10 mg/mL	0.019 mL
HYDROMORPHONE	IV/SQ	> 6 mo	0.015 mg/kg	0.57 mg	10 mg/mL	0.057 mL
REMIFENTANIL	IV	0.5 mcg/kg		1 mcg	50 mcg/mL	0.02 mL
SUFENTANIL	IV	0.5 mcg/kg		19 mcg	50 mcg/mL	0.38 mL
REVERSALS						
ATROPINE	IV	0.02 mg/kg		0.5 mg	0.4 mg/mL	1.25 mL
EDROPHONIUM	IV	neonate	0.1 mg single dose		10 mg/mL	0.01 mL
EDROPHONIUM	IV	> 2 mo	0.04 mg/kg	1.52 mg	10 mg/mL	0.152 mL
FLUMAZENIL	IV	> 1 y	0.01 mg/kg	0.6 mg	0.1 mg/mL	2 mL
NALOXONE	IM	< 5 y; < 20 kg	0.1 mg/kg	2 mg	0.4 mg/mL	5 mL
NALOXONE	IV/IM	> 5 y; > 20 kg	2 mg per dose		0.4 mg/mL	5 mL
NALOXONE	ETT	0.3 mg/kg		11.4 mg	0.4 mg/mL	28.5 mL

additional pediatric drugs		route	dose	mg to pt	supplied	mL to give
ANTIBIOTICS						
AMPICILLIN	<6 y	IV	50 mg/kg	300 mg		
AMPICILLIN	>6 y	IV	50 mg/kg	1,900 mg		
AMPICILLIN & SULBACTUM	>1 mo	IV	50 mg/kg	1,900 mg		
CEFAZOLIN		IV	25 mg/kg	950 mg		
CLINDAMYCIN		IV	10 mg/kg	380 mg		
ERTAPENEM	3 mo-12 y	IV	15 mg/kg	570 mg		
ERTAPENEM	>12 y	IV	1 Gm	per dose		
GENTAMICIN		IV	2 mg/kg	76 mg		
LEVOFLOXACIN		IV	10 mg/kg	380 mg		
METRONIDAZOLE		IV	10 mg/kg	380 mg		
PIPERACILLIN & TAZOBACTAM	<40 kg & 2-9 mo	IV	80 mg/kg	3,040 mg		
PIPERACILLIN & TAZOBACTAM	<40 kg & >9 mo	IV	100 mg/kg	3,375 mg		
PIPERACILLIN & TAZOBACTAM	>40 kg	IV	3.375 Gm per dose			
VANCOMYCIN		IV	15 mg/kg	570 mg		
ANTINAUSEA						
METOCLOPROMIDE		IV	0.2 mg/kg	7.6 mg	5 mg/mL	1.52 mL
DIPHENHYDRAMINE		IV/IM	1.25 mg/kg	47.5 mg	50 mg/mL	0.95 mL
SCOPOLAMINE		IV/IM	6 mcg/kg	228 mcg	400 mcg/mL	0.57 mL
MISCELLANEOUS MEDS						
AMINOCAPROIC ACID		IV	100 mg/kg	3,800 mg	250 mg/mL	15.2 mL
DESMOPRESSIN		IV/SQ	0.3 mcg/kg	11.4 mcg	4 mcg/mL	2.85 mL
DEXAMETHASONE	croup	IV	0.6 mg/kg	16 mg	4 mg/mL	4 mL
HYDROCORTISONE		IV/IO	3 mg/kg	100 mg	100 mg/mL	1 mL

38 KG

1 year ← 13 kg and up

Ventilation: trained rescuer	1 breath q 6-8 sec (8-10 breaths/minute) about 1 second/ breath-visible chest rise; if intubated, continuous compressions without pause for ventilations
Pulse check	carotid or femoral
Compression	heel of 1 hand or both hands one atop the other-lower half of sternum between nipples
Depth	2 inches (5 cm) or at least 1/3 chest depth
Rate	at least 100 compressions per minute
Compress/vent ratio	30:2 single rescuer 15:2 2 healthcare providers
Foreign body obstruction	Heimlich maneuver Never perform a blind finger-sweep. Open the mouth and look for object; if you see it, remove it.

sync cardioversion	0.5 J/kg	19 J	
	repeat	1 J/kg	38 J
defibrillation	2 J/kg	76 J	
	repeat	4 J/kg	152 J

IV Bolus Drugs		dose	mg to pt	supplied	mL to give
ADENOSINE	IV	0.1 mg/kg	3.8 mg	3 mg/mL	1.27 mL
ADENOSINE repeat dose	IV	0.2 mg/kg	7.6 mg	3 mg/mL	2.53 mL
AMIODARONE	IV/IO	5 mg/kg	190 mg	50 mg/mL	3.80 mL
ATROPINE	IV/IM	0.02 mg/kg	0.5 mg	0.4 mg/mL	1.25 mL
ATROPINE	ETT	0.04 mg/kg	1.52 mg	0.4 mg/mL	3.80 mL
CALCIUM CHLORIDE	IV	20 mg/kg	760 mg	100 mg/mL	7.60 mL
CALCIUM GLUCONATE	IV/IO	60 mg/kg	800 mg	100 mg/mL	8.00 mL
DANTROLENE	IV	2.5 mg/kg	30 mg		
EPHEDRINE	IV	0.15 mg/kg	5.7 mg	10 mg/mL	0.57 mL
EPINEPHRINE (1:10,000)	IV/IO	0.01 mg/kg	0.38 mg	0.1 mg/mL	3.80 mL
EPINEPHRINE (1:1,000)	ETT	0.1 mg/kg	2.5 mg	1 mg/mL	2.50 mL
ESMOLOL	IV	0.5 mg/kg	19 mg	10 mg/mL	1.90 mL
LABETALOL	IV	0.2 mg/kg	7.6 mg	5 mg/mL	1.52 mL
LIDOCAINE	IV/IO	1 mg/kg	38 mg	20 mg/mL	1.90 mL
NEOSYNEPHRINE	IV	5 mcg/kg	190 mcg	100 mcg/mL	1.90 mL
ROMAZICON	IV	0.01 mg/kg	0.2 mg	0.1 mg/mL	2.00 mL
VASOPRESSIN	IV/IO	0.4 unit/kg	15.2 units	20 u/mL	0.76 mL

39 KG MAINTENANCE IV FLUIDS: 79 ML/HR

common pediatric drugs		route	dose	mg to pt	supplied	mL to give
ATROPINE	vagolytic	IV	0.02 mg/kg	0.5 mg	0.4 mg/mL	1.25 mL
GLYCOPYRROLATE	vagolytic	IV	0.004 mg/kg	0.156 mg	0.2 mg/mL	0.78 mL
MIDAZOLAM		IV	0.05 mg/kg	0.6 mg	1 mg/mL	0.6 mL
MIDAZOLAM		PO	0.5 mg/kg	19.5 mg	1 mg/mL	19.5 mL
MIDAZOLAM		IN	0.2 mg/kg	7.8 mg	1 mg/mL	7.8 mL
SUCCINYLCHOLINE		IV	2 mg/kg	78 mg	20 mg/mL	3.9 mL
SUCCINYLCHOLINE		IM	4 mg/kg	156 mg	20 mg/mL	7.8 mL
PROPOFOL		IV	3 mg/kg	117 mg	10 mg/mL	11.7 mL
ETOMIDATE	>10 y	IV	0.3 mg/kg	11.7 mg	2 mg/mL	5.85 mL
FENTANYL		IV	1 mcg/kg	39 mcg	50 mcg/mL	0.78 mL
FENTANYL		IN	2 mcg/kg	78 mcg	50 mcg/mL	1.56 mL
MORPHINE	<6 mo	IV/IM	0.05 mg/kg	1.95 mg	10 mg/mL	0.195 mL
MORPHINE	>6 mo	IV/IM	0.1 mg/kg	3.9 mg	10 mg/mL	0.39 mL
TORADOL	>2-16 y	IV	0.5 mg/kg	15 mg	30 mg/mL	0.5 mL
TORADOL	>2-16 y	IM	1 mg/kg	30 mg	30 mg/mL	1 mL
ACETAMINOPHEN		PR	20 mg/kg	780 mg		
ACETAMINOPHEN	2-12 y	IV	15 mg/kg	585 mg	10 mg/mL	58.5 mL
CISATRACURIUM		IV	0.1 mg/kg	3.9 mg	2 mg/mL	1.95 mL
PANCURONIUM	<1 mo	IV	0.02 mg/kg	0.78 mg	1 mg/mL	0.78 mL
PANCURONIUM	>1 mo	IV	0.1 mg/kg	3.9 mg	1 mg/mL	3.9 mL
ROCURONIUM		IV	0.6 mg/kg	23.4 mg	10 mg/mL	2.34 mL
ROCURONIUM	RSI	IV	1.2 mg/kg	46.8 mg	10 mg/mL	4.68 mL
VECURONIUM		IV	0.1 mg/kg	3.9 mg	1 mg/mL	3.9 mL
GLYCOPYRROLATE	reversal	IV	0.007 mg/kg	0.273 mg	0.2 mg/mL	1.365 mL
NEOSTIGMINE		IV	0.07 mg/kg	2.73 mg	1 mg/mL	2.73 mL
DEXAMETHASONE		IV	0.25 mg/kg	9.75 mg	10 mg/mL	0.975 mL
ONDANSETRON		IV	0.15 mg/kg	4 mg	2 mg/mL	2 mL

additional pediatric drugs	route	dose	mg to pt	supplied	mL to give
PREMED/SEDATION; VAGOLYTIC/ANTISIALAGOGUE; GIVE IM 30-60 MIN PREOP					
ATROPINE	IM	0.02 mg/kg	0.5 mg	0.4 mg/mL	1.25 mL
GLYCOPYRROLATE	IM	0.004 mg/kg	0.009 mg	0.2 mg/mL	0.045 mL
MIDAZOLAM	IM	0.1 mg/kg	0.5 mg	1 mg/mL	0.5 mL
DEXMEDETOMIDINE	IV	0.5 mcg/kg load dose	1 mcg	4 mcg/mL	0.25 mL
INDUCTION					
KETAMINE	IV	2 mg/kg	78 mg	10 mg/mL	7.8 mL
KETAMINE	IM/PR	5 mg/kg	195 mg	10 mg/mL	19.5 mL
OPIOIDS/NONOPIOIDS					
FENTANYL	IV	4 mcg/kg high dose	156 mcg	50 mcg/mL	3.12 mL
FENTANYL	IV	10 mcg/kg cardiac	390 mcg	50 mcg/mL	7.8 mL
HYDROMORPHONE	IV/SQ	<6 mo 0.005 mg/kg	0.195 mg	10 mg/mL	0.0195 mL
HYDROMORPHONE	IV/SQ	>6 mo 0.015 mg/kg	0.585 mg	10 mg/mL	0.0585 mL
REMIFENTANIL	IV	0.5 mcg/kg	1 mcg	50 mcg/mL	0.02 mL
SUFENTANIL	IV	0.5 mcg/kg	19.5 mcg	50 mcg/mL	0.39 mL
REVERSALS					
ATROPINE	IV	0.02 mg/kg	0.5 mg	0.4 mg/mL	1.25 mL
EDROPHONIUM	IV	neonate 0.1 mg single dose		10 mg/mL	0.01 mL
EDROPHONIUM	IV	>2 mo 0.04 mg/kg	1.56 mg	10 mg/mL	0.156 mL
FLUMAZENIL	IV	>1 y 0.01 mg/kg	0.2 mg	0.1 mg/mL	2 mL
NALOXONE	IM/IV	<5 y; <20 kg 0.1 mg/kg	2 mg	0.4 mg/mL	5 mL
NALOXONE	IM/IV	>5 y; >20 kg 2 mg per dose		0.4 mg/mL	5 mL
NALOXONE	ETT	0.3 mg/kg	11.7 mg	0.4 mg/mL	29.25 mL

additional pediatric drugs		route	dose	mg to pt	supplied	mL to give
ANTIBIOTICS						
AMPICILLIN	<6 y	IV	50 mg/kg	300 mg		
AMPICILLIN	>6 y	IV	50 mg/kg	1,950 mg		
AMPICILLIN & SULBACTUM	>1 mo	IV	50 mg/kg	1,950 mg		
CEFAZOLIN		IV	25 mg/kg	975 mg		
CLINDAMYCIN		IV	10 mg/kg	390 mg		
ERTAPENEM	3 mo-12 y	IV	15 mg/kg	585 mg		
ERTAPENEM	>12 y	IV	1 Gm	per dose		
GENTAMICIN		IV	2 mg/kg	78 mg		
LEVOFLOXACIN		IV	10 mg/kg	390 mg		
METRONIDAZOLE		IV	10 mg/kg	390 mg		
PIPERACILLIN & TAZOBACTAM	<40 kg & 2-9 mo	IV	80 mg/kg	3,120 mg		
PIPERACILLIN & TAZOBACTAM	<40 kg & >9 mo	IV	100 mg/kg	3,375 mg		
PIPERACILLIN & TAZOBACTAM	>40 kg	IV	3.375 Gm per dose			
VANCOMYCIN		IV	15 mg/kg	585 mg		
ANTINAUSEA						
METOCLOPROMIDE		IV	0.2 mg/kg	7.8 mg	5 mg/mL	1.56 mL
DIPHENHYDRAMINE		IV/IM	1.25 mg/kg	48.75 mg	50 mg/mL	0.975 mL
SCOPOLAMINE		IV/IM	6 mcg/kg	234 mcg	400 mcg/mL	0.585 mL
MISCELLANEOUS MEDS						
AMINOCAPROIC ACID		IV	100 mg/kg	3,900 mg	250 mg/mL	15.6 mL
DESMOPRESSIN		IV/SQ	0.3 mcg/kg	11.7 mcg	4 mcg/mL	2.925 mL
DEXAMETHASONE	croup	IV	0.6 mg/kg	16 mg	4 mg/mL	4 mL
HYDROCORTISONE		IV/IO	3 mg/kg	100 mg	100 mg/mL	1 mL

39 KG

1 year ← 13 kg and up

Ventilation: trained rescuer	1 breath q 6-8 sec (8-10 breaths/minute) about 1 second/ breath-visible chest rise; if intubated, continuous compressions without pause for ventilations
Pulse check	carotid or femoral
Compression	heel of 1 hand or both hands one atop the other–lower half of sternum between nipples
Depth	2 inches (5 cm) or at least 1/3 chest depth
Rate	at least 100 compressions per minute
Compress/vent ratio	30:2 single rescuer 15:2 2 healthcare providers
Foreign body obstruction	Heimlich maneuver Never perform a blind finger-sweep. Open the mouth and look for object; if you see it, remove it.

	dose			supplied
sync cardioversion	0.5 J/kg	19.5 J		
defibrillation	1 J/kg	39 J	repeat	
	2 J/kg	78 J		
	4 J/kg	156 J	repeat	

IV Bolus Drugs		dose	mg to pt	supplied	mL to give
ADENOSINE	IV	0.1 mg/kg	3.9 mg	3 mg/mL	1.30 mL
ADENOSINE repeat dose	IV	0.2 mg/kg	7.8 mg	3 mg/mL	2.60 mL
AMIODARONE	IV/IO	5 mg/kg	195 mg	50 mg/mL	3.90 mL
ATROPINE	IM/IV	0.02 mg/kg	0.5 mg	0.4 mg/mL	1.25 mL
ATROPINE	ETT	0.04 mg/kg	1.56 mg	0.4 mg/mL	3.90 mL
CALCIUM CHLORIDE	IV	20 mg/kg	780 mg	100 mg/mL	7.80 mL
CALCIUM GLUCONATE	IV/IO	60 mg/kg	800 mg	100 mg/mL	8.00 mL
DANTROLENE	IV	2.5 mg/kg	30 mg		
			5.85 mg/kg	0.15 mg/kg	
DANTROLENE	IV	2.5 mg/kg	5.85 mg	10 mg/mL	0.59 mL
EPHEDRINE	IV	0.15 mg/kg	5.85 mg	10 mg/mL	0.59 mL
EPINEPHRINE (1:10,000)	IV/IO	0.01 mg/kg	0.39 mg	0.1 mg/mL	3.90 mL
EPINEPHRINE (1:1,000)	ETT	0.1 mg/kg	2.5 mg	1 mg/mL	2.50 mL
ESMOLOL	IV	0.5 mg/kg	19.5 mg	10 mg/mL	1.95 mL
LABETALOL	IV	0.2 mg/kg	7.8 mg	5 mg/mL	1.56 mL
LIDOCAINE	IV/IO	1 mg/kg	39 mg	100 mcg/mL	1.95 mL
NEOSYNEPHRINE	IV	5 mcg/kg	195 mcg	100 mcg/mL	1.95 mL
ROMAZICON	IV	0.01 mg/kg	0.2 mg	0.1 mg/mL	2.00 mL
VASOPRESSIN	IV/IO	0.4 unit/kg	15.6 units	20 u/mL	0.78 mL

40 KG MAINTENANCE IV FLUIDS: 80 ML/HR

common pediatric drugs		route	dose	mg to pt	supplied	mL to give
ATROPINE	vagolytic	IV	0.02 mg/kg	0.5 mg	0.4 mg/mL	1.25 mL
GLYCOPYRROLATE	vagolytic	IV	0.004 mg/kg	0.16 mg	0.2 mg/mL	0.8 mL
MIDAZOLAM		IV	0.05 mg/kg	0.6 mg	1 mg/mL	0.6 mL
MIDAZOLAM		PO	0.5 mg/kg	20 mg	1 mg/mL	20 mL
MIDAZOLAM		IN	0.2 mg/kg	8 mg	1 mg/mL	8 mL
SUCCINYLCHOLINE		IV	2 mg/kg	80 mg	20 mg/mL	4 mL
SUCCINYLCHOLINE		IM	4 mg/kg	160 mg	20 mg/mL	8 mL
PROPOFOL		IV	3 mg/kg	120 mg	10 mg/mL	12 mL
ETOMIDATE	>10 y	IV	0.3 mg/kg	12 mg	2 mg/mL	6 mL
FENTANYL		IV	1 mcg/kg	40 mcg	50 mcg/mL	0.8 mL
FENTANYL		IN	2 mcg/kg	80 mcg	50 mcg/mL	1.6 mL
MORPHINE	<6 mo	IV/IM	0.05 mg/kg	2 mg	10 mg/mL	0.2 mL
MORPHINE	>6 mo	IV/IM	0.1 mg/kg	4 mg	10 mg/mL	0.4 mL
TORADOL	>2-16 y	IV	0.5 mg/kg	15 mg	30 mg/mL	0.5 mL
TORADOL	>2-16 y	IM	1 mg/kg	30 mg	30 mg/mL	1 mL
ACETAMINOPHEN		PR	20 mg/kg	800 mg		
ACETAMINOPHEN	2-12 y	IV	15 mg/kg	600 mg	10 mg/mL	60 mL
CISATRACURIUM		IV	0.1 mg/kg	4 mg	2 mg/mL	2 mL
PANCURONIUM	<1 mo	IV	0.02 mg/kg	0.8 mg	1 mg/mL	0.8 mL
PANCURONIUM	>1 mo	IV	0.1 mg/kg	4 mg	1 mg/mL	4 mL
ROCURONIUM		IV	0.6 mg/kg	24 mg	10 mg/mL	2.4 mL
ROCURONIUM	RSI	IV	1.2 mg/kg	48 mg	10 mg/mL	4.8 mL
VECURONIUM		IV	0.1 mg/kg	4 mg	1 mg/mL	4 mL
GLYCOPYRROLATE	reversal	IV	0.007 mg/kg	0.28 mg	0.2 mg/mL	1.4 mL
NEOSTIGMINE		IV	0.07 mg/kg	2.8 mg	1 mg/mL	2.8 mL
DEXAMETHASONE		IV	0.25 mg/kg	10 mg	10 mg/mL	1 mL
ONDANSETRON		IV	0.15 mg/kg	4 mg	2 mg/mL	2 mL

additional pediatric drugs	route	dose	mg to pt	supplied	mL to give
PREMED/SEDATION; VAGOLYTIC/ANTISIALAGOGUE; GIVE IM 30-60 MIN PREOP					
ATROPINE	IM	0.02 mg/kg	0.5 mg	0.4 mg/mL	1.25 mL
GLYCOPYRROLATE	IM	0.004 mg/kg	0.009 mg	0.2 mg/mL	0.045 mL
MIDAZOLAM	IM	0.1 mg/kg	0.5 mg	1 mg/mL	0.5 mL
DEXMEDETOMIDINE load dose	IV	0.5 mcg/kg	1 mcg	4 mcg/mL	0.25 mL
INDUCTION					
KETAMINE	IV	2 mg/kg	80 mg	10 mg/mL	8 mL
KETAMINE	IM/PR	5 mg/kg	200 mg	10 mg/mL	20 mL
OPIOIDS/NONOPIOIDS					
FENTANYL high dose	IV	4 mcg/kg	160 mcg	50 mcg/mL	3.2 mL
FENTANYL cardiac	IV	10 mcg/kg	400 mcg	50 mcg/mL	8 mL
HYDROMORPHONE <6 mo	IV/SQ	0.005 mg/kg	0.2 mg	10 mg/mL	0.02 mL
HYDROMORPHONE >6 mo	IV/SQ	0.015 mg/kg	0.6 mg	10 mg/mL	0.06 mL
REMIFENTANIL	IV	0.5 mcg/kg	1 mcg	50 mcg/mL	0.02 mL
SUFENTANIL	IV	0.5 mcg/kg	20 mcg	50 mcg/mL	0.4 mL
REVERSALS					
ATROPINE	IV	0.02 mg/kg	0.5 mg	0.4 mg/mL	1.25 mL
EDROPHONIUM neonate	IV	0.1 mg single dose		10 mg/mL	0.01 mL
EDROPHONIUM >2 mo	IV	0.04 mg/kg	1.6 mg	10 mg/mL	0.16 mL
FLUMAZENIL <1 y	IV	0.01 mg/kg	0.2 mg	0.1 mg/mL	2 mL
NALOXONE <5 y; <20 kg	IV/IM	0.1 mg/kg	2 mg	0.4 mg/mL	5 mL
NALOXONE <5 y; >20 kg	IV/IM	2 mg per dose		0.4 mg/mL	5 mL
NALOXONE	ETT	0.3 mg/kg	12 mg	0.4 mg/mL	30 mL

additional pediatric drugs		route	dose	mg to pt	supplied	mL to give
ANTIBIOTICS						
AMPICILLIN	<6 y	IV	50 mg/kg	300 mg		
AMPICILLIN	>6 y	IV	50 mg/kg	2,000 mg		
AMPICILLIN & SULBACTUM	>1 mo	IV	50 mg/kg	2,000 mg		
CEFAZOLIN		IV	25 mg/kg	1,000 mg		
CLINDAMYCIN		IV	10 mg/kg	400 mg		
ERTAPENEM	3 mo-12 y	IV	15 mg/kg	600 mg		
ERTAPENEM	>12 y	IV	1 Gm	per dose		
GENTAMICIN		IV	2 mg/kg	80 mg		
LEVOFLOXACIN		IV	10 mg/kg	400 mg		
METRONIDAZOLE		IV	10 mg/kg	400 mg		
PIPERACILLIN & TAZOBACTAM	<40 kg & 2-9 mo	IV	80 mg/kg	3,200 mg		
PIPERACILLIN & TAZOBACTAM	<40 kg & >9 mo	IV	100 mg/kg	3,375 mg		
PIPERACILLIN & TAZOBACTAM	>40 kg	IV	3.375 Gm per dose			
VANCOMYCIN		IV	15 mg/kg	600 mg		
ANTINAUSEA						
METOCLOPROMIDE		IV	0.2 mg/kg	8 mg	5 mg/mL	1.6 mL
DIPHENHYDRAMINE		IV/IM	1.25 mg/kg	50 mg	50 mg/mL	1 mL
SCOPOLAMINE		IV/IM	6 mcg/kg	240 mcg	400 mcg/mL	0.6 mL
MISCELLANEOUS MEDS						
AMINOCAPROIC ACID		IV	100 mg/kg	4,000 mg	250 mg/mL	16 mL
DESMOPRESSIN		IV/SQ	0.3 mcg/kg	12 mcg	4 mcg/mL	3 mL
DEXAMETHASONE	croup	IV	0.6 mg/kg	16 mg	4 mg/mL	4 mL
HYDROCORTISONE		IV/IO	3 mg/kg	100 mg	100 mg/mL	1 mL

40 KG

1 year ← 13 year and up

Ventilation: trained rescuer	1 breath q 6-8 sec (8-10 breaths/minute) about 1 second/breath-visible chest rise; if intubated, continuous compressions without pause for ventilations
Pulse check	carotid or femoral
Compression	heel of 1 hand or both hands atop the other-lower half of sternum between nipples
Depth	2 inches (5 cm) or at least 1/3 chest depth
Rate	at least 100 compressions per minute
Compress/vent ratio	30:2 single rescuer / 15:2 2 healthcare providers
Foreign body obstruction	Heimlich maneuver. Never perform a blind finger-sweep. Open the mouth and look for object; if you see it, remove it.

sync cardioversion	0.5 J/kg	20 J
	1 J/kg repeat	40 J
defibrillation	2 J/kg	80 J
	4 J/kg repeat	160 J

IV Bolus Drugs		dose	mg to pt	supplied	mL to give
ADENOSINE	IV	0.1 mg/kg	4 mg	3 mg/mL	1.33 mL
ADENOSINE repeat dose	IV	0.2 mg/kg	8 mg	3 mg/mL	2.67 mL
AMIODARONE	IV/IO	5 mg/kg	200 mg	50 mg/mL	4.00 mL
ATROPINE	IV/IM	0.02 mg/kg	0.5 mg	0.4 mg/mL	1.25 mL
ATROPINE	ETT	0.04 mg/kg	1.6 mg	0.4 mg/mL	4.00 mL
CALCIUM CHLORIDE	IV	20 mg/kg	800 mg	100 mg/mL	8.00 mL
CALCIUM GLUCONATE	IV/IO	60 mg/kg	800 mg	100 mg/mL	8.00 mL
DANTROLENE	IV	2.5 mg/kg	30 mg		
EPHEDRINE	IV	0.15 mg/kg	6 mg	10 mg/mL	0.60 mL
EPINEPHRINE (1:10,000)	IV/IO	0.01 mg/kg	0.4 mg	0.1 mg/mL	4.00 mL
EPINEPHRINE (1:1,000)	ETT	0.1 mg/kg	2.5 mg	1 mg/mL	2.50 mL
ESMOLOL	IV	0.5 mg/kg	20 mg	10 mg/mL	2.00 mL
LABETALOL	IV	0.2 mg/kg	8 mg	5 mg/mL	1.60 mL
LIDOCAINE	IV/IO	1 mg/kg	40 mg	20 mg/mL	2.00 mL
NEOSYNEPHRINE	IV	5 mcg/kg	200 mcg	100 mcg/mL	2.00 mL
ROMAZICON	IV	0.01 mg/kg	0.2 mg	0.1 mg/mL	2.00 mL
VASOPRESSIN	IV/IO	0.4 unit/kg	16 units	20 u/mL	0.80 mL

41 KG MAINTENANCE IV FLUIDS: 81 ML/HR

common pediatric drugs		route	dose	mg to pt	supplied	mL to give
ATROPINE	vagolytic	IV	0.02 mg/kg	0.5 mg	0.4 mg/mL	1.25 mL
GLYCOPYRROLATE	vagolytic	IV	0.004 mg/kg	0.164 mg	0.2 mg/mL	0.82 mL
MIDAZOLAM		IV	0.05 mg/kg	0.6 mg	1 mg/mL	0.6 mL
MIDAZOLAM		PO	0.5 mg/kg	20 mg	1 mg/mL	20 mL
MIDAZOLAM		IN	0.2 mg/kg	8.2 mg	1 mg/mL	8.2 mL
SUCCINYLCHOLINE		IV	2 mg/kg	82 mg	20 mg/mL	4.1 mL
SUCCINYLCHOLINE		IM	4 mg/kg	164 mg	20 mg/mL	8.2 mL
PROPOFOL		IV	3 mg/kg	123 mg	10 mg/mL	12.3 mL
ETOMIDATE	>10 y	IV	0.3 mg/kg	12.3 mg	2 mg/mL	6.15 mL
FENTANYL		IV	1 mcg/kg	41 mcg	50 mcg/mL	0.82 mL
FENTANYL		IN	2 mcg/kg	82 mcg	50 mcg/mL	1.64 mL
MORPHINE	<6 mo	IV/IM	0.05 mg/kg	2.05 mg	10 mg/mL	0.205 mL
MORPHINE	>6 mo	IV/IM	0.1 mg/kg	4.1 mg	10 mg/mL	0.41 mL
TORADOL	>2-16 y	IV	0.5 mg/kg	15 mg	30 mg/mL	0.5 mL
TORADOL	>2-16 y	IM	1 mg/kg	30 mg	30 mg/mL	1 mL
ACETAMINOPHEN		PR	20 mg/kg	820 mg		
ACETAMINOPHEN	2-12 y	IV	15 mg/kg	615 mg	10 mg/mL	61.5 mL
CISATRACURIUM		IV	0.1 mg/kg	4.1 mg	2 mg/mL	2.05 mL
PANCURONIUM	<1 mo	IV	0.02 mg/kg	0.82 mg	1 mg/mL	0.82 mL
PANCURONIUM	>1 mo	IV	0.1 mg/kg	4.1 mg	1 mg/mL	4.1 mL
ROCURONIUM		IV	0.6 mg/kg	24.6 mg	10 mg/mL	2.46 mL
ROCURONIUM	RSI	IV	1.2 mg/kg	49.2 mg	10 mg/mL	4.92 mL
VECURONIUM		IV	0.1 mg/kg	4.1 mg	1 mg/mL	4.1 mL
GLYCOPYRROLATE	reversal	IV	0.007 mg/kg	0.287 mg	0.2 mg/mL	1.435 mL
NEOSTIGMINE		IV	0.07 mg/kg	2.87 mg	1 mg/mL	2.87 mL
DEXAMETHASONE		IV	0.25 mg/kg	10 mg	10 mg/mL	1 mL
ONDANSETRON		IV	0.15 mg/kg	4 mg	2 mg/mL	2 mL

additional pediatric drugs	route	dose	mg to pt	supplied	mL to give
PREMED/SEDATION; VAGOLYTIC/ANTISIALAGOGUE; GIVE IM 30-60 MIN PREOP					
ATROPINE	IM	0.02 mg/kg	0.5 mg	0.4 mg/mL	1.25 mL
GLYCOPYRROLATE	IM	0.004 mg/kg	0.009 mg	0.2 mg/mL	0.045 mL
MIDAZOLAM	IM	0.1 mg/kg	0.5 mg	1 mg/mL	0.5 mL
DEXMEDETOMIDINE load dose	IV	0.5 mcg/kg	1 mcg	4 mcg/mL	0.25 mL
INDUCTION					
KETAMINE	IV	2 mg/kg	82 mg	10 mg/mL	8.2 mL
KETAMINE	IM/PR	5 mg/kg	205 mg	10 mg/mL	20.5 mL
OPIOIDS/NONOPIOIDS					
FENTANYL	IV	high dose 4 mcg/kg	164 mcg	50 mcg/mL	3.28 mL
FENTANYL	IV	cardiac 10 mcg/kg	410 mcg	50 mcg/mL	8.2 mL
HYDROMORPHONE < 6 mo	IV/SQ	0.005 mg/kg	0.205 mg	10 mg/mL	0.0205 mL
HYDROMORPHONE > 6 mo	IV/SQ	0.015 mg/kg	0.615 mg	10 mg/mL	0.0615 mL
REMIFENTANIL	IV	0.5 mcg/kg	1 mcg	50 mcg/mL	0.02 mL
SUFENTANIL	IV	0.5 mcg/kg	20 mcg	50 mcg/mL	0.4 mL
REVERSALS					
ATROPINE	IV	0.02 mg/kg	0.5 mg	0.4 mg/mL	1.25 mL
EDROPHONIUM neonate	IV	0.1 mg single dose	10 mg	10 mg/mL	0.01 mL
EDROPHONIUM > 2 mo	IV	0.04 mg/kg	1.64 mg	10 mg/mL	0.164 mL
FLUMAZENIL > 1 y	IV	0.01 mg/kg	0.2 mg	0.1 mg/mL	2 mL
NALOXONE < 5 y; < 20 kg	IM/IV	0.1 mg/kg	2 mg	0.4 mg/mL	5 mL
NALOXONE > 5 y; > 20 kg	IM/IV	2 mg per dose		0.4 mg/mL	5 mL
NALOXONE	ETT	0.3 mg/kg	12.3 mg	0.4 mg/mL	30.75 mL

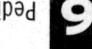

additional pediatric drugs		route	dose	mg to pt	supplied	mL to give
ANTIBIOTICS						
AMPICILLIN	<6 y	IV	50 mg/kg	300 mg		
AMPICILLIN	>6 y	IV	50 mg/kg	2,000 mg		
AMPICILLIN & SULBACTUM	>1 mo	IV	50 mg/kg	2,050 mg		
CEFAZOLIN		IV	25 mg/kg	1,000 mg		
CLINDAMYCIN		IV	10 mg/kg	410 mg		
ERTAPENEM	3 mo-12 y	IV	15 mg/kg	615 mg		
ERTAPENEM	>12 y	IV	1 Gm	per dose		
GENTAMICIN		IV	2 mg/kg	82 mg		
LEVOFLOXACIN		IV	10 mg/kg	410 mg		
METRONIDAZOLE		IV	10 mg/kg	410 mg		
PIPERACILLIN & TAZOBACTAM	<40 kg & 2-9 mo	IV	80 mg/kg	3,280 mg		
PIPERACILLIN & TAZOBACTAM	<40 kg & >9 mo	IV	100 mg/kg	3,375 mg		
PIPERACILLIN & TAZOBACTAM	>40 kg	IV	3.375 Gm per dose			
VANCOMYCIN		IV	15 mg/kg	615 mg		
ANTINAUSEA						
METOCLOPROMIDE		IV	0.2 mg/kg	8.2 mg	5 mg/mL	1.64 mL
DIPHENHYDRAMINE		IV/IM	1.25 mg/kg	51.25 mg	50 mg/mL	1.025 mL
SCOPOLAMINE		IV/IM	6 mcg/kg	246 mcg	400 mcg/mL	0.615 mL
MISCELLANEOUS MEDS						
AMINOCAPROIC ACID		IV	100 mg/kg	4,100 mg	250 mg/mL	16.4 mL
DESMOPRESSIN		IV/SQ	0.3 mcg/kg	12.3 mcg	4 mcg/mL	3.075 mL
DEXAMETHASONE	croup	IV	0.6 mg/kg	16 mg	4 mg/mL	4 mL
HYDROCORTISONE		IV/IO	3 mg/kg	100 mg	100 mg/mL	1 mL

41 KG

1 year → 13 kg and up

Ventilation: trained rescuer	1 breath q 6-8 sec (8-10 breaths/minute) about 1 second/ breath-visible chest rise; if intubated, continuous compressions without pause for ventilations
Pulse check	carotid or femoral
Compression	heel of 1 hand or both hands one atop the other-lower half of sternum between nipples
Depth	2 inches (5 cm) or at least 1/3 chest depth
Rate	at least 100 compressions per minute
Compress/vent ratio	30:2 single rescuer 15:2 2 healthcare providers
Foreign body obstruction	Heimlich maneuver Never perform a blind finger-sweep. Open the mouth and look for object; if you see it, remove it.

sync cardioversion	0.5 J/kg	20.5 J
defibrillation	1 J/kg	41 J
repeat	2 J/kg	82 J
repeat	4 J/kg	164 J

IV Bolus Drugs		dose	mg to pt	supplied	mL to give
ADENOSINE	IV	0.1 mg/kg	4.1 mg	3 mg/mL	1.37 mL
ADENOSINE repeat dose	IV	0.2 mg/kg	8.2 mg	3 mg/mL	2.73 mL
AMIODARONE	IV/IO	5 mg/kg	205 mg	50 mg/mL	4.10 mL
ATROPINE	IV/IM	0.02 mg/kg	0.5 mg	0.4 mg/mL	1.25 mL
ATROPINE	ETT	0.04 mg/kg	1.64 mg	0.4 mg/mL	4.10 mL
CALCIUM CHLORIDE	IV	20 mg/kg	820 mg	100 mg/mL	8.20 mL
CALCIUM GLUCONATE	IV/IO	60 mg/kg	800 mg	100 mg/mL	8.00 mL
DANTROLENE	IV	2.5 mg/kg	30 mg		
EPHEDRINE	IV	0.15 mg/kg	6.15 mg	10 mg/mL	0.62 mL
EPINEPHRINE (1:10,000)	IV/IO	0.01 mg/kg	0.41 mg	0.1 mg/mL	4.10 mL
EPINEPHRINE (1:1,000)	ETT	0.1 mg/kg	2.5 mg	1 mg/mL	2.50 mL
ESMOLOL	IV	0.5 mg/kg	20.5 mg	10 mg/mL	2.05 mL
LABETALOL	IV	0.2 mg/kg	8.2 mg	5 mg/mL	1.64 mL
LIDOCAINE	IV/IO	1 mg/kg	41 mg	100 mcg/mL	2.05 mL
NEOSYNEPHRINE	IV	5 mcg/kg	205 mcg	100 mcg/mL	2.05 mL
ROMAZICON	IV	0.01 mg/kg	0.2 mg	0.1 mg/mL	2.00 mL
VASOPRESSIN	IV/IO	0.4 unit/kg	16.4 units	20 u/mL	0.82 mL

42 KG MAINTENANCE IV FLUIDS: 82 ML/HR

common pediatric drugs		route	dose	mg to pt	supplied	mL to give
ATROPINE	vagolytic	IV	0.02 mg/kg	0.5 mg	0.4 mg/mL	1.25 mL
GLYCOPYRROLATE	vagolytic	IV	0.004 mg/kg	0.168 mg	0.2 mg/mL	0.84 mL
MIDAZOLAM		IV	0.05 mg/kg	0.6 mg	1 mg/mL	0.6 mL
MIDAZOLAM		PO	0.5 mg/kg	20 mg	1 mg/mL	20 mL
MIDAZOLAM		IN	0.2 mg/kg	8.4 mg	1 mg/mL	8.4 mL
SUCCINYLCHOLINE		IV	2 mg/kg	84 mg	20 mg/mL	4.2 mL
SUCCINYLCHOLINE		IM	4 mg/kg	168 mg	20 mg/mL	8.4 mL
PROPOFOL		IV	3 mg/kg	126 mg	10 mg/mL	12.6 mL
ETOMIDATE	>10 y	IV	0.3 mg/kg	12.6 mg	2 mg/mL	6.3 mL
FENTANYL		IV	1 mcg/kg	42 mcg	50 mcg/mL	0.84 mL
FENTANYL		IN	2 mcg/kg	84 mcg	50 mcg/mL	1.68 mL
MORPHINE	<6 mo	IV/IM	0.05 mg/kg	2.1 mg	10 mg/mL	0.21 mL
MORPHINE	>6 mo	IV/IM	0.1 mg/kg	4.2 mg	10 mg/mL	0.42 mL
TORADOL	>2-16 y	IV	0.5 mg/kg	15 mg	30 mg/mL	0.5 mL
TORADOL	>2-16 y	IM	1 mg/kg	30 mg	30 mg/mL	1 mL
ACETAMINOPHEN		PR	20 mg/kg	840 mg		
ACETAMINOPHEN	2-12 y	IV	15 mg/kg	630 mg	10 mg/mL	63 mL
CISATRACURIUM		IV	0.1 mg/kg	4.2 mg	2 mg/mL	2.1 mL
PANCURONIUM	<1 mo	IV	0.02 mg/kg	0.84 mg	1 mg/mL	0.84 mL
PANCURONIUM	>1 mo	IV	0.1 mg/kg	4.2 mg	1 mg/mL	4.2 mL
ROCURONIUM		IV	0.6 mg/kg	25.2 mg	10 mg/mL	2.52 mL
ROCURONIUM	RSI	IV	1.2 mg/kg	50.4 mg	10 mg/mL	5.04 mL
VECURONIUM		IV	0.1 mg/kg	4.2 mg	1 mg/mL	4.2 mL
GLYCOPYRROLATE	reversal	IV	0.007 mg/kg	0.294 mg	0.2 mg/mL	1.47 mL
NEOSTIGMINE		IV	0.07 mg/kg	2.94 mg	1 mg/mL	2.94 mL
DEXAMETHASONE		IV	0.25 mg/kg	10 mg	10 mg/mL	1 mL
ONDANSETRON		IV	0.15 mg/kg	4 mg	2 mg/mL	2 mL

additional pediatric drugs	route	dose	mg to pt	supplied	mL to give
PREMED/SEDATION; VAGOLYTIC/ANTISIALAGOGUE; GIVE IM 30-60 MIN PREOP					
ATROPINE	IM	0.02 mg/kg	0.5 mg	0.4 mg/mL	1.25 mL
GLYCOPYRROLATE	IM	0.004 mg/kg	0.009 mg	0.2 mg/mL	0.045 mL
MIDAZOLAM	IM	0.1 mg/kg	0.5 mg	1 mg/mL	0.5 mL
DEXMEDETOMIDINE load dose	IV	0.5 mcg/kg	1 mcg	4 mcg/mL	0.25 mL
INDUCTION					
KETAMINE	IV	2 mg/kg	84 mg	10 mg/mL	8.4 mL
KETAMINE	IM/PR	5 mg/kg	210 mg	10 mg/mL	21 mL
OPIOIDS/NONOPIOIDS					
FENTANYL	IV	high dose 4 mcg/kg	168 mcg	50 mcg/mL	3.36 mL
FENTANYL	IV	cardiac 10 mcg/kg	420 mcg	50 mcg/mL	8.4 mL
HYDROMORPHONE <6 mo	IV/SQ	0.005 mg/kg	0.21 mg	10 mg/mL	0.021 mL
HYDROMORPHONE >6 mo	IV/SQ	0.015 mg/kg	0.63 mg	10 mg/mL	0.063 mL
REMIFENTANIL	IV	0.5 mcg/kg	1 mcg	50 mcg/mL	0.02 mL
SUFENTANIL	IV	0.5 mcg/kg	20 mcg	50 mcg/mL	0.4 mL
REVERSALS					
ATROPINE	IV	0.02 mg/kg	0.5 mg	0.4 mg/mL	1.25 mL
EDROPHONIUM neonate	IV	0.1 mg single dose		10 mg/mL	0.01 mL
EDROPHONIUM >2 mo	IV	0.04 mg/kg	1.68 mg	10 mg/mL	0.168 mL
FLUMAZENIL >1 y	IV	0.01 mg/kg	0.2 mg	0.1 mg/mL	2 mL
NALOXONE <5 y; <20 kg	IV/IM	0.1 mg/kg	2 mg	0.4 mg/mL	5 mL
NALOXONE <5 y; >20 kg	IV/IM	2 mg per dose		0.4 mg/mL	5 mL
NALOXONE	ETT	0.3 mg/kg	12.6 mg	0.4 mg/mL	31.5 mL

additional pediatric drugs		route	dose	mg to pt	supplied	mL to give
ANTIBIOTICS						
AMPICILLIN	<6 y	IV	50 mg/kg	300 mg		
AMPICILLIN	>6 y	IV	50 mg/kg	2,000 mg		
AMPICILLIN & SULBACTUM	>1 mo	IV	50 mg/kg	2,100 mg		
CEFAZOLIN		IV	25 mg/kg	1,000 mg		
CLINDAMYCIN		IV	10 mg/kg	420 mg		
ERTAPENEM	3 mo-12 y	IV	15 mg/kg	630 mg		
ERTAPENEM	>12 y	IV	1 Gm	per dose		
GENTAMICIN		IV	2 mg/kg	84 mg		
LEVOFLOXACIN		IV	10 mg/kg	420 mg		
METRONIDAZOLE		IV	10 mg/kg	420 mg		
PIPERACILLIN & TAZOBACTAM	<40 kg & 2-9 mo	IV	80 mg/kg	3,360 mg		
PIPERACILLIN & TAZOBACTAM	<40 kg & >9 mo	IV	100 mg/kg	3,375 mg		
PIPERACILLIN & TAZOBACTAM	>40 kg	IV	3.375 Gm per dose			
VANCOMYCIN		IV	15 mg/kg	630 mg		
ANTINAUSEA						
METOCLOPROMIDE		IV	0.2 mg/kg	8.4 mg	5 mg/mL	1.68 mL
DIPHENHYDRAMINE		IV/IM	1.25 mg/kg	52.5 mg	50 mg/mL	1.05 mL
SCOPOLAMINE		IV/IM	6 mcg/kg	252 mcg	400 mcg/mL	0.63 mL
MISCELLANEOUS MEDS						
AMINOCAPROIC ACID		IV	100 mg/kg	4,200 mg	250 mg/mL	16.8 mL
DESMOPRESSIN		IV/SQ	0.3 mcg/kg	12.6 mcg	4 mcg/mL	3.15 mL
DEXAMETHASONE	croup	IV	0.6 mg/kg	16 mg	4 mg/mL	4 mL
HYDROCORTISONE		IV/IO	3 mg/kg	100 mg	100 mg/mL	1 mL

42 KG
1 year → 13 kg and up

Ventilation: trained rescuer	1 breath q 6-8 sec (8-10 breaths/minute) about 1 second/ breath-visible chest rise; if intubated, continuous compressions without pause for ventilations
Pulse check	carotid or femoral
Compression	heel of 1 hand or both hands one atop the other-lower half of sternum between nipples
Depth	2 inches (5 cm) or at least 1/3 chest depth
Rate	at least 100 compressions per minute
Compress/vent ratio	30:2 single rescuer 15:2 2 healthcare providers
Foreign body obstruction	Heimlich maneuver Never perform a blind finger-sweep. Open the mouth and look for object; if you see it, remove it.

sync cardioversion	0.5 J/kg	21 J
defibrillation	1 J/kg	42 J
repeat	2 J/kg	84 J
repeat	4 J/kg	168 J

IV Bolus Drugs		dose	mg to pt	supplied	mL to give
ADENOSINE	IV	0.1 mg/kg	4.2 mg	3 mg/mL	1.40 mL
ADENOSINE repeat dose	IV	0.2 mg/kg	8.4 mg	3 mg/mL	2.80 mL
AMIODARONE	IV/IO	5 mg/kg	210 mg	50 mg/mL	4.20 mL
ATROPINE	IM/IV	0.02 mg/kg	0.5 mg	0.5 mg/mL	1.25 mL
ATROPINE	ETT	0.04 mg/kg	1.68 mg	0.4 mg/mL	4.20 mL
CALCIUM CHLORIDE	IV	20 mg/kg	840 mg	100 mg/mL	8.40 mL
CALCIUM GLUCONATE	IV/IO	60 mg/kg	800 mg	100 mg/mL	8.00 mL
DANTROLENE	IV	2.5 mg/kg	30 mg		
EPHEDRINE	IV	0.15 mg/kg	6.3 mg	10 mg/mL	0.63 mL
EPINEPHRINE (1:10,000)	IV/IO	0.01 mg/kg	0.42 mg	0.1 mg/mL	4.20 mL
EPINEPHRINE (1:1,000)	ETT	0.1 mg/kg	2.5 mg	1 mg/mL	2.50 mL
ESMOLOL	IV	0.5 mg/kg	21 mg	10 mg/mL	2.10 mL
LABETALOL	IV	0.2 mg/kg	8.4 mg	5 mg/mL	1.68 mL
LIDOCAINE	IV/IO	1 mg/kg	42 mg	20 mg/mL	2.10 mL
NEOSYNEPHRINE	IV	5 mcg/kg	210 mcg	100 mcg/mL	2.10 mL
ROMAZICON	IV	0.01 mg/kg	0.2 mg	0.1 mg/mL	2.00 mL
VASOPRESSIN	IV/IO	0.4 unit/kg	16.8 units	20 u/mL	0.84 mL

43 KG MAINTENANCE IV FLUIDS: 83 ML/HR

common pediatric drugs		route	dose	mg to pt	supplied	mL to give
ATROPINE	vagolytic	IV	0.02 mg/kg	0.5 mg	0.4 mg/mL	1.25 mL
GLYCOPYRROLATE	vagolytic	IV	0.004 mg/kg	0.172 mg	0.2 mg/mL	0.86 mL
MIDAZOLAM		IV	0.05 mg/kg	0.6 mg	1 mg/mL	0.6 mL
MIDAZOLAM		PO	0.5 mg/kg	20 mg	1 mg/mL	20 mL
MIDAZOLAM		IN	0.2 mg/kg	8.6 mg	1 mg/mL	8.6 mL
SUCCINYLCHOLINE		IV	2 mg/kg	86 mg	20 mg/mL	4.3 mL
SUCCINYLCHOLINE		IM	4 mg/kg	172 mg	20 mg/mL	8.6 mL
PROPOFOL		IV	3 mg/kg	129 mg	10 mg/mL	12.9 mL
ETOMIDATE	>10 y	IV	0.3 mg/kg	12.9 mg	2 mg/mL	6.45 mL
FENTANYL		IV	1 mcg/kg	43 mcg	50 mcg/mL	0.86 mL
FENTANYL		IN	2 mcg/kg	86 mcg	50 mcg/mL	1.72 mL
MORPHINE	<6 mo	IV/IM	0.05 mg/kg	2.15 mg	10 mg/mL	0.215 mL
MORPHINE	>6 mo	IV/IM	0.1 mg/kg	4.3 mg	10 mg/mL	0.43 mL
TORADOL	>2-16 y	IV	0.5 mg/kg	15 mg	30 mg/mL	0.5 mL
TORADOL	>2-16 y	IM	1 mg/kg	30 mg	30 mg/mL	1 mL
ACETAMINOPHEN		PR	20 mg/kg	860 mg		
ACETAMINOPHEN	2-12 y	IV	15 mg/kg	645 mg	10 mg/mL	64.5 mL
CISATRACURIUM		IV	0.1 mg/kg	4.3 mg	2 mg/mL	2.15 mL
PANCURONIUM	<1 mo	IV	0.02 mg/kg	0.86 mg	1 mg/mL	0.86 mL
PANCURONIUM	>1 mo	IV	0.1 mg/kg	4.3 mg	1 mg/mL	4.3 mL
ROCURONIUM		IV	0.6 mg/kg	25.8 mg	10 mg/mL	2.58 mL
ROCURONIUM	RSI	IV	1.2 mg/kg	51.6 mg	10 mg/mL	5.16 mL
VECURONIUM		IV	0.1 mg/kg	4.3 mg	1 mg/mL	4.3 mL
GLYCOPYRROLATE	reversal	IV	0.007 mg/kg	0.301 mg	0.2 mg/mL	1.505 mL
NEOSTIGMINE		IV	0.07 mg/kg	3.01 mg	1 mg/mL	3.01 mL
DEXAMETHASONE		IV	0.25 mg/kg	10 mg	10 mg/mL	1 mL
ONDANSETRON		IV	0.15 mg/kg	4 mg	2 mg/mL	2 mL

additional pediatric drugs	route	dose	mg to pt	supplied	mL to give
PREMED/SEDATION; VAGOLYTIC/ANTISIALAGOGUE; GIVE IM 30–60 MIN PREOP					
ATROPINE	IM	0.02 mg/kg	0.5 mg	0.4 mg/mL	1.25 mL
GLYCOPYRROLATE	IM	0.004 mg/kg	0.009 mg	0.2 mg/mL	0.045 mL
MIDAZOLAM	IM	0.1 mg/kg	0.5 mg	1 mg/mL	0.5 mL
DEXMEDETOMIDINE load dose	IV	0.5 mcg/kg	1 mcg	4 mcg/mL	0.25 mL
INDUCTION					
KETAMINE	IV	2 mg/kg	86 mg	10 mg/mL	8.6 mL
KETAMINE	IM/PR	5 mg/kg	215 mg	10 mg/mL	21.5 mL
OPIOIDS/NONOPIOIDS					
FENTANYL high dose	IV	4 mcg/kg	172 mcg	50 mcg/mL	3.44 mL
FENTANYL cardiac	IV	10 mcg/kg	430 mcg	50 mcg/mL	8.6 mL
HYDROMORPHONE < 6 mo	IV/SQ	0.005 mg/kg	0.215 mg	10 mg/mL	0.0215 mL
HYDROMORPHONE > 6 mo	IV/SQ	0.015 mg/kg	0.645 mg	10 mg/mL	0.0645 mL
REMIFENTANIL	IV	0.5 mcg/kg	1 mcg	50 mcg/mL	0.02 mL
SUFENTANIL	IV	0.5 mcg/kg	20 mcg	50 mcg/mL	0.4 mL
REVERSALS					
ATROPINE	IV	0.02 mg/kg	0.5 mg	0.4 mg/mL	1.25 mL
EDROPHONIUM neonate	IV	0.1 mg single dose		10 mg/mL	0.01 mL
EDROPHONIUM > 2 mo	IV	0.04 mg/kg	1.72 mg	10 mg/mL	0.172 mL
FLUMAZENIL > 1 y	IV	0.01 mg/kg	0.2 mg	0.1 mg/mL	2 mL
NALOXONE < 5 y; < 20 kg	IM	0.1 mg/kg	2 mg	0.4 mg/mL	5 mL
NALOXONE < 5 y; > 20 kg	IV/IM	2 mg per dose		0.4 mg/mL	5 mL
NALOXONE	ETT	0.3 mg/kg	12.9 mg	0.4 mg/mL	32.25 mL

additional pediatric drugs		route	dose	mg to pt	supplied	mL to give
ANTIBIOTICS						
AMPICILLIN	<6 y	IV	50 mg/kg	300 mg		
AMPICILLIN	>6 y	IV	50 mg/kg	2,000 mg		
AMPICILLIN & SULBACTUM	>1 mo	IV	50 mg/kg	2,150 mg		
CEFAZOLIN		IV	25 mg/kg	1,000 mg		
CLINDAMYCIN		IV	10 mg/kg	430 mg		
ERTAPENEM	3 mo-12 y	IV	15 mg/kg	645 mg		
ERTAPENEM	>12 y	IV	1 Gm	per dose		
GENTAMICIN		IV	2 mg/kg	86 mg		
LEVOFLOXACIN		IV	10 mg/kg	430 mg		
METRONIDAZOLE		IV	10 mg/kg	430 mg		
PIPERACILLIN & TAZOBACTAM	<40 kg & 2-9 mo	IV	80 mg/kg	3,375 mg		
PIPERACILLIN & TAZOBACTAM	<40 kg & >9 mo	IV	100 mg/kg	3,375 mg		
PIPERACILLIN & TAZOBACTAM	>40 kg	IV	3.375 Gm per dose			
VANCOMYCIN		IV	15 mg/kg	645 mg		
ANTINAUSEA						
METOCLOPROMIDE		IV	0.2 mg/kg	8.6 mg	5 mg/mL	1.72 mL
DIPHENHYDRAMINE		IV/IM	1.25 mg/kg	53.75 mg	50 mg/mL	1.075 mL
SCOPOLAMINE		IV/IM	6 mcg/kg	258 mcg	400 mcg/mL	0.645 mL
MISCELLANEOUS MEDS						
AMINOCAPROIC ACID		IV	100 mg/kg	4,300 mg	250 mg/mL	17.2 mL
DESMOPRESSIN		IV/SQ	0.3 mcg/kg	12.9 mcg	4 mcg/mL	3.225 mL
DEXAMETHASONE	croup	IV	0.6 mg/kg	16 mg	4 mg/mL	4 mL
HYDROCORTISONE		IV/IO	3 mg/kg	100 mg	100 mg/mL	1 mL

43 KG

1 year ← 13 kg and up

Ventilation: trained rescuer	1 breath q 6-8 sec (8-10 breaths/minute) about 1 second/ breath-visible chest rise; if intubated, continuous compressions without pause for ventilations
Pulse check	carotid or femoral
Compression	heel of 1 hand or both hands one atop the other-lower half of sternum between nipples
Depth	2 inches (5 cm) or at least 1/3 chest depth
Rate	at least 100 compressions per minute
Compress/vent ratio	30:2 single rescuer / 15:2 2 healthcare providers
Foreign body obstruction	Heimlich maneuver - Never perform a blind finger-sweep. Open the mouth and look for object; if you see it, remove it.

sync cardioversion	0.5 J/kg	21.5 J	
defibrillation	1 J/kg	43 J	repeat
	2 J/kg	86 J	
repeat	4 J/kg	172 J	

IV Bolus Drugs		dose	mg to pt	supplied	mL to give
ADENOSINE	IV	0.1 mg/kg	4.3 mg	3 mg/mL	1.43 mL
ADENOSINE repeat dose	IV	0.2 mg/kg	8.6 mg	3 mg/mL	2.87 mL
AMIODARONE	IV/IO	5 mg/kg	215 mg	50 mg/mL	4.30 mL
ATROPINE	IM/IV	0.02 mg/kg	0.5 mg	0.4 mg/mL	1.25 mL
ATROPINE	ETT	0.04 mg/kg	1.72 mg	0.4 mg/mL	4.30 mL
CALCIUM CHLORIDE	IV	20 mg/kg	860 mg	100 mg/mL	8.60 mL
CALCIUM GLUCONATE	IV/IO	60 mg/kg	800 mg	100 mg/mL	8.00 mL
DANTROLENE	IV	2.5 mg/kg		30 mg	
EPHEDRINE	IV	0.15 mg/kg	6.45 mg	10 mg/mL	0.65 mL
EPINEPHRINE (1:10,000)	IV/IO	0.01 mg/kg	0.43 mg	0.1 mg/mL	4.30 mL
EPINEPHRINE (1:1,000)	ETT	0.1 mg/kg	2.5 mg	1 mg/mL	2.50 mL
ESMOLOL	IV	0.5 mg/kg	21.5 mg	10 mg/mL	2.15 mL
LABETALOL	IV	0.2 mg/kg	8.6 mg	5 mg/mL	1.72 mL
LIDOCAINE	IV/IO	1 mg/kg	43 mg	20 mg/mL	2.15 mL
NEOSYNEPHRINE	IV	5 mcg/kg	215 mcg	100 mcg/mL	2.15 mL
ROMAZICON	IV	0.01 mg/kg	0.2 mg	0.1 mg/mL	2.00 mL
VASOPRESSIN	IV/IO	0.4 unit/kg	17.2 units	20 u/mL	0.86 mL

44 KG MAINTENANCE IV FLUIDS: 84 ML/HR

common pediatric drugs		route	dose	mg to pt	supplied	mL to give
ATROPINE	vagolytic	IV	0.02 mg/kg	0.5 mg	0.4 mg/mL	1.25 mL
GLYCOPYRROLATE	vagolytic	IV	0.004 mg/kg	0.176 mg	0.2 mg/mL	0.88 mL
MIDAZOLAM		IV	0.05 mg/kg	0.6 mg	1 mg/mL	0.6 mL
MIDAZOLAM		PO	0.5 mg/kg	20 mg	1 mg/mL	20 mL
MIDAZOLAM		IN	0.2 mg/kg	8.8 mg	1 mg/mL	8.8 mL
SUCCINYLCHOLINE		IV	2 mg/kg	88 mg	20 mg/mL	4.4 mL
SUCCINYLCHOLINE		IM	4 mg/kg	176 mg	20 mg/mL	8.8 mL
PROPOFOL		IV	3 mg/kg	132 mg	10 mg/mL	13.2 mL
ETOMIDATE	>10 y	IV	0.3 mg/kg	13.2 mg	2 mg/mL	6.6 mL
FENTANYL		IV	1 mcg/kg	44 mcg	50 mcg/mL	0.88 mL
FENTANYL		IN	2 mcg/kg	88 mcg	50 mcg/mL	1.76 mL
MORPHINE	<6 mo	IV/IM	0.05 mg/kg	2.2 mg	10 mg/mL	0.22 mL
MORPHINE	>6 mo	IV/IM	0.1 mg/kg	4.4 mg	10 mg/mL	0.44 mL
TORADOL	>2-16 y	IV	0.5 mg/kg	15 mg	30 mg/mL	0.5 mL
TORADOL	>2-16 y	IM	1 mg/kg	30 mg	30 mg/mL	1 mL
ACETAMINOPHEN		PR	20 mg/kg	880 mg		
ACETAMINOPHEN	2-12 y	IV	15 mg/kg	660 mg	10 mg/mL	66 mL
CISATRACURIUM		IV	0.1 mg/kg	4.4 mg	2 mg/mL	2.2 mL
PANCURONIUM	<1 mo	IV	0.02 mg/kg	0.88 mg	1 mg/mL	0.88 mL
PANCURONIUM	>1 mo	IV	0.1 mg/kg	4.4 mg	1 mg/mL	4.4 mL
ROCURONIUM		IV	0.6 mg/kg	26.4 mg	10 mg/mL	2.64 mL
ROCURONIUM	RSI	IV	1.2 mg/kg	52.8 mg	10 mg/mL	5.28 mL
VECURONIUM		IV	0.1 mg/kg	4.4 mg	1 mg/mL	4.4 mL
GLYCOPYRROLATE	reversal	IV	0.007 mg/kg	0.308 mg	0.2 mg/mL	1.54 mL
NEOSTIGMINE		IV	0.07 mg/kg	3.08 mg	1 mg/mL	3.08 mL
DEXAMETHASONE		IV	0.25 mg/kg	10 mg	10 mg/mL	1 mL
ONDANSETRON		IV	0.15 mg/kg	4 mg	2 mg/mL	2 mL

additional pediatric drugs	route	dose	mg to pt	supplied	mL to give
PREMED/SEDATION; VAGOLYTIC/ANTISIALAGOGUE; GIVE IM 30–60 MIN PREOP					
ATROPINE	IM	0.02 mg/kg	0.5 mg	0.4 mg/mL	1.25 mL
GLYCOPYRROLATE	IM	0.004 mg/kg	0.009 mg	0.2 mg/mL	0.045 mL
MIDAZOLAM	IM	0.1 mg/kg	0.5 mg	1 mg/mL	0.5 mL
DEXMEDETOMIDINE load dose	IV	0.5 mcg/kg	1 mcg	4 mcg/mL	0.25 mL
INDUCTION					
KETAMINE	IV	2 mg/kg	88 mg	10 mg/mL	8.8 mL
KETAMINE	IM/PR	5 mg/kg	220 mg	10 mg/mL	22 mL
OPIOIDS/NONOPIOIDS					
FENTANYL	IV	high dose	4 mcg/kg	176 mcg	50 mcg/mL	3.52 mL
FENTANYL	IV	cardiac	10 mcg/kg	440 mcg	50 mcg/mL	8.8 mL
HYDROMORPHONE	<6 mo	IV/SQ	0.005 mg/kg	0.22 mg	10 mg/mL	0.022 mL
HYDROMORPHONE	>6 mo	IV/SQ	0.015 mg/kg	0.66 mg	10 mg/mL	0.066 mL
REMIFENTANIL	IV	0.5 mcg/kg	1 mcg	50 mcg/mL	0.02 mL
SUFENTANIL	IV	0.5 mcg/kg	20 mcg	50 mcg/mL	0.4 mL
REVERSALS					
ATROPINE	IV	0.02 mg/kg	0.5 mg	0.4 mg/mL	1.25 mL
EDROPHONIUM	neonate	IV	0.1 mg single dose	10 mg/mL	0.01 mL
EDROPHONIUM	>2 mo	IV	0.04 mg/kg	1.76 mg	10 mg/mL	0.176 mL
FLUMAZENIL	>1 y	IV	0.01 mg/kg	0.2 mg	1 mg/mL	2 mL
NALOXONE	<5 y; <20 kg	IM/IV	0.1 mg/kg	2 mg	0.4 mg/mL	5 mL
NALOXONE	>5 y; >20 kg	IM/IV	2 mg per dose	0.4 mg/mL	5 mL
NALOXONE	ETT	0.3 mg/kg	13.2 mg	0.4 mg/mL	33 mL

additional pediatric drugs		route	dose	mg to pt	supplied	mL to give
ANTIBIOTICS						
AMPICILLIN	<6 y	IV	50 mg/kg	300 mg		
AMPICILLIN	>6 y	IV	50 mg/kg	2,000 mg		
AMPICILLIN & SULBACTUM	>1 mo	IV	50 mg/kg	2,200 mg		
CEFAZOLIN		IV	25 mg/kg	1,000 mg		
CLINDAMYCIN		IV	10 mg/kg	440 mg		
ERTAPENEM	3 mo-12 y	IV	15 mg/kg	660 mg		
ERTAPENEM	>12 y	IV	1 Gm	per dose		
GENTAMICIN		IV	2 mg/kg	88 mg		
LEVOFLOXACIN		IV	10 mg/kg	440 mg		
METRONIDAZOLE		IV	10 mg/kg	440 mg		
PIPERACILLIN & TAZOBACTAM	<40 kg & 2-9 mo	IV	80 mg/kg	3,375 mg		
PIPERACILLIN & TAZOBACTAM	<40 kg & >9 mo	IV	100 mg/kg	3,375 mg		
PIPERACILLIN & TAZOBACTAM	>40 kg	IV	3.375 Gm per dose			
VANCOMYCIN		IV	15 mg/kg	660 mg		
ANTINAUSEA						
METOCLOPROMIDE		IV	0.2 mg/kg	8.8 mg	5 mg/mL	1.76 mL
DIPHENHYDRAMINE		IV/IM	1.25 mg/kg	55 mg	50 mg/mL	1.1 mL
SCOPOLAMINE		IV/IM	6 mcg/kg	264 mcg	400 mcg/mL	0.66 mL
MISCELLANEOUS MEDS						
AMINOCAPROIC ACID		IV	100 mg/kg	4,400 mg	250 mg/mL	17.6 mL
DESMOPRESSIN		IV/SQ	0.3 mcg/kg	13.2 mcg	4 mcg/mL	3.3 mL
DEXAMETHASONE	croup	IV	0.6 mg/kg	16 mg	4 mg/mL	4 mL
HYDROCORTISONE		IV/IO	3 mg/kg	100 mg	100 mg/mL	1 mL

44 KG

1 year → 13 kg and up

Ventilation: trained rescuer	1 breath q 6-8 sec (8-10 breaths/minute) about 1 second/breath-visible chest rise; if intubated, continuous compressions without pause for ventilations
Pulse check	carotid or femoral
Compression	heel of 1 hand or both hands one atop the other—lower half of sternum between nipples
Depth	2 inches (5 cm) or at least 1/3 chest depth
Rate	at least 100 compressions per minute
Compress/vent ratio	30:2 single rescuer 15:2 2 healthcare providers
Foreign body obstruction	Heimlich maneuver Never perform a blind finger-sweep. Open the mouth and look for object; if you see it, remove it.

sync cardioversion	0.5 J/kg	22 J
repeat	1 J/kg	44 J
defibrillation	2 J/kg	88 J
repeat	4 J/kg	176 J

IV Bolus Drugs		dose	mg to pt	supplied	mL to give
ADENOSINE	IV	0.1 mg/kg	4.4 mg	3 mg/mL	1.47 mL
ADENOSINE repeat dose	IV	0.2 mg/kg	8.8 mg	3 mg/mL	2.93 mL
AMIODARONE	IV/IO	5 mg/kg	220 mg	50 mg/mL	4.40 mL
ATROPINE	IM/IV	0.02 mg/kg	0.5 mg	0.4 mg/mL	1.25 mL
ATROPINE	ETT	0.04 mg/kg	1.76 mg	0.4 mg/mL	4.40 mL
CALCIUM CHLORIDE	IV	20 mg/kg	880 mg	100 mg/mL	8.80 mL
CALCIUM GLUCONATE	IV/IO	60 mg/kg	800 mg	100 mg/mL	8.00 mL
DANTROLENE	IV	2.5 mg/kg	30 mg		
EPHEDRINE	IV	0.15 mg/kg	6.6 mg	10 mg/mL	0.66 mL
EPINEPHRINE (1:10,000)	IV/IO	0.01 mg/kg	0.44 mg	0.1 mg/mL	4.40 mL
EPINEPHRINE (1:1,000)	ETT	0.1 mg/kg	2.5 mg	1 mg/mL	2.50 mL
ESMOLOL	IV	0.5 mg/kg	22 mg	10 mg/mL	2.20 mL
LABETALOL	IV	0.2 mg/kg	8.8 mg	5 mg/mL	1.76 mL
LIDOCAINE	IV/IO	1 mg/kg	44 mg	100 mcg/mL	2.20 mL
NEOSYNEPHRINE	IV	5 mcg/kg	220 mcg	100 mcg/mL	2.20 mL
ROMAZICON	IV	0.01 mg/kg	0.2 mg	0.1 mg/mL	2.00 mL
VASOPRESSIN	IV/IO	0.4 unit/kg	17.6 units	20 u/mL	0.88 mL

45 KG MAINTENANCE IV FLUIDS: 84 ML/HR

common pediatric drugs		route	dose	mg to pt	supplied	mL to give
ATROPINE	vagolytic	IV	0.02 mg/kg	0.5 mg	0.4 mg/mL	1.25 mL
GLYCOPYRROLATE	vagolytic	IV	0.004 mg/kg	0.18 mg	0.2 mg/mL	0.9 mL
MIDAZOLAM		IV	0.05 mg/kg	0.6 mg	1 mg/mL	0.6 mL
MIDAZOLAM		PO	0.5 mg/kg	20 mg	1 mg/mL	20 mL
MIDAZOLAM		IN	0.2 mg/kg	9 mg	1 mg/mL	9 mL
SUCCINYLCHOLINE		IV	2 mg/kg	90 mg	20 mg/mL	4.5 mL
SUCCINYLCHOLINE		IM	4 mg/kg	180 mg	20 mg/mL	9 mL
PROPOFOL		IV	3 mg/kg	135 mg	10 mg/mL	13.5 mL
ETOMIDATE	>10 y	IV	0.3 mg/kg	13.5 mg	2 mg/mL	6.75 mL
FENTANYL		IV	1 mcg/kg	45 mcg	50 mcg/mL	0.9 mL
FENTANYL		IN	2 mcg/kg	90 mcg	50 mcg/mL	1.8 mL
MORPHINE	<6 mo	IV/IM	0.05 mg/kg	2.25 mg	10 mg/mL	0.225 mL
MORPHINE	>6 mo	IV/IM	0.1 mg/kg	4.5 mg	10 mg/mL	0.45 mL
TORADOL	>2-16 y	IV	0.5 mg/kg	15 mg	30 mg/mL	0.5 mL
TORADOL	>2-16 y	IM	1 mg/kg	30 mg	30 mg/mL	1 mL
ACETAMINOPHEN		PR	20 mg/kg	900 mg		
ACETAMINOPHEN	2-12 y	IV	15 mg/kg	675 mg	10 mg/mL	67.5 mL
CISATRACURIUM		IV	0.1 mg/kg	4.5 mg	2 mg/mL	2.25 mL
PANCURONIUM	<1 mo	IV	0.02 mg/kg	0.9 mg	1 mg/mL	0.9 mL
PANCURONIUM	>1 mo	IV	0.1 mg/kg	4.5 mg	1 mg/mL	4.5 mL
ROCURONIUM		IV	0.6 mg/kg	27 mg	10 mg/mL	2.7 mL
ROCURONIUM	RSI	IV	1.2 mg/kg	54 mg	10 mg/mL	5.4 mL
VECURONIUM		IV	0.1 mg/kg	4.5 mg	1 mg/mL	4.5 mL
GLYCOPYRROLATE	reversal	IV	0.007 mg/kg	0.315 mg	0.2 mg/mL	1.575 mL
NEOSTIGMINE		IV	0.07 mg/kg	3.15 mg	1 mg/mL	3.15 mL
DEXAMETHASONE		IV	0.25 mg/kg	10 mg	10 mg/mL	1 mL
ONDANSETRON		IV	0.15 mg/kg	4 mg	2 mg/mL	2 mL

additional pediatric drugs	route	dose	mg to pt	supplied	mL to give
PREMED/SEDATION, VAGOLYTIC/ANTISIALAGOGUE; GIVE IM 30-60 MIN PREOP					
ATROPINE	IM	0.02 mg/kg	0.5 mg	0.4 mg/mL	1.25 mL
GLYCOPYRROLATE	IM	0.004 mg/kg	0.009 mg	0.2 mg/mL	0.045 mL
MIDAZOLAM	IM	0.1 mg/kg	0.5 mg	1 mg/mL	0.5 mL
DEXMEDETOMIDINE load dose	IV	0.5 mcg/kg	1 mcg	4 mcg/mL	0.25 mL
INDUCTION					
KETAMINE	IV	2 mg/kg	90 mg	10 mg/mL	9 mL
KETAMINE	IM/PR	5 mg/kg	225 mg	10 mg/mL	22.5 mL
OPIOIDS/NONOPIOIDS					
FENTANYL high dose	IV	4 mcg/kg	180 mcg	50 mcg/mL	3.6 mL
FENTANYL cardiac	IV	10 mcg/kg	450 mcg	50 mcg/mL	9 mL
HYDROMORPHONE <6 mo	IV/SQ	0.005 mg/kg	0.225 mg	10 mg/mL	0.0225 mL
HYDROMORPHONE >6 mo	IV/SQ	0.015 mg/kg	0.675 mg	10 mg/mL	0.0675 mL
REMIFENTANIL	IV	0.5 mcg/kg	1 mcg	50 mcg/mL	0.02 mL
SUFENTANIL	IV	0.5 mcg/kg	20 mcg	50 mcg/mL	0.4 mL
REVERSALS					
ATROPINE	IV	0.02 mg/kg	0.5 mg	0.4 mg/mL	1.25 mL
EDROPHONIUM neonate	IV	0.1 mg single dose		10 mg/mL	0.01 mL
EDROPHONIUM >2 mo	IV	0.04 mg/kg	1.8 mg	10 mg/mL	0.18 mL
FLUMAZENIL >1 y	IV	0.01 mg/kg	0.2 mg	0.1 mg/mL	2 mL
NALOXONE <5 y; <20 kg	IV/IM	0.1 mg/kg	2 mg	0.4 mg/mL	5 mL
NALOXONE >5 y; >20 kg	IV/IM	2 mg per dose		0.4 mg/mL	5 mL
NALOXONE	ETT	0.3 mg/kg	13.5 mg	0.4 mg/mL	33.75 mL

additional pediatric drugs		route	dose	mg to pt	supplied	mL to give
ANTIBIOTICS						
AMPICILLIN	<6 y	IV	50 mg/kg	300 mg		
AMPICILLIN	>6 y	IV	50 mg/kg	2,000 mg		
AMPICILLIN & SULBACTUM	>1 mo	IV	50 mg/kg	2,250 mg		
CEFAZOLIN		IV	25 mg/kg	1,000 mg		
CLINDAMYCIN		IV	10 mg/kg	450 mg		
ERTAPENEM	3 mo-12 y	IV	15 mg/kg	675 mg		
ERTAPENEM	>12 y	IV	1 Gm	per dose		
GENTAMICIN		IV	2 mg/kg	90 mg		
LEVOFLOXACIN		IV	10 mg/kg	450 mg		
METRONIDAZOLE		IV	10 mg/kg	450 mg		
PIPERACILLIN & TAZOBACTAM	<40 kg & 2-9 mo	IV	80 mg/kg	3,375 mg		
PIPERACILLIN & TAZOBACTAM	<40 kg & >9 mo	IV	100 mg/kg	3,375 mg		
PIPERACILLIN & TAZOBACTAM	>40 kg	IV	3.375 Gm per dose			
VANCOMYCIN		IV	15 mg/kg	675 mg		
ANTINAUSEA						
METOCLOPROMIDE		IV	0.2 mg/kg	9 mg	5 mg/mL	1.8 mL
DIPHENHYDRAMINE		IV/IM	1.25 mg/kg	56.25 mg	50 mg/mL	1.125 mL
SCOPOLAMINE		IV/IM	6 mcg/kg	270 mcg	400 mcg/mL	0.675 mL
MISCELLANEOUS MEDS						
AMINOCAPROIC ACID		IV	100 mg/kg	4,500 mg	250 mg/mL	18 mL
DESMOPRESSIN		IV/SQ	0.3 mcg/kg	13.5 mcg	4 mcg/mL	3.375 mL
DEXAMETHASONE	croup	IV	0.6 mg/kg	16 mg	4 mg/mL	4 mL
HYDROCORTISONE		IV/IO	3 mg/kg	100 mg	100 mg/mL	1 mL

45 KG

1 year ← 13 kg and up

Ventilation: trained rescuer	1 breath q 6-8 sec (8-10 breaths/minute) about 1 second/ breath-visible chest rise; if intubated, continuous compressions without pause for ventilations
Pulse check	carotid or femoral
Compression	heel of 1 hand or both hands one atop the other-lower half of sternum between nipples
Depth	2 inches (5 cm) or at least 1/3 chest depth
Rate	at least 100 compressions per minute
Compress/vent ratio	30:2 single rescuer 15:2 2 healthcare providers
Foreign body obstruction	Heimlich maneuver Never perform a blind finger-sweep. Open the mouth and look for object; if you see it, remove it.

sync cardioversion	0.5 J/kg	22.5 J	
	1 J/kg	45 J	repeat
defibrillation	2 J/kg	90 J	
	4 J/kg	180 J	repeat

IV Bolus Drugs		dose	mg to pt	supplied	mL to give
ADENOSINE	IV	0.1 mg/kg	4.5 mg	3 mg/mL	1.50 mL
ADENOSINE repeat dose	IV	0.2 mg/kg	9 mg	3 mg/mL	3.00 mL
AMIODARONE	IV/IO	5 mg/kg	225 mg	50 mg/mL	4.50 mL
ATROPINE	IM/IV	0.02 mg/kg	0.5 mg	0.4 mg/mL	1.25 mL
ATROPINE	ETT	0.04 mg/kg	1.8 mg	0.4 mg/mL	4.50 mL
CALCIUM CHLORIDE	IV	20 mg/kg	900 mg	100 mg/mL	9.00 mL
CALCIUM GLUCONATE	IV/IO	60 mg/kg	800 mg	100 mg/mL	8.00 mL
DANTROLENE	IV	2.5 mg/kg	30 mg		
EPHEDRINE	IV	0.15 mg/kg	6.75 mg	10 mg/mL	0.68 mL
EPINEPHRINE (1:10,000)	IV/IO	0.01 mg/kg	0.45 mg	0.1 mg/mL	4.50 mL
EPINEPHRINE (1:1,000)	ETT	0.1 mg/kg	2.5 mg	1 mg/mL	2.50 mL
ESMOLOL	IV	0.5 mg/kg	22.5 mg	10 mg/mL	2.25 mL
LABETALOL	IV	0.2 mg/kg	9 mg	5 mg/mL	1.80 mL
LIDOCAINE	IV/IO	1 mg/kg	45 mg	20 mg/mL	2.25 mL
NEOSYNEPHRINE	IV	5 mcg/kg	225 mcg	100 mcg/mL	2.25 mL
ROMAZICON	IV	0.01 mg/kg	0.2 mg	0.1 mg/mL	2.00 mL
VASOPRESSIN	IV/IO	0.4 unit/kg	18 units	20 u/mL	0.90 mL

46 KG MAINTENANCE IV FLUIDS: 86 ML/HR

common pediatric drugs		route	dose	mg to pt	supplied	mL to give
ATROPINE	vagolytic	IV	0.02 mg/kg	0.5 mg	0.4 mg/mL	1.25 mL
GLYCOPYRROLATE	vagolytic	IV	0.004 mg/kg	0.184 mg	0.2 mg/mL	0.92 mL
MIDAZOLAM		IV	0.05 mg/kg	0.6 mg	1 mg/mL	0.6 mL
MIDAZOLAM		PO	0.5 mg/kg	20 mg	1 mg/mL	20 mL
MIDAZOLAM		IN	0.2 mg/kg	9.2 mg	1 mg/mL	9.2 mL
SUCCINYLCHOLINE		IV	2 mg/kg	92 mg	20 mg/mL	4.6 mL
SUCCINYLCHOLINE		IM	4 mg/kg	184 mg	20 mg/mL	9.2 mL
PROPOFOL		IV	3 mg/kg	138 mg	10 mg/mL	13.8 mL
ETOMIDATE	>10 y	IV	0.3 mg/kg	13.8 mg	2 mg/mL	6.9 mL
FENTANYL		IV	1 mcg/kg	46 mcg	50 mcg/mL	0.92 mL
FENTANYL		IN	2 mcg/kg	92 mcg	50 mcg/mL	1.84 mL
MORPHINE	<6 mo	IV/IM	0.05 mg/kg	2.3 mg	10 mg/mL	0.23 mL
MORPHINE	>6 mo	IV/IM	0.1 mg/kg	4.6 mg	10 mg/mL	0.46 mL
TORADOL	>2-16 y	IV	0.5 mg/kg	15 mg	30 mg/mL	0.5 mL
TORADOL	>2-16 y	IM	1 mg/kg	30 mg	30 mg/mL	1 mL
ACETAMINOPHEN		PR	20 mg/kg	920 mg		
ACETAMINOPHEN	2-12 y	IV	15 mg/kg	690 mg	10 mg/mL	69 mL
CISATRACURIUM		IV	0.1 mg/kg	4.6 mg	2 mg/mL	2.3 mL
PANCURONIUM	<1 mo	IV	0.02 mg/kg	0.92 mg	1 mg/mL	0.92 mL
PANCURONIUM	>1 mo	IV	0.1 mg/kg	4.6 mg	1 mg/mL	4.6 mL
ROCURONIUM		IV	0.6 mg/kg	27.6 mg	10 mg/mL	2.76 mL
ROCURONIUM	RSI	IV	1.2 mg/kg	55.2 mg	10 mg/mL	5.52 mL
VECURONIUM		IV	0.1 mg/kg	4.6 mg	1 mg/mL	4.6 mL
GLYCOPYRROLATE	reversal	IV	0.007 mg/kg	0.322 mg	0.2 mg/mL	1.61 mL
NEOSTIGMINE		IV	0.07 mg/kg	3.22 mg	1 mg/mL	3.22 mL
DEXAMETHASONE		IV	0.25 mg/kg	10 mg	10 mg/mL	1 mL
ONDANSETRON		IV	0.15 mg/kg	4 mg	2 mg/mL	2 mL

additional pediatric drugs	route	dose	mg to pt	supplied	mL to give
PREMED/SEDATION; VAGOLYTIC/ANTISIALAGOGUE; GIVE IM 30-60 MIN PREOP					
ATROPINE	IM	0.02 mg/kg	0.5 mg	0.4 mg/mL	1.25 mL
GLYCOPYRROLATE	IM	0.004 mg/kg	0.009 mg	0.2 mg/mL	0.045 mL
MIDAZOLAM	IM	0.1 mg/kg	0.5 mg	1 mg/mL	0.5 mL
DEXMEDETOMIDINE load dose	IV	0.5 mcg/kg	1 mcg	4 mcg/mL	0.25 mL
INDUCTION					
KETAMINE	IV	2 mg/kg	92 mg	10 mg/mL	9.2 mL
KETAMINE	IM/PR	5 mg/kg	230 mg	10 mg/mL	23 mL
OPIOIDS/NONOPIOIDS					
FENTANYL high dose	IV	4 mcg/kg	184 mcg	50 mcg/mL	3.68 mL
FENTANYL cardiac	IV	10 mcg/kg	460 mcg	50 mcg/mL	9.2 mL
HYDROMORPHONE <6 mo	IV/SQ	0.005 mg/kg	0.23 mg	10 mg/mL	0.023 mL
HYDROMORPHONE >6 mo	IV/SQ	0.015 mg/kg	0.69 mg	10 mg/mL	0.069 mL
REMIFENTANIL	IV	0.5 mcg/kg	1 mcg	50 mcg/mL	0.02 mL
SUFENTANIL	IV	0.5 mcg/kg	20 mcg	50 mcg/mL	0.4 mL
REVERSALS					
ATROPINE	IV	0.02 mg/kg	0.5 mg	0.4 mg/mL	1.25 mL
EDROPHONIUM neonate	IV	0.1 mg single dose		10	0.01 mL
EDROPHONIUM <2 mo	IV	0.04 mg/kg	1.84 mg	10	0.184 mL
FLUMAZENIL >1 y	IV		0.2 mg	0.1 mg/mL	2 mL
NALOXONE <5 y; <20 kg	IM/IV	0.1 mg/kg	2 mg	0.4 mg/mL	5 mL
NALOXONE >5 y; <20 kg	IM/IV	2 mg per dose		0.4 mg/mL	5 mL
NALOXONE	ETT	0.3 mg/kg	13.8 mg	0.4 mg/mL	34.5 mL

additional pediatric drugs		route	dose	mg to pt	supplied	mL to give
ANTIBIOTICS						
AMPICILLIN	<6 y	IV	50 mg/kg	300 mg		
AMPICILLIN	>6 y	IV	50 mg/kg	2,000 mg		
AMPICILLIN & SULBACTUM	>1 mo	IV	50 mg/kg	2,300 mg		
CEFAZOLIN		IV	25 mg/kg	1,000 mg		
CLINDAMYCIN		IV	10 mg/kg	460 mg		
ERTAPENEM	3 mo-12 y	IV	15 mg/kg	690 mg		
ERTAPENEM	>12 y	IV	1 Gm	per dose		
GENTAMICIN		IV	2 mg/kg	92 mg		
LEVOFLOXACIN		IV	10 mg/kg	460 mg		
METRONIDAZOLE		IV	10 mg/kg	460 mg		
PIPERACILLIN & TAZOBACTAM	<40 kg & 2-9 mo	IV	80 mg/kg	3,375 mg		
PIPERACILLIN & TAZOBACTAM	<40 kg & >9 mo	IV	100 mg/kg	3,375 mg		
PIPERACILLIN & TAZOBACTAM	>40 kg	IV	3.375 Gm per dose			
VANCOMYCIN		IV	15 mg/kg	690 mg		
ANTINAUSEA						
METOCLOPROMIDE		IV	0.2 mg/kg	9.2 mg	5 mg/mL	1.84 mL
DIPHENHYDRAMINE		IV/IM	1.25 mg/kg	57.5 mg	50 mg/mL	1.15 mL
SCOPOLAMINE		IV/IM	6 mcg/kg	276 mcg	400 mcg/mL	0.69 mL
MISCELLANEOUS MEDS						
AMINOCAPROIC ACID		IV	100 mg/kg	4,600 mg	250 mg/mL	18.4 mL
DESMOPRESSIN		IV/SQ	0.3 mcg/kg	13.8 mcg	4 mcg/mL	3.45 mL
DEXAMETHASONE	croup	IV	0.6 mg/kg	16 mg	4 mg/mL	4 mL
HYDROCORTISONE		IV/IO	3 mg/kg	100 mg	100 mg/mL	1 mL

46 KG

1 year ← 13 kg and up

Ventilation: trained rescuer	1 breath q 6-8 sec (8-10 breaths/minute) about 1 second/ breath-visible chest rise; if intubated, continuous compressions without pause for ventilations
Pulse check	carotid or femoral
Compression	heel of 1 hand or both hands one atop the other-lower half of sternum between nipples
Depth	2 inches (5 cm) or at least 1/3 chest depth
Rate	at least 100 compressions per minute
Compress/vent ratio	30:2 single rescuer 15:2 2 healthcare providers
Foreign body obstruction	Heimlich maneuver Never perform a blind finger-sweep. Open the mouth and look for object; if you see it, remove it.

sync cardioversion	0.5 J/kg	23 J
repeat	1 J/kg	46 J
defibrillation	2 J/kg	92 J
repeat	4 J/kg	184 J

IV Bolus Drugs		dose	mg to pt	supplied	mL to give
ADENOSINE	IV	0.1 mg/kg	4.6 mg	3 mg/mL	1.53 mL
ADENOSINE repeat dose	IV	0.2 mg/kg	9.2 mg	3 mg/mL	3.07 mL
AMIODARONE	IV/IO	5 mg/kg	230 mg	50 mg/mL	4.60 mL
ATROPINE	IM/IV	0.02 mg/kg	0.5 mg	0.4 mg/mL	1.25 mL
ATROPINE	ETT	0.04 mg/kg	1.84 mg	0.4 mg/mL	4.60 mL
CALCIUM CHLORIDE	IV	20 mg/kg	920 mg	100 mg/mL	9.20 mL
CALCIUM GLUCONATE	IV/IO	60 mg/kg	800 mg	100 mg/mL	8.00 mL
DANTROLENE	IV	2.5 mg/kg	30 mg		
EPHEDRINE	IV	0.15 mg/kg	6.9 mg	10 mg/mL	0.69 mL
EPINEPHRINE (1:10,000)	IV/IO	0.01 mg/kg	0.46 mg	0.1 mg/mL	4.60 mL
EPINEPHRINE (1:1,000)	ETT	0.1 mg/kg	2.5 mg	1 mg/mL	2.50 mL
ESMOLOL	IV	0.5 mg/kg	23 mg	10 mg/mL	2.30 mL
LABETALOL	IV	0.2 mg/kg	9.2 mg	5 mg/mL	1.84 mL
LIDOCAINE	IV/IO	1 mg/kg	46 mg	20 mg/mL	2.30 mL
NEOSYNEPHRINE	IV	5 mcg/kg	230 mcg	100 mcg/mL	2.30 mL
ROMAZICON	IV	0.01 mg/kg	0.2 mg	0.1 mg/mL	2.00 mL
VASOPRESSIN	IV/IO	0.4 unit/kg	18.4 units	20 u/mL	0.92 mL

47 KG MAINTENANCE IV FLUIDS: 87 ML/HR

common pediatric drugs		route	dose	mg to pt	supplied	mL to give
ATROPINE	vagolytic	IV	0.02 mg/kg	0.5 mg	0.4 mg/mL	1.25 mL
GLYCOPYRROLATE	vagolytic	IV	0.004 mg/kg	0.188 mg	0.2 mg/mL	0.94 mL
MIDAZOLAM		IV	0.05 mg/kg	0.6 mg	1 mg/mL	0.6 mL
MIDAZOLAM		PO	0.5 mg/kg	20 mg	1 mg/mL	20 mL
MIDAZOLAM		IN	0.2 mg/kg	9.4 mg	1 mg/mL	9.4 mL
SUCCINYLCHOLINE		IV	2 mg/kg	94 mg	20 mg/mL	4.7 mL
SUCCINYLCHOLINE		IM	4 mg/kg	188 mg	20 mg/mL	9.4 mL
PROPOFOL		IV	3 mg/kg	141 mg	10 mg/mL	14.1 mL
ETOMIDATE	>10 y	IV	0.3 mg/kg	14.1 mg	2 mg/mL	7.05 mL
FENTANYL		IV	1 mcg/kg	47 mcg	50 mcg/mL	0.94 mL
FENTANYL		IN	2 mcg/kg	94 mcg	50 mcg/mL	1.88 mL
MORPHINE	<6 mo	IV/IM	0.05 mg/kg	2.35 mg	10 mg/mL	0.235 mL
MORPHINE	>6 mo	IV/IM	0.1 mg/kg	4.7 mg	10 mg/mL	0.47 mL
TORADOL	>2-16 y	IV	0.5 mg/kg	15 mg	30 mg/mL	0.5 mL
TORADOL	>2-16 y	IM	1 mg/kg	30 mg	30 mg/mL	1 mL
ACETAMINOPHEN		PR	20 mg/kg	940 mg		
ACETAMINOPHEN	2-12 y	IV	15 mg/kg	705 mg	10 mg/mL	70.5 mL
CISATRACURIUM		IV	0.1 mg/kg	4.7 mg	2 mg/mL	2.35 mL
PANCURONIUM	<1 mo	IV	0.02 mg/kg	0.94 mg	1 mg/mL	0.94 mL
PANCURONIUM	>1 mo	IV	0.1 mg/kg	4.7 mg	1 mg/mL	4.7 mL
ROCURONIUM		IV	0.6 mg/kg	28.2 mg	10 mg/mL	2.82 mL
ROCURONIUM	RSI	IV	1.2 mg/kg	56.4 mg	10 mg/mL	5.64 mL
VECURONIUM		IV	0.1 mg/kg	4.7 mg	1 mg/mL	4.7 mL
GLYCOPYRROLATE	reversal	IV	0.007 mg/kg	0.329 mg	0.2 mg/mL	1.645 mL
NEOSTIGMINE		IV	0.07 mg/kg	3.29 mg	1 mg/mL	3.29 mL
DEXAMETHASONE		IV	0.25 mg/kg	10 mg	10 mg/mL	1 mL
ONDANSETRON		IV	0.15 mg/kg	4 mg	2 mg/mL	2 mL

additional pediatric drugs		route	dose	mg to pt	supplied	mL to give
PREMED/SEDATION; VAGOLYTIC/ANTISIALAGOGUE; GIVE IM 30-60 MIN PREOP						
ATROPINE		IM	0.02 mg/kg	0.5 mg	0.4 mg/mL	1.25 mL
GLYCOPYRROLATE		IM	0.004 mg/kg	0.009 mg	0.2 mg/mL	0.045 mL
MIDAZOLAM		IM	0.1 mg/kg	0.5 mg	1 mg/mL	0.5 mL
DEXMEDETOMIDINE load dose		IV	0.5 mcg/kg	1 mcg	4 mcg/mL	0.25 mL
INDUCTION						
KETAMINE		IV	2 mg/kg	94 mg	10 mg/mL	9.4 mL
KETAMINE		IM/PR	5 mg/kg	235 mg	10 mg/mL	23.5 mL
OPIOIDS/NONOPIOIDS						
FENTANYL	high dose	IV	4 mcg/kg	188 mcg	50 mcg/mL	3.76 mL
FENTANYL	cardiac	IV	10 mcg/kg	470 mcg	50 mcg/mL	9.4 mL
HYDROMORPHONE	< 6 mo	IV/SQ	0.005 mg/kg	0.235 mg	10 mg/mL	0.0235 mL
HYDROMORPHONE	> 6 mo	IV/SQ	0.015 mg/kg	0.705 mg	10 mg/mL	0.0705 mL
REMIFENTANIL		IV	0.5 mcg/kg	1 mcg	50 mcg/mL	0.02 mL
SUFENTANIL		IV	0.5 mcg/kg	20 mcg	50 mcg/mL	0.4 mL
REVERSALS						
ATROPINE		IV	0.02 mg/kg	0.5 mg	0.4 mg/mL	1.25 mL
EDROPHONIUM	neonate	IV	0.1 mg single dose		10 mg/mL	0.01 mL
EDROPHONIUM	> 2 mo	IV	0.04 mg/kg	1.88 mg	10 mg/mL	0.188 mL
FLUMAZENIL		IV	0.01 mg/kg	0.2 mg	0.1 mg/mL	2 mL
NALOXONE	< 5 y; < 20 kg	IM/IV	0.1 mg/kg	2 mg	0.4 mg/mL	5 mL
NALOXONE	< 5 y; > 20 kg	IM/IV	2 mg per dose		0.4 mg/mL	5 mL
NALOXONE	ETT		0.3 mg/kg	14.1 mg	0.4 mg/mL	35.25 mL

additional pediatric drugs	route		dose	mg to pt	supplied	mL to give
ANTIBIOTICS						
AMPICILLIN	<6 y	IV	50 mg/kg	300 mg		
AMPICILLIN	>6 y	IV	50 mg/kg	2,000 mg		
AMPICILLIN & SULBACTUM	>1 mo	IV	50 mg/kg	2,350 mg		
CEFAZOLIN		IV	25 mg/kg	1,000 mg		
CLINDAMYCIN		IV	10 mg/kg	470 mg		
ERTAPENEM	3 mo-12 y	IV	15 mg/kg	705 mg		
ERTAPENEM	>12 y	IV	1 Gm	per dose		
GENTAMICIN		IV	2 mg/kg	94 mg		
LEVOFLOXACIN		IV	10 mg/kg	470 mg		
METRONIDAZOLE		IV	10 mg/kg	470 mg		
PIPERACILLIN & TAZOBACTAM	<40 kg & 2-9 mo	IV	80 mg/kg	3,375 mg		
PIPERACILLIN & TAZOBACTAM	<40 kg & >9 mo	IV	100 mg/kg	3,375 mg		
PIPERACILLIN & TAZOBACTAM	>40 kg	IV	3.375 Gm per dose			
VANCOMYCIN		IV	15 mg/kg	705 mg		
ANTINAUSEA						
METOCLOPROMIDE		IV	0.2 mg/kg	9.4 mg	5 mg/mL	1.88 mL
DIPHENHYDRAMINE		IV/IM	1.25 mg/kg	58.75 mg	50 mg/mL	1.175 mL
SCOPOLAMINE		IV/IM	6 mcg/kg	282 mcg	400 mcg/mL	0.705 mL
MISCELLANEOUS MEDS						
AMINOCAPROIC ACID		IV	100 mg/kg	4,700 mg	250 mg/mL	18.8 mL
DESMOPRESSIN		IV/SQ	0.3 mcg/kg	14.1 mcg	4 mcg/mL	3.525 mL
DEXAMETHASONE	croup	IV	0.6 mg/kg	16 mg	4 mg/mL	4 mL
HYDROCORTISONE		IV/IO	3 mg/kg	100 mg	100 mg/mL	1 mL

47 KG

1 year ← 13 kg and up

Ventilation: trained rescuer	1 breath q 6-8 sec (8-10 breaths/minute) about 1 second/ breath-visible chest rise; if intubated, continuous compressions without pause for ventilations
Pulse check	carotid or femoral
Compression	heel of 1 hand or both hands one atop the other-lower half of sternum between nipples
Depth	2 inches (5 cm) or at least 1/3 chest depth
Rate	at least 100 compressions per minute
Compress/vent ratio	30:2 single rescuer 15:2 2 healthcare providers
Foreign body obstruction	Heimlich maneuver Never perform a blind finger-sweep. Open the mouth and look for object; if you see it, remove it.

sync cardioversion	0.5 J/kg	23.5 J
repeat	1 J/kg	47 J
defibrillation	2 J/kg	94 J
repeat	4 J/kg	188 J

IV Bolus Drugs		dose	mg to pt	supplied	mL to give
ADENOSINE	IV	0.1 mg/kg	4.7 mg	3 mg/mL	1.57 mL
ADENOSINE repeat dose	IV	0.2 mg/kg	9.4 mg	3 mg/mL	3.13 mL
AMIODARONE	IV/IO	5 mg/kg	235 mg	50 mg/mL	4.70 mL
ATROPINE	IV/IM	0.02 mg/kg	0.5 mg	0.4 mg/mL	1.25 mL
ATROPINE	ETT	0.04 mg/kg	1.88 mg	0.4 mg/mL	4.70 mL
CALCIUM CHLORIDE	IV	20 mg/kg	940 mg	100 mg/mL	9.40 mL
CALCIUM GLUCONATE	IV/IO	60 mg/kg	800 mg	100 mg/mL	8.00 mL
DANTROLENE	IV	2.5 mg/kg	30 mg		
EPHEDRINE	IV	0.15 mg/kg	7.05 mg	10 mg/mL	0.71 mL
EPINEPHRINE (1:10,000)	IV/IO	0.01 mg/kg	0.47 mg	0.1 mg/mL	4.70 mL
EPINEPHRINE (1:1,000)	ETT	0.1 mg/kg	2.5 mg	1 mg/mL	2.50 mL
ESMOLOL	IV	0.5 mg/kg	23.5 mg	10 mg/mL	2.35 mL
LABETALOL	IV	0.2 mg/kg	9.4 mg	5 mg/mL	1.88 mL
LIDOCAINE	IV/IO	1 mg/kg	47 mg	20 mg/mL	2.35 mL
NEOSYNEPHRINE	IV	5 mcg/kg	235 mcg	100 mcg/mL	2.35 mL
ROMAZICON	IV	0.01 mg/kg	0.2 mg	0.1 mg/mL	2.00 mL
VASOPRESSIN	IV/IO	0.4 unit/kg	18.8 units	20 u/mL	0.94 mL

48 KG MAINTENANCE IV FLUIDS: 88 ML/HR

common pediatric drugs		route	dose	mg to pt	supplied	mL to give
ATROPINE	vagolytic	IV	0.02 mg/kg	0.5 mg	0.4 mg/mL	1.25 mL
GLYCOPYRROLATE	vagolytic	IV	0.004 mg/kg	0.192 mg	0.2 mg/mL	0.96 mL
MIDAZOLAM		IV	0.05 mg/kg	0.6 mg	1 mg/mL	0.6 mL
MIDAZOLAM		PO	0.5 mg/kg	20 mg	1 mg/mL	20 mL
MIDAZOLAM		IN	0.2 mg/kg	9.6 mg	1 mg/mL	9.6 mL
SUCCINYLCHOLINE		IV	2 mg/kg	96 mg	20 mg/mL	4.8 mL
SUCCINYLCHOLINE		IM	4 mg/kg	192 mg	20 mg/mL	9.6 mL
PROPOFOL		IV	3 mg/kg	144 mg	10 mg/mL	14.4 mL
ETOMIDATE	>10 y	IV	0.3 mg/kg	14.4 mg	2 mg/mL	7.2 mL
FENTANYL		IV	1 mcg/kg	48 mcg	50 mcg/mL	0.96 mL
FENTANYL		IN	2 mcg/kg	96 mcg	50 mcg/mL	1.92 mL
MORPHINE	<6 mo	IV/IM	0.05 mg/kg	2.4 mg	10 mg/mL	0.24 mL
MORPHINE	>6 mo	IV/IM	0.1 mg/kg	4.8 mg	10 mg/mL	0.48 mL
TORADOL	<2-16 y	IV	0.5 mg/kg	15 mg	30 mg/mL	0.5 mL
TORADOL	>2-16 y	IM	1 mg/kg	30 mg	30 mg/mL	1 mL
ACETAMINOPHEN		PR	20 mg/kg	960 mg		
ACETAMINOPHEN	2-12 y	IV	15 mg/kg	720 mg	10 mg/mL	72 mL
CISATRACURIUM		IV	0.1 mg/kg	4.8 mg	2 mg/mL	2.4 mL
PANCURONIUM	<1 mo	IV	0.02 mg/kg	0.96 mg	1 mg/mL	0.96 mL
PANCURONIUM	>1 mo	IV	0.1 mg/kg	4.8 mg	1 mg/mL	4.8 mL
ROCURONIUM		IV	0.6 mg/kg	28.8 mg	10 mg/mL	2.88 mL
ROCURONIUM	RSI	IV	1.2 mg/kg	57.6 mg	10 mg/mL	5.76 mL
VECURONIUM		IV	0.1 mg/kg	4.8 mg	1 mg/mL	4.8 mL
GLYCOPYRROLATE	reversal	IV	0.007 mg/kg	0.336 mg	0.2 mg/mL	1.68 mL
NEOSTIGMINE		IV	0.07 mg/kg	3.36 mg	1 mg/mL	3.36 mL
DEXAMETHASONE		IV	0.25 mg/kg	10 mg	10 mg/mL	1 mL
ONDANSETRON		IV	0.15 mg/kg	4 mg	2 mg/mL	2 mL

additional pediatric drugs	route	dose	mg to pt	supplied	mL to give
PREMED/SEDATION; VAGOLYTIC/ANTISIALAGOGUE; GIVE IM 30-60 MIN PREOP					
ATROPINE	IM	0.02 mg/kg	0.5 mg	0.4 mg/mL	1.25 mL
GLYCOPYRROLATE	IM	0.004 mg/kg	0.009 mg	0.2 mg/mL	0.045 mL
MIDAZOLAM	IM	0.1 mg/kg	0.5 mg	1 mg/mL	0.5 mL
DEXMEDETOMIDINE load dose	IV	0.5 mcg/kg	1 mcg	4 mcg/mL	0.25 mL
INDUCTION					
KETAMINE	IV	2 mg/kg	96 mg	10 mg/mL	9.6 mL
KETAMINE	IM/PR	5 mg/kg	240 mg	10 mg/mL	24 mL
OPIOIDS/NONOPIOIDS					
FENTANYL high dose	IV	4 mcg/kg	192 mcg	50 mcg/mL	3.84 mL
FENTANYL cardiac	IV	10 mcg/kg	480 mcg	50 mcg/mL	9.6 mL
HYDROMORPHONE <6 mo	IV/SQ	0.005 mg/kg	0.24 mg	10 mg/mL	0.024 mL
HYDROMORPHONE >6 mo	IV/SQ	0.015 mg/kg	0.72 mg	10 mg/mL	0.072 mL
REMIFENTANIL	IV	0.5 mcg/kg	1 mcg	50 mcg/mL	0.02 mL
SUFENTANIL	IV	0.5 mcg/kg	20 mcg	50 mcg/mL	0.4 mL
REVERSALS					
ATROPINE	IV	0.02 mg/kg	0.5 mg	0.4 mg/mL	1.25 mL
EDROPHONIUM neonate	IV	0.1 mg single dose		10 mg/mL	0.01 mL
EDROPHONIUM >2 mo	IV	0.04 mg/kg	1.92 mg	10 mg/mL	0.192 mL
FLUMAZENIL >1 y	IV	0.01 mg/kg	0.2 mg	0.1 mg/mL	2 mL
NALOXONE <5 y; <20 kg	IV/IM	0.1 mg/kg	2 mg	0.4 mg/mL	5 mL
NALOXONE <5 y; >20 kg	IM	2 mg per dose		0.4 mg/mL	5 mL
NALOXONE	ETT	0.3 mg/kg	14.4 mg	0.4 mg/mL	36 mL

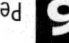

additional pediatric drugs		route	dose	mg to pt	supplied	mL to give
ANTIBIOTICS						
AMPICILLIN	<6 y	IV	50 mg/kg	300 mg		
AMPICILLIN	>6 y	IV	50 mg/kg	2,000 mg		
AMPICILLIN & SULBACTUM	>1 mo	IV	50 mg/kg	2,400 mg		
CEFAZOLIN		IV	25 mg/kg	1,000 mg		
CLINDAMYCIN		IV	10 mg/kg	480 mg		
ERTAPENEM	3 mo-12 y	IV	15 mg/kg	720 mg		
ERTAPENEM	>12 y	IV	1 Gm	per dose		
GENTAMICIN		IV	2 mg/kg	96 mg		
LEVOFLOXACIN		IV	10 mg/kg	480 mg		
METRONIDAZOLE		IV	10 mg/kg	480 mg		
PIPERACILLIN & TAZOBACTAM	<40 kg & 2-9 mo	IV	80 mg/kg	3,375 mg		
PIPERACILLIN & TAZOBACTAM	<40 kg & >9 mo	IV	100 mg/kg	3,375 mg		
PIPERACILLIN & TAZOBACTAM	>40 kg	IV	3.375 Gm per dose			
VANCOMYCIN		IV	15 mg/kg	720 mg		
ANTINAUSEA						
METOCLOPROMIDE		IV	0.2 mg/kg	9.6 mg	5 mg/mL	1.92 mL
DIPHENHYDRAMINE		IV/IM	1.25 mg/kg	60 mg	50 mg/mL	1.2 mL
SCOPOLAMINE		IV/IM	6 mcg/kg	288 mcg	400 mcg/mL	0.72 mL
MISCELLANEOUS MEDS						
AMINOCAPROIC ACID		IV	100 mg/kg	4,800 mg	250 mg/mL	19.2 mL
DESMOPRESSIN		IV/SQ	0.3 mcg/kg	14.4 mcg	4 mcg/mL	3.6 mL
DEXAMETHASONE	croup	IV	0.6 mg/kg	16 mg	4 mg/mL	4 mL
HYDROCORTISONE		IV/IO	3 mg/kg	100 mg	100 mg/mL	1 mL

48 KG

1 year ← 13 kg and up

Ventilation:	1 breath q 6–8 sec (8–10 breaths/minute) about 1 second/
trained rescuer	breath-visible chest rise; if intubated, continuous compressions
	without pause for ventilations
Pulse check	carotid or femoral
Compression	heel of 1 hand or both hands one atop the other–lower
	half of sternum between nipples
Depth	2 inches (5 cm) or at least 1/3 chest depth
Rate	at least 100 compressions per minute
Compress/vent ratio	30:2 single rescuer
	15:2 2 healthcare providers
Foreign body obstruction	Heimlich maneuver
	Never perform a blind finger-sweep. Open the mouth
	and look for object; if you see it, remove it.

sync cardioversion	0.5 J/kg	24 J	
defibrillation	1 J/kg	48 J	repeat
	2 J/kg	96 J	
	4 J/kg	192 J	repeat

IV Bolus Drugs		dose	mg to pt	supplied	mL to give
ADENOSINE	IV	0.1 mg/kg	4.8 mg	3 mg/mL	1.60 mL
ADENOSINE	IV	0.2 mg/kg	9.6 mg	3 mg/mL	3.20 mL
repeat dose					
AMIODARONE	IV/IO	5 mg/kg	240 mg	50 mg/mL	4.80 mL
ATROPINE	IM/IV	0.02 mg/kg	0.96 mg	0.4 mg/mL	1.25 mL
ATROPINE	ETT	0.04 mg/kg	1.92 mg	0.4 mg/mL	4.80 mL
CALCIUM CHLORIDE	IV	20 mg/kg	960 mg	100 mg/mL	9.60 mL
CALCIUM GLUCONATE	IV/IO	60 mg/kg	800 mg	100 mg/mL	8.00 mL
DANTROLENE	IV	2.5 mg/kg	30 mg		
			120 mg		
EPHEDRINE	IV	0.15 mg/kg	7.2 mg	10 mg/mL	0.72 mL
EPINEPHRINE (1:10,000)	IV/IO	0.01 mg/kg	0.48 mg	0.1 mg/mL	4.80 mL
EPINEPHRINE (1:1,000)	ETT	0.1 mg/kg	2.5 mg	1 mg/mL	2.50 mL
ESMOLOL	IV	0.5 mg/kg	24 mg	10 mg/mL	2.40 mL
LABETALOL	IV	0.2 mg/kg	9.6 mg	5 mg/mL	1.92 mL
LIDOCAINE	IV/IO	1 mg/kg	48 mg	20 mg/mL	2.40 mL
NEOSYNEPHRINE	IV	5 mcg/kg	240 mcg	100 mcg/mL	2.40 mL
ROMAZICON	IV	0.01 mg/kg	0.2 mg	0.1 mg/mL	2.00 mL
VASOPRESSIN	IV/IO	0.4 unit/kg	19.2 units	20 u/mL	0.96 mL

49 KG MAINTENANCE IV FLUIDS: 89 ML/HR

common pediatric drugs		route	dose	mg to pt	supplied	mL to give
ATROPINE	vagolytic	IV	0.02 mg/kg	0.5 mg	0.4 mg/mL	1.25 mL
GLYCOPYRROLATE	vagolytic	IV	0.004 mg/kg	0.196 mg	0.2 mg/mL	0.98 mL
MIDAZOLAM		IV	0.05 mg/kg	0.6 mg	1 mg/mL	0.6 mL
MIDAZOLAM		PO	0.5 mg/kg	20 mg	1 mg/mL	20 mL
MIDAZOLAM		IN	0.2 mg/kg	9.8 mg	1 mg/mL	9.8 mL
SUCCINYLCHOLINE		IV	2 mg/kg	98 mg	20 mg/mL	4.9 mL
SUCCINYLCHOLINE		IM	4 mg/kg	196 mg	20 mg/mL	9.8 mL
PROPOFOL		IV	3 mg/kg	147 mg	10 mg/mL	14.7 mL
ETOMIDATE	>10 y	IV	0.3 mg/kg	14.7 mg	2 mg/mL	7.35 mL
FENTANYL		IV	1 mcg/kg	49 mcg	50 mcg/mL	0.98 mL
FENTANYL		IN	2 mcg/kg	98 mcg	50 mcg/mL	1.96 mL
MORPHINE	<6 mo	IV/IM	0.05 mg/kg	2.45 mg	10 mg/mL	0.245 mL
MORPHINE	>6 mo	IV/IM	0.1 mg/kg	4.9 mg	10 mg/mL	0.49 mL
TORADOL	>2-16 y	IV	0.5 mg/kg	15 mg	30 mg/mL	0.5 mL
TORADOL	>2-16 y	IM	1 mg/kg	30 mg	30 mg/mL	1 mL
ACETAMINOPHEN		PR	20 mg/kg	980 mg		
ACETAMINOPHEN	2-12 y	IV	15 mg/kg	735 mg	10 mg/mL	73.5 mL
CISATRACURIUM		IV	0.1 mg/kg	4.9 mg	2 mg/mL	2.45 mL
PANCURONIUM	<1 mo	IV	0.02 mg/kg	0.98 mg	1 mg/mL	0.98 mL
PANCURONIUM	>1 mo	IV	0.1 mg/kg	4.9 mg	1 mg/mL	4.9 mL
ROCURONIUM		IV	0.6 mg/kg	29.4 mg	10 mg/mL	2.94 mL
ROCURONIUM	RSI	IV	1.2 mg/kg	58.8 mg	10 mg/mL	5.88 mL
VECURONIUM		IV	0.1 mg/kg	4.9 mg	1 mg/mL	4.9 mL
GLYCOPYRROLATE	reversal	IV	0.007 mg/kg	0.343 mg	0.2 mg/mL	1.715 mL
NEOSTIGMINE		IV	0.07 mg/kg	3.43 mg	1 mg/mL	3.43 mL
DEXAMETHASONE		IV	0.25 mg/kg	10 mg	10 mg/mL	1 mL
ONDANSETRON		IV	0.15 mg/kg	4 mg	2 mg/mL	2 mL

additional pediatric drugs	route		dose	mg to pt	supplied	mL to give
PREMED/SEDATION; VAGOLYTIC/ANTISIALAGOGUE; GIVE IM 30–60 MIN PREOP						
ATROPINE	IM		0.02 mg/kg	0.5 mg	0.4 mg/mL	1.25 mL
GLYCOPYRROLATE	IM		0.004 mg/kg	0.009 mg	0.2 mg/mL	0.045 mL
MIDAZOLAM	IM		0.1 mg/kg	0.5 mg	1 mg/mL	0.5 mL
DEXMEDETOMIDINE load dose	IV		0.5 mcg/kg	1 mcg	4 mcg/mL	0.25 mL
INDUCTION						
KETAMINE	IV		2 mg/kg	98 mg	10 mg/mL	9.8 mL
KETAMINE	IM/PR		5 mg/kg	245 mg	10 mg/mL	24.5 mL
OPIOIDS/NONOPIOIDS						
FENTANYL	IV	high dose	4 mcg/kg	196 mcg	50 mcg/mL	3.92 mL
FENTANYL	IV	cardiac	10 mcg/kg	490 mcg	50 mcg/mL	9.8 mL
HYDROMORPHONE	IV/SO	< 6 mo	0.005 mg/kg	0.245 mg	10 mg/mL	0.0245 mL
HYDROMORPHONE	IV/SO	> 6 mo	0.015 mg/kg	0.735 mg	10 mg/mL	0.0735 mL
REMIFENTANIL	IV		0.5 mcg/kg	1 mcg	50 mcg/mL	0.02 mL
SUFENTANIL	IV		0.5 mcg/kg	20 mcg	50 mcg/mL	0.4 mL
REVERSALS						
ATROPINE	IV		0.02 mg/kg	0.5 mg	0.4 mg/mL	1.25 mL
EDROPHONIUM	IV	neonate	0.1 mg single dose		10 mg/mL	0.01 mL
EDROPHONIUM	IV	< 2 mo	0.04 mg/kg	1.96 mg	10 mg/mL	0.196 mL
FLUMAZENIL	IV	> 1 y	0.01 mg/kg	2 mg	0.1 mg/mL	2 mL
NALOXONE	IM/IV	< 5 y; < 20 kg	0.1 mg/kg	2 mg	0.4 mg/mL	5 mL
NALOXONE	IM/IV	< 5 y; > 20 kg	2 mg per dose		0.4 mg/mL	5 mL
NALOXONE	ETT		0.3 mg/kg	14.7 mg	0.4 mg/mL	36.75 mL

additional pediatric drugs		route	dose	mg to pt	supplied	mL to give
ANTIBIOTICS						
AMPICILLIN	<6 y	IV	50 mg/kg	300 mg		
AMPICILLIN	>6 y	IV	50 mg/kg	2,000 mg		
AMPICILLIN & SULBACTUM	>1 mo	IV	50 mg/kg	2,450 mg		
CEFAZOLIN		IV	25 mg/kg	1,000 mg		
CLINDAMYCIN		IV	10 mg/kg	490 mg		
ERTAPENEM	3 mo-12 y	IV	15 mg/kg	735 mg		
ERTAPENEM	>12 y	IV	1 Gm	per dose		
GENTAMICIN		IV	2 mg/kg	98 mg		
LEVOFLOXACIN		IV	10 mg/kg	490 mg		
METRONIDAZOLE		IV	10 mg/kg	490 mg		
PIPERACILLIN & TAZOBACTAM	<40 kg & 2-9 mo	IV	80 mg/kg	3,375 mg		
PIPERACILLIN & TAZOBACTAM	<40 kg & >9 mo	IV	100 mg/kg	3,375 mg		
PIPERACILLIN & TAZOBACTAM	>40 kg	IV	3.375 Gm per dose			
VANCOMYCIN		IV	15 mg/kg	735 mg		
ANTINAUSEA						
METOCLOPROMIDE		IV	0.2 mg/kg	9.8 mg	5 mg/mL	1.96 mL
DIPHENHYDRAMINE		IV/IM	1.25 mg/kg	61.25 mg	50 mg/mL	1.225 mL
SCOPOLAMINE		IV/IM	6 mcg/kg	294 mcg	400 mcg/mL	0.735 mL
MISCELLANEOUS MEDS						
AMINOCAPROIC ACID		IV	100 mg/kg	4,900 mg	250 mg/mL	19.6 mL
DESMOPRESSIN		IV/SQ	0.3 mcg/kg	14.7 mcg	4 mcg/mL	3.675 mL
DEXAMETHASONE	croup	IV	0.6 mg/kg	16 mg	4 mg/mL	4 mL
HYDROCORTISONE		IV/IO	3 mg/kg	100 mg	100 mg/mL	1 mL

49 KG

1 year ← 13 kg and up

Ventilation: trained rescuer	1 breath q 6-8 sec (8-10 breaths/minute) about 1 second/breath-visible chest rise; if intubated, continuous compressions without pause for ventilations
Pulse check	carotid or femoral
Compression	heel of 1 hand or both hands one atop the other–lower half of sternum between nipples
Depth	2 inches (5 cm) or at least 1/3 chest depth
Rate	at least 100 compressions per minute
Compress/vent ratio	30:2 single rescuer 15:2 healthcare providers
Foreign body obstruction	Helmlich maneuver Never perform a blind finger-sweep. Open the mouth and look for object; if you see it, remove it.

sync cardioversion	0.5 J/kg	24.5 J
repeat	1 J/kg	49 J
defibrillation	2 J/kg	98 J
repeat	4 J/kg	196 J

IV Bolus Drugs		dose	mg to pt	supplied	mL to give
ADENOSINE	IV	0.1 mg/kg	4.9 mg	3 mg/mL	1.63 mL
ADENOSINE repeat dose	IV	0.2 mg/kg	9.8 mg	3 mg/mL	3.27 mL
AMIODARONE	IV/IO	5 mg/kg	245 mg	50 mg/mL	4.90 mL
ATROPINE	IV/IM	0.02 mg/kg	0.5 mg	0.4 mg/mL	1.25 mL
ATROPINE	ETT	0.04 mg/kg	1.96 mg	0.4 mg/mL	4.90 mL
CALCIUM CHLORIDE	IV	20 mg/kg	980 mg	100 mg/mL	9.80 mL
CALCIUM GLUCONATE	IV/IO	60 mg/kg	800 mg	100 mg/mL	8.00 mL
DANTROLENE	IV	2.5 mg/kg	30 mg		
EPHEDRINE	IV	0.15 mg/kg	7.35 mg	10 mg/mL	0.74 mL
EPINEPHRINE (1:10,000)	IV/IO	0.01 mg/kg	0.49 mg	0.1 mg/mL	4.90 mL
EPINEPHRINE (1:1,000)	ETT	0.1 mg/kg	2.5 mg	1 mg/mL	2.50 mL
ESMOLOL	IV	0.5 mg/kg	24.5 mg	10 mg/mL	2.45 mL
LABETALOL	IV	0.2 mg/kg	9.8 mg	5 mg/mL	1.96 mL
LIDOCAINE	IV/IO	1 mg/kg	49 mg	20 mg/mL	2.45 mL
NEOSYNEPHRINE	IV	5 mcg/kg	245 mcg	100 mcg/mL	2.45 mL
ROMAZICON	IV	0.01 mg/kg	0.2 mg	0.1 mg/mL	2.00 mL
VASOPRESSIN	IV/IO	0.4 unit/kg	19.6 units	20 u/mL	0.98 mL

50 KG MAINTENANCE IV FLUIDS: 90 ML/HR

common pediatric drugs		route	dose	mg to pt	supplied	mL to give
ATROPINE	vagolytic	IV	0.02 mg/kg	0.5 mg	0.4 mg/mL	1.25 mL
GLYCOPYRROLATE	vagolytic	IV	0.004 mg/kg	0.2 mg	0.2 mg/mL	1 mL
MIDAZOLAM		IV	0.05 mg/kg	0.6 mg	1 mg/mL	0.6 mL
MIDAZOLAM		PO	0.5 mg/kg	20 mg	1 mg/mL	20 mL
MIDAZOLAM		IN	0.2 mg/kg	10 mg	1 mg/mL	10 mL
SUCCINYLCHOLINE		IV	2 mg/kg	100 mg	20 mg/mL	5 mL
SUCCINYLCHOLINE		IM	4 mg/kg	200 mg	20 mg/mL	10 mL
PROPOFOL		IV	3 mg/kg	150 mg	10 mg/mL	15 mL
ETOMIDATE	>10 y	IV	0.3 mg/kg	15 mg	2 mg/mL	7.5 mL
FENTANYL		IV	1 mcg/kg	50 mcg	50 mcg/mL	1 mL
FENTANYL		IN	2 mcg/kg	100 mcg	50 mcg/mL	2 mL
MORPHINE	<6 mo	IV/IM	0.05 mg/kg	2.5 mg	10 mg/mL	0.25 mL
MORPHINE	>6 mo	IV/IM	0.1 mg/kg	5 mg	10 mg/mL	0.5 mL
TORADOL	>2-16 y	IV	0.5 mg/kg	15 mg	30 mg/mL	0.5 mL
TORADOL	>2-16 y	IM	1 mg/kg	30 mg	30 mg/mL	1 mL
ACETAMINOPHEN		PR	20 mg/kg	1,000 mg		
ACETAMINOPHEN	2-12 y	IV	15 mg/kg	750 mg	10 mg/mL	75 mL
CISATRACURIUM		IV	0.1 mg/kg	5 mg	2 mg/mL	2.5 mL
PANCURONIUM	<1 mo	IV	0.02 mg/kg	1 mg	1 mg/mL	1 mL
PANCURONIUM	>1 mo	IV	0.1 mg/kg	5 mg	1 mg/mL	5 mL
ROCURONIUM		IV	0.6 mg/kg	30 mg	10 mg/mL	3 mL
ROCURONIUM	RSI	IV	1.2 mg/kg	60 mg	10 mg/mL	6 mL
VECURONIUM		IV	0.1 mg/kg	5 mg	1 mg/mL	5 mL
GLYCOPYRROLATE	reversal	IV	0.007 mg/kg	0.35 mg	0.2 mg/mL	1.75 mL
NEOSTIGMINE		IV	0.07 mg/kg	3.5 mg	1 mg/mL	3.5 mL
DEXAMETHASONE		IV	0.25 mg/kg	10 mg	10 mg/mL	1 mL
ONDANSETRON		IV	0.15 mg/kg	4 mg	2 mg/mL	2 mL

additional pediatric drugs	route	dose	mg to pt	supplied	mL to give
PREMED/SEDATION; VAGOLYTIC/ANTISIALAGOGUE; GIVE IM 30–60 MIN PREOP					
ATROPINE	IM	0.02 mg/kg	0.5 mg	0.4 mg/mL	1.25 mL
GLYCOPYRROLATE	IM	0.004 mg/kg	0.009 mg	0.2 mg/mL	0.045 mL
MIDAZOLAM	IM	0.1 mg/kg	0.5 mg	1 mg/mL	0.5 mL
DEXMEDETOMIDINE load dose	IV	0.5 mcg/kg	1 mcg	4 mcg/mL	0.25 mL
INDUCTION					
KETAMINE	IV	2 mg/kg	100 mg	10 mg/mL	10 mL
KETAMINE	IM/PR	5 mg/kg	250 mg	10 mg/mL	25 mL
OPIOIDS/NONOPIOIDS					
FENTANYL	IV high dose	4 mcg/kg	200 mcg	50 mcg/mL	4 mL
FENTANYL	IV cardiac	10 mcg/kg	500 mcg	50 mcg/mL	10 mL
HYDROMORPHONE < 6 mo	IV/SQ	0.005 mg/kg	0.25 mg	10 mg/mL	0.025 mL
HYDROMORPHONE > 6 mo	IV/SQ	0.015 mg/kg	0.75 mg	10 mg/mL	0.075 mL
REMIFENTANIL	IV	0.5 mcg/kg	1 mcg	50 mcg/mL	0.02 mL
SUFENTANIL	IV	0.5 mcg/kg	20 mcg	50 mcg/mL	0.4 mL
REVERSALS					
ATROPINE	IV	0.02 mg/kg	0.5 mg	0.4 mg/mL	1.25 mL
EDROPHONIUM neonate	IV	0.1 mg single dose		10 mg/mL	0.01 mL
EDROPHONIUM < 2 mo	IV	0.04 mg/kg	2 mg	10 mg/mL	0.2 mL
FLUMAZENIL	IV	0.02 mg/kg	0.2 mg	0.1 mg/mL	2 mL
NALOXONE < 5 y; < 20 kg	IV/IM	0.1 mg/kg	2 mg	0.4 mg/mL	5 mL
NALOXONE > 5 y; > 20 kg	IM	2 mg per dose		0.4 mg/mL	5 mL
NALOXONE	ETT	0.3 mg/kg	15 mg	0.4 mg/mL	37.5 mL

additional pediatric drugs		route	dose	mg to pt	supplied	mL to give
ANTIBIOTICS						
AMPICILLIN	<6 y	IV	50 mg/kg	300 mg		
AMPICILLIN	>6 y	IV	50 mg/kg	2,000 mg		
AMPICILLIN & SULBACTUM	>1 mo	IV	50 mg/kg	2,500 mg		
CEFAZOLIN		IV	25 mg/kg	1,000 mg		
CLINDAMYCIN		IV	10 mg/kg	500 mg		
ERTAPENEM	3 mo-12 y	IV	15 mg/kg	750 mg		
ERTAPENEM	>12 y	IV	1 Gm	per dose		
GENTAMICIN		IV	2 mg/kg	100 mg		
LEVOFLOXACIN		IV	10 mg/kg	500 mg		
METRONIDAZOLE		IV	10 mg/kg	500 mg		
PIPERACILLIN & TAZOBACTAM	<40 kg & 2-9 mo	IV	80 mg/kg	3,375 mg		
PIPERACILLIN & TAZOBACTAM	<40 kg & >9 mo	IV	100 mg/kg	3,375 mg		
PIPERACILLIN & TAZOBACTAM	>40 kg	IV	3.375 Gm per dose			
VANCOMYCIN		IV	15 mg/kg	750 mg		
ANTINAUSEA						
METOCLOPROMIDE		IV	0.2 mg/kg	10 mg	5 mg/mL	2 mL
DIPHENHYDRAMINE		IV/IM	1.25 mg/kg	62.5 mg	50 mg/mL	1.25 mL
SCOPOLAMINE		IV/IM	6 mcg/kg	300 mcg	400 mcg/mL	0.75 mL
MISCELLANEOUS MEDS						
AMINOCAPROIC ACID		IV	100 mg/kg	5,000 mg	250 mg/mL	20 mL
DESMOPRESSIN		IV/SQ	0.3 mcg/kg	15 mcg	4 mcg/mL	3.75 mL
DEXAMETHASONE	croup	IV	0.6 mg/kg	16 mg	4 mg/mL	4 mL
HYDROCORTISONE		IV/IO	3 mg/kg	100 mg	100 mg/mL	1 mL

50 KG

1 year ← 13 kg and up

Ventilation: trained rescuer	1 breath q 6-8 sec (8-10 breaths/minute) about 1 second/ breath-visible chest rise; if intubated, continuous compressions without pause for ventilations
Pulse check	carotid or femoral
Compression	heel of 1 hand or both hands one atop the other–lower half of sternum between nipples
Depth	2 inches (5 cm) or at least 1/3 chest depth
Rate	at least 100 compressions per minute
Compress/vent ratio	30:2 single rescuer 15:2 2 healthcare providers
Foreign body obstruction	Heimlich maneuver Never perform a blind finger-sweep. Open the mouth and look for object; if you see it, remove it.

sync cardioversion	0.5 J/kg	25 J
repeat	1 J/kg	50 J
defibrillation	2 J/kg	100 J
repeat	4 J/kg	200 J

IV Bolus Drugs		dose	mg to pt	supplied	mL to give
ADENOSINE	IV	0.1 mg/kg	5 mg	3 mg/mL	1.67 mL
ADENOSINE repeat dose	IV	0.2 mg/kg	10 mg	3 mg/mL	3.33 mL
AMIODARONE	IV/IO	5 mg/kg	250 mg	50 mg/mL	5.00 mL
ATROPINE	IM/IV	0.02 mg/kg	0.5 mg	0.4 mg/mL	1.25 mL
ATROPINE	ETT	0.04 mg/kg	2 mg	0.4 mg/mL	5.00 mL
CALCIUM CHLORIDE	IV	20 mg/kg	1,000 mg	100 mg/mL	10.00 mL
CALCIUM GLUCONATE	IV/IO	60 mg/kg	800 mg	100 mg/mL	8.00 mL
DANTROLENE	IV	2.5 mg/kg	30 mg		
EPHEDRINE	IV	0.15 mg/kg	7.5 mg	10 mg/mL	0.75 mL
EPINEPHRINE (1:10,000)	IV/IO	0.01 mg/kg	0.5 mg	0.1 mg/mL	5.00 mL
EPINEPHRINE (1:1,000)	ETT	0.1 mg/kg	2.5 mg	1 mg/mL	2.50 mL
ESMOLOL	IV	0.5 mg/kg	25 mg	5 mg/mL	5.00 mL
LABETALOL	IV	0.2 mg/kg	10 mg	5 mg/mL	2.00 mL
LIDOCAINE	IV/IO	1 mg/kg	50 mg	20 mg/mL	2.50 mL
NEOSYNEPHRINE	IV	5 mcg/kg	250 mcg	100 mcg/mL	2.50 mL
ROMAZICON	IV	0.01 mg/kg	0.2 mg	0.1 mg/mL	2.00 mL
VASOPRESSIN	IV/IO	0.4 unit/kg	20 units	20 u/mL	1.00 mL

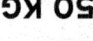

7

Neonatal Pearls, Diseases, Emergencies, and Procedures

■ Neonatal pearls (age 1–28 days)

Understanding the physiologic changes that occur in cardiovascular, pulmonary, hepatic, and renal systems during the transition from fetal to neonatal life is crucial to the anesthetic management of the neonate.

Hypoxia, hypercarbia, acidosis, and hypothermia can cause the newborn to revert to fetal circulation (also known as persistent pulmonary hypertension of newborn) and induce right-to-left shunting through the foramen ovale and ductus arteriosus, accompanied by an increased right ventricular pressure and pulmonary vascular resistance in the neonate.

Neonate: Volume Status

Assessment of the severity of dehydration and volume status are similar as in the older child, but in the neonate an additional check is as follows:

■ Anterior skull fontanel to see if membranes are sunken, indicating low volume

See "Pediatric: Volume Status" for more information.

Neonate: Cardiovascular

Fetal circulation is characterized by high pulmonary vascular resistance, low systemic vascular resistance, and right-to-left shunting of blood through the foramen ovale and ductus arteriosus. The onset of spontaneous ventilation at birth is associated with decreased pulmonary vascular resistance and increased pulmonary blood flow.

Three fetal cardiac shunts may occur:

- Connection between the right and left atria via the **foramen ovale**. The foramen ovale closes within 5–10 days secondary to increased systemic vascular resistance and a decrease in pulmonary vascular resistance.

- Connection between the pulmonary artery and the proximal descending aorta via the **ductus arteriosus**. The ductus arteriosus closes physiologically at 10–15 hours due to increased levels of oxygen, decreased prostaglandin levels, and a normal acid–base balance; it closes anatomically at 2–3 weeks.

- The **ductus venosus** shunts a portion of umbilical venous blood around the liver directly to the inferior vena cava. The ductus venosus closes by constriction from increased oxygen levels.

Heart rate is the main factor of cardiac output in the neonate; cardiac output cannot be escalated by increased contractility.

Stroke volume is relatively fixed by a noncompliant and poorly developed left ventricle in neonates and infants. Thus, cardiac output is very dependent on heart rate.

Ventricles are stiff due to the high percentage of noncontractile proteins. A decreased heart rate does not allow for increased filling.

Neonates have an immature baroreceptor reflect and have a limited capacity to increase heart rate in response to hypotension.

The parasympathetic nervous system is fully functional at birth. The sympathetic nervous system develops around 4 months. Until then, stress causes bradycardia and apnea.

Neonates have increased vagal tone and are prone to bradycardia. Major causes of bradycardia include the following:

- Hypoxia
- Vagal stimulation
- Inhaled anesthetics

Treatment of bradycardia:

- Give 100% FiO_2 as long as necessary for an O_2 saturation between 85% and 95%. *Lower FiO_2 levels of oxygen should be used to prevent retinopathy.*
- If bradycardia is caused by vagal stimulation, give atropine 10–20 mcg/kg IV; may repeat q 5 min to max 1.0 mg. The ETT dose of atropine is 2–3 × IV/IO dose.
- *Hypotension/hypovolemia: IVF bolus LR 10–20 mL/kg.*

Neonate: Hematology

Neonates have 60–90% fetal hemoglobin (HbF). The characteristics of HbF influence oxygen transfer as HbF has a decreased concentration of 2,3-diphosphoglycerate (2,3-DPG), resulting in a left shift of the oxyhemoglobin curve and making hemoglobin have a high affinity for oxygen. In short, HbF binds oxygen to the hemoglobin molecule with greater affinity, thereby decreasing the release of oxygen to peripheral tissues. The decreased release of oxygen to the tissues is offset by the increased oxygen delivery provided by the increased hemoglobin concentration characteristic of a neonate (1 day: 19 Gm/dL; 2 weeks: 17 Gm/dL; 1 month: 14 Gm/dL; 2 months: 11 Gm/dL; 6 months: 12 Gm/dL; 1 year: 12 Gm/dL).

After birth, the total hemoglobin level decreases rapidly as the proportion of HbF diminishes, reaching its lowest level by 2–3 months of age (referred to as physiologic anemia of infancy).

The PaO_2 at which hemoglobin is 50% saturated is called the P_{50}.

- Fetal hemoglobin has a P_{50} of 19 mm Hg.
- Adult hemoglobin has a P_{50} of 26 mm Hg.

While the hemoglobin drops in the first few months of infancy, the P_{50} increases, exceeding adult values by 4–6 months of age.

Neonate: Respiratory
Airway
Infants are obligate nasal breathers until 3–5 months; occlusion of the nares can cause complete airway obstruction.

- Glottis corresponds to:
  - **C3: premature infant**
  - **C3–C4: newborn**
  - **C4: children**
- Length of trachea is approximately 4 cm.
- The narrowest portion of the neonatal airway is the cricoid cartilage, just below the vocal cords.

Intubation
In preparing the pediatric patient for intubation, it is important to note that the neck is flexed because of a prominent occiput when the child lies on a flat surface. This predisposes sleeping children to airway obstruction.

The sniffing position is best for airway management. A rolled towel under the shoulders helps to gently extend the infant's large head to achieve a more neutral position of the neck and open up the airway, thus improving intubating conditions.

- Large tongue obstructs the airway more easily
- Floppy, "U"-shaped epiglottis
- High, anterior cords
- Smaller airway

A Miller blade was designed to directly lift the epiglottis, which may assist in intubating small children. If using a Macintosh blade, place it in the far right side of the mouth, scooping the tongue up and to the left to improve visualization of the larynx.

- Endotracheal tube size for neonates roughly corresponds to 1/10 of gestational age rounded down to the nearest size:
  - A 32-week preemie would get a 3.0 ETT.
  - A 28-week preemie would get a 2.5 ETT.
- Uncuffed tube size can also be calculated $= \text{age} + 16/4$ or $\text{age}/4 + 4$.
- Use of an uncuffed endotracheal tube is more common in neonates.
- Air leak should be 20–25 cm H_2O.

Lungs

- High closing volumes reflect the volume of gas remaining in the lungs when the small airways begin to close during a controlled maximum exhalation. Due to normal tidal volumes with higher closing volumes in the neonate and infant, atelectasis and hypoxia develop more easily.

- Hypoxia and hypercarbia will depress respirations in neonates (but stimulate respirations in adults). The ventilation response to hypoxia is biphasic.

  1. Initial hyperpnea—lasts around 2 minutes (abolished by hypothermia and low levels of anesthetic gas)
  2. Depression of respiration

  By 3 weeks of age, hypoxia produces sustained hyperventilation.

- Once hypoxia ensues, apnea occurs much more quickly than in an adult.

- Neonates' oxygen requirements are 150 mL/min/m^2 – 6 mL/kg (adults: 3 mL/kg): 2–3 times that of an adult. A warm environment will help to minimize oxygen consumption.

- Although tidal volumes are proportionately the same as adults (6 mL/kg), the respiratory rate in infants is much higher, leading to a higher alveolar ventilation in relation to function residual capacity (5:1 in infants versus 1.4:1 in adults). This results in a faster inhalational induction and emergence.
- Work of breathing is higher in neonates than in older children.
- Intrinsic PEEP keeps lungs from collapsing; therefore, + 4 cm PEEP should be given to every infant or child less than 2 years old. When awake, a baby will terminate expiratory phase before reaching FRC. Once anesthetized, this protective mechanism is abolished.
- There is a high ratio of minute ventilation in neonates: 100–150 mL/kg/min (compared to 60 mL/kg/min in adults).
- Chest wall compliance is high and tends to collapse inward during spontaneous inspiration, due to the neonate's cartilaginous ribs and limited thoracic muscle mass.

- Neonates are more prone to atelectasis and respiratory insufficiency, especially under general anesthesia.
- Neonates are more prone to severe obstruction of upper and lower airways due to immaturity of respiratory muscles.
- Neonates have increased sensitivity to superior laryngeal nerve stimulus, causing ventilatory depression or apnea.
- Infants younger than 60 weeks post-conceptual age are at risk for apnea after general anesthesia. Apnea of infancy: respiratory pauses > 20 seconds and/or accompanied by bradycardia or cyanosis.

Neonate: Renal

- Renal function at birth depends on post conceptual age. By 34 weeks, all nephrons are developed. In the first several days of life, there is a decreased ability to concentrate urine due to a low glomerular filtration rate at birth. Normal neonate creatinine: 0.8–1.2 mg/dL.
- There is inadequate sodium conservation due to immature neonatal tubules. Neonates do not completely reabsorb sodium under the simulation of aldosterone;

they are called obligate sodium losers. Neonate urine sodium: 20–25 mEq/L. Replacement fluids for the neonate **must** contain sodium.

- IV fluids: D_5.2NS for maintenance IV fluids. Lactated Ringer's is given for deficit replacement (third-space and insensible losses).

Neonate: Hepatic
- Hepatic enzymes start to mature at birth.
- Neonates require lower doses of anesthetic drugs due to an immature blood–brain barrier and decreased ability to hepatically metabolize these drugs.

Neonate: Temperature
See "Pediatric: Temperature" for more information on pediatric temperature concerns.

Premature infants can lose 15 times more heat than full-term babies. To compensate for increased heat losses, the sympathetic nervous system constricts peripheral blood vessels, thereby centralizing body heat (the most consistent response). The cost of this is a two- to three-fold increase in oxygen consumption and cell metabolism.

Like pediatric patients, neonates lose heat through conduction, convection, evaporation, and radiation. Neonates have a much smaller muscle mass and maintain body temperature through nonshivering thermogenesis (NST) mediated by brown fat (fatty acid) metabolism. Infants born before the third trimester have less ability to initiate NST and are more prone to hypothermia.

Aggressive prevention of temperature loss is needed in neonates to prevent reversion to fetal circulation (helps to prevent an increase in PVR and a decrease in pulmonary blood flow causing a right-to-left shunt and increased blood flow through the patent ductus arteriosus). Hypoventilation, along with inadequate oxygen delivery and acidosis, followed by cardiovascular collapse, can occur when a neonate cannot maintain a warm temperature.

■ Common neonatal emergencies and anesthetic management

- Congenital diaphragmatic hernia (CDH)
- Gastroschisis
- Myelomeningocele
- Omphalocele
- Patent ductus arteriosus (PDA)
- Pyloric stenosis
- Tracheoesophageal fistula (TEF)

Congenital Diaphragmatic Hernia

CDH is a congenital malformation of the diaphragm occurring primarily on the left side (can occur bilaterally, which is usually fatal) during fetal development. This diaphragmatic hole allows abdominal contents to herniate into the chest, occupying that space and preventing the lung from growing to normal size, resulting in pulmonary hypoplasia. A left diaphragmatic hernia usually presents with a mediastinal shift to the right.

While only one lung is usually affected, both lungs can be abnormal, having decreased numbers and function of their alveoli. Functionally, lungs are noncompliant and cannot be inflated with volumes in excess of normal. Many alveoli remain closed even at increased airway pressures, and ventilating with increased pressures reaches only the already open alveoli, resulting in rupture and pneumothoraces.

This condition has a mortality rate of 40–55%. If the infant survives, the ipsilateral lung expands with decompression of abdominal contents and becomes functional, although it remains small with fewer than normal alveoli.

There is a one in three chance that an infant with CDH will have other birth defects; these infants are often seen with dextrocardia.

Presentation includes significant hypoxia, cyanosis, dyspnea, scaphoid abdomen, barrel chest, and bowel sounds in the chest.

Persistent fetal circulation is often present due to acidosis, hypoxia, and hypercarbia, with increased pulmonary vascular resistance. A diagnosis of fetal circulation can be confirmed by measuring the PaO_2 in blood obtained simultaneously from a pre-ductal (right radial) artery and a post-ductal (umbilical, posterior tibial, or dorsalis pedis) artery. A difference of greater than 20 mm Hg verifies the diagnosis.

Treatment

Immediate intervention includes:

- Insert an orogastric tube to decompress the bowel (distention would worsen intrathoracic pressure).
- Avoid positive-pressure mask ventilations so as not to distend the bowel.
- Immediately intubate; avoid high peak inspiratory pressures (keep < 25 cm H_2O). High-frequency jet ventilation or extracorporeal membrane oxygenation (ECMO) may be required.
- Correct acid–base imbalance and increase pulmonary perfusion.
- Before surgery, optimizing oxygenation without worsening persistent pulmonary hypertension of the newborn (PPHN) and pulmonary hypoplasia is crucial. (*See the later discussion of PPHN for more information.*)

- Worsening hemodynamics and a sudden increase in cyanosis can indicate a pneumothorax. Immediate chest tube insertion and decompression on the contralateral side must be done.

Anesthetic Management

- IV access is best in the upper extremities (inferior vena cava compression from increased intra-abdominal pressures will limit venous return from lower extremities).
- Intubate with the baby fully awake.
- Consider pre- (right hand) and post-ductal (foot) pulse oximetry.
- The use of supplemental oxygen should be limited to that required to maintain the oxygen saturation between 85% and 95% to prevent retinopathy of prematurity.
- Nitric oxide can be given to decrease pulmonary hypertension.
- Increased respiratory rate with decreased tidal volumes is best; avoid positive-pressure ventilation or airway pressures > 25 cm H_2O to avoid danger of pneumothorax. Hand-ventilation is often required.

- During surgery, insert nasogastric tube to decompress the stomach if not already done.
- Ensure normothermia.
- Place an arterial line for cardiovascular or respiratory problems.
- Watch peak inspiratory pressure levels during abdominal closure. Tight closure can lead to vascular insufficiency, compression of the inferior vena cava, and respiratory insufficiency. The abdomen may need to be left open with a plastic covering with the plan for future surgical closure.
- Do not attempt to reinflate the hypoplastic lung following hernia reduction and diaphragm repair—this can lead to pneumothorax on the contralateral lung.
- The neonate should remain intubated postoperatively. $PaCO_2$ is a good predictor of outcome.

Gastroschisis
Similar to omphalocele but with important differences.

Gastroschisis has an idiopathic etiology. It is not an umbilical defect, but rather an abdominal wall defect in which the intestines are not "midline" (often being off to the right). The intestines are external; there is an increased risk of infection because the bowel is not encased in the peritoneum but instead is exposed. Gastroschisis is considered a surgical emergency.

This abdominal defect is more common than omphalocele but less commonly associated with other congenital abnormalities.

- These babies have a greater fluid loss due to exposed viscera and require higher amounts of fluid resuscitation.
- Hypothermia is an increased risk in these babies. It is important to keep baby and exposed viscera warm. The bowel should be covered with warm, saline-soaked gauze and wrapped in plastic until surgery.
- Infection prevention is crucial; peritonitis is a potential problem. Give antibiotics.

Anesthetic Management
- IV access is best in the upper extremities (inferior vena cava compression from increased intra-abdominal pressures will limit venous return from the lower extremities).

- Fluid resuscitation with crystalloids (6–10 mL/kg/hr) and albumin is needed for hypovolemia. Urinary output of 1–2 mL/kg/hr indicates adequate hydration, although fluid management can be guided by central venous pressure monitoring.
- If not already placed immediately after birth, an orogastric or nasogastric tube should be placed before induction.
- Perform rapid-sequence induction for intubation.
- The use of supplemental oxygen should be limited to that required to maintain the oxygen saturation between 85% and 95% to prevent retinopathy of prematurity.
- Avoid nitrous oxide.
- High-dose narcotics and muscle relaxants (pancuronium) are the mainstay anesthetics.
- The goal is to close the defect; complete muscle relaxation is needed to facilitate return of the eviscerated bowel into the abdominal cavity.
- Ventilatory requirements often change once the bowel is placed in the abdomen; it is best to hand-ventilate during this time. Notify the surgeon of increased peak airway pressures (>40 cm H_2O).

- It may be necessary to leave the abdomen open if the viscera are too large for the abdominal cavity. Tight closure can lead to vascular insufficiency, compression of the inferior vena cava, and respiratory insufficiency. The abdomen may need to be left open with a plastic covering for future surgical closure.
- A pulse oximeter probe on the foot helps to detect compromised venous return or blood from viscera too large for the abdominal cavity.
- The neonate should remain intubated postoperatively.

Myelodysplasia

This congenital failure of the middle or caudal end of the neural tube results in spina bifida, meningocele, or myelomeningocele. These patients are prone to infection and sepsis.

- **Meningocele:** sac at the lower spine contains *only* cerebrospinal fluid; neural function is intact. The spinal cord is tethered by the sacral nerve roots. If unrepaired, a meningocele results in orthopedic and/or urologic symptoms below the level of the lesion.

- **Myelomeningocele:** sac usually at lower spine contains neural components—spinal cord. Varying degrees of sensory and motor deficits are present. Dilation of the upper urinary tract occurs, along with spasticity and scoliosis. These babies often have hydrocephalus and Arnold-Chiari malformations. The defect must be sterilely covered as soon as possible after birth to prevent infection and fluid losses prior to surgery.

Anesthetic Management
Surgical repair is done the first day of life.

- Good intravenous access is required. The neonate needs fluid resuscitation, and may be hypovolemic due to seepage of cerebrospinal fluid (CSF). There is a potential for intraoperative blood loss.
- Avoid pressure on the sac during induction. The baby can be positioned supine on a foam or gel doughnut with the defect down in the center hole, or intubation may need to be done in a lateral decubitus position to avoid pressure on sac.

- Take special care to not extend the head and compress the cervical spinal cord with possible congenital malformations.
- Awake intubation may be needed for suspected difficult airway.
- The use of supplemental oxygen should be limited to that required to maintain the oxygen saturation between 85% and 95% to prevent retinopathy of prematurity.
- Succinylcholine does not produce a hyperkalemic response and can be used.
- Avoid muscle relaxants initially; neurophysiologic monitoring (SSEPs) may be used.
- Hypothermia is a greater concern than normal with abnormal autonomic control below the level of the lesion.
- Surgical closure of the myelomeningocele sac must be tight enough to prevent leakage of CSF; the surgeon may ask for Valsalva maneuver with positive airway pressures initiated and briefly maintained close to 40 mm Hg to test for leaking.
- Postoperatively, the baby should be maintained in a lateral decubitus or prone position.

Omphalocele

In this umbilical defect, the intestines are herniated into the base of the umbilical cord and are outside the body. The bowel is completely covered with membranes and has less fluid and electrolyte difficulties than with gastroschisis. Cover the defect with warm, saline-soaked gauze to prevent infection and maintain body warmth.

This abdominal defect is less common than gastroschisis but is associated with more congenital defects (e.g., mental retardation, urologic, metabolic, and cardiac [tetralogy of Fallot] abnormalities).

Anesthetic Management

- Immediately after birth and diagnosis, provide for IV access and fluid resuscitation.
- IV access is best in the upper extremities (inferior vena cava compression from increased intra-abdominal pressures will limit venous return from the lower extremities).
- Heat loss, rapid dehydration, and infection are added problems. It is important to keep the baby and exposed hernia warm. Give antibiotics.

- Orogastric or nasogastric tube insertion is performed to decompress the stomach if not already done.
- Perform rapid-sequence induction or awake intubation.
- High-dose narcotics and pancuronium are the mainstay anesthetics. Complete muscle relaxation facilitates reduction of the eviscerated bowel back into the abdomen.
- Avoid nitrous oxide.
- The use of supplemental oxygen should be limited to that required to maintain the oxygen saturation between 85% and 95% to prevent retinopathy of prematurity.
- It may be necessary to leave the abdomen open if the viscera are too large for the abdominal cavity. Tight closure can lead to vascular insufficiency, compression of the inferior vena cava, and respiratory insufficiency. The abdomen may need to be left open for future surgical closure.
- A pulse oximeter probe on the foot helps to detect compromised venous return or blood from viscera too large for the abdominal cavity.
- Healthy babies with a small closure often can be extubated immediately postoperatively.

Patent Ductus Arteriosus

The ductus arteriosus (DA) is a normal fetal blood vessel connecting the pulmonary artery to the descending aorta. It allows most of the fetal blood ejected from the right ventricle to bypass the lungs and is essential in fetal systemic perfusion in utero. Usually, the DA functionally closes within 72 hours after birth in response to increased oxygen tensions. Anatomic closure occurs over the next several days.

One of the most common congenital heart defects, a PDA allows a persistent communication from the aorta (higher pressure) to the pulmonary vasculature. Fluid overload, respiratory distress syndrome, severe illness, acidosis, hypoxia, and hypercarbia may reopen a functionally closed DA.

- Symptoms: hemodynamically significant PDA signs and symptoms include respiratory distress from pulmonary overload, and congestive heart failure from a left-to-right shunt as the pulmonary vascular resistance falls.

- Treatment: pharmacologic or surgical. Indomethacin or ibuprofen can be given in attempt to block cyclooxygenase (which inhibits prostaglandin synthesis, thereby facilitating ductal closure). Other medical management includes fluid restriction and diuretics.

Anesthetic Management

Surgical approach is usually via a small left posterolateral thoracotomy, but a video-assisted thoracoscopic clip ligation technique can also be used. The main consideration during surgery is to balance the pulmonary vascular resistance (PVR) with the systemic vascular resistance (SVR). It is important to maintain PVR, SVR, and myocardial contractility.

- Perform pre-ductal (right hand) and post-ductal (foot) pulse oximetry.
- Capnography is useful for detecting inadvertent pulmonary artery ligation.
- Measure blood pressure in the right arm (preferable) and a lower extremity.
- Although blood loss is usually minimal, be prepared for hemorrhage: Have good intravenous access, with albumin and packed red blood cells immediately available.

- Clear air bubbles meticulously from the IV tubing.
- Ensure normothermia.
- High-dose narcotics and pancuronium are the mainstay anesthetics.
- The use of supplemental oxygen should be limited to that required to maintain the oxygen saturation between 85% and 95% to prevent retinopathy of prematurity.
- Surgical dissection and lung retraction may be necessary to expose the duct, which can result in hypoxemia, hypercarbia, bradycardia, and hypotension. Higher levels of oxygen may be necessary during lung retraction.
- Avoid nitrous oxide.
- After ligation, there is an acute increase in blood pressure and LV afterload (SVR). Inotropic support may be necessary for the severely dysfunctional ventricle.
- Postoperative chest X-ray is done to check for pneumothorax.
- Neonates may require postoperative mechanical ventilation.

Pyloric Stenosis

This gross thickening of the circular smooth muscle of the pylorus results in gradual obstruction of the gastric outlet. Persistent vomiting leads to loss of acidic gastric juices rich in hydrogen and chloride ions and, to a lesser extent, sodium and potassium ions. The kidneys begin secreting potassium ions in exchange for hydrogen in an attempt to maintain a normal pH.

Presentation occurs between 2 and 8 weeks of age, with symptoms consisting of forceful, projectile, nonbilous vomiting. Severe cases result in a dehydrated infant with a hypokalemic, hypochloremic metabolic alkalosis.

Diagnosis is made by palpation of an olive-sized mass in the upper aspect of the abdomen. Many cases are verified by upper GI series with barium.

This is a medical—not surgical—emergency. Treat dehydration and correct electrolyte disturbances prior to surgery. IVF: $D_5.2NS$ with 40 mEq potassium chloride at $3L/m^2$ for 12–48 hours preoperatively.

Surgical pyloromyotomy is curative and usually lasts less than 30 minutes with an experienced surgeon.

Anesthetic Management

- Aspiration of gastric contents is the primary concern and is due to obstructed pylorus and associated vomiting.

- Suction the stomach through a nasogastric or orogastric tube at least three times before induction; give oxygen in between passes of the suction catheter. This greatly reduces the chance of regurgitation during induction (but does not completely eliminate the possibility).

- Ensure proper preoxygenation and monitoring. The use of supplemental oxygen should be limited to that required to maintain the oxygen saturation between 85% and 95% to prevent retinopathy of prematurity.

- This condition is considered a "full stomach" case. Rapid-sequence induction is also needed to prevent aspiration.

- Perform induction with an IV in place.

- After induction, an NG tube is reinserted and left in place during the operation. To test the integrity of the pyloric wall after pyloromyotomy, a small volume of air is injected down the nasogastric tube by syringe; the surgeon manipulates the air bubble into the duodenum to occlude the bowel lumen both proximal and distal to the incision. Mucosal perforation is indicated if air leakage occurs.

- Narcotics are rarely indicated; they may prolong emergence. Local anesthesia is given at the incision site.

- Use short-acting muscle relaxants, if any at all; some surgeons can do this procedure in as little as 10–15 minutes. If such drugs are given, muscle relaxation is reversed at the end of the procedure.

- Try to maintain CO_2 in the low 40s.

- These babies will be prone to postoperative respiratory depression on emergence due to preexisting central alkalosis (CSF); apnea will not raise CO_2.

- Watch for facial grimacing and hip flexion; safely extubate the neonate when awake and with intact protective airway reflexes.

- Lethargy and drowsiness are not unusual postoperatively.

Tracheoesophageal Fistula

TEF is caused by a failure of the lung buds to separate from the foregut in utero. Several different types of TEF can occur, though most often (90%) a fistula exists between the trachea (just above the carina) and the lower esophageal segment, while the upper esophagus ends in a blind pouch.

TEF diagnosis is confirmed by the inability to pass a soft suction catheter into the stomach.

Presentation consists of polyhydramnios in utero (esophageal obstruction prevents swallowing of amniotic fluid), prematurity, excessive oral secretions, inability to feed, and regurgitation of saliva and feeding attempts.

TEF can accompany other congenital abnormalities. Approximately 25% of affected neonates have congenital heart disease; often with VACTERL syndromes:

- Vertebral anomalies
- Anus, imperforate or atresia
- Cardiac abnormalities
- Tracheoesophageal fistula

- Esophageal atresia
- Renal or radial abnormalities
- Limb abnormalities

Treatment consists of surgical ligation of the TEF and anastomosis of the esophagus, done through a right thoracotomy. The surgery can be done extrapleurally (fewer postoperative complications), although this procedure is technically more difficult. If there is isolated esophageal atresia, treat with gastrostomy and esophagostomy at 6 months of age; a jejunal substitution is done at 1 year.

Anesthetic Management

- A gastrostomy tube may need to be placed prior to induction if the neonate is in respiratory distress. If a gastrostomy tube is already present, it can be "vented" to release stomach air.
- Positive-pressure mask ventilation can distend the stomach.
- A blood pressure cuff is placed on right upper arm. The precordial stethoscope taped in place; no esophageal stethoscope can be used.

- With an IV in place, perform oropharyngeal and proximal esophageal suctioning.
- Induction with an awake intubation is preferred; spontaneous respiration decreases gastric distention.
- Insert the endotracheal tube (ETT), without a Murphy eye side hole, deeply into the right main stem, and gradually withdraw it until the fistula is occluded but both lungs are being ventilated and bilateral breath sounds are heard. Auscultate the stomach to ensure it is not overinflated. If a Murphy eye is present on the ETT, position the ETT bevel anteriorly to avoid ventilation of the fistula. Positioning the ETT properly can be quite difficult depending on where the fistula is located in the trachea.
- Hand-ventilate to pick up changes in vent pressures. The trachea can become kinked or the ETT can easily become dislodged.
- Antibiotics are needed with sepsis or aspiration pneumonia.
- Position the neonate in left lateral position for right-sided thoracotomy.
- An arterial line is needed for cardiovascular or respiratory problems.

- Mix the oxygen/air with sevoflurane or isoflurane to whatever is tolerated; go easy on the narcotics so that extubation is an option.

- Keep O_2 saturation at 85–95% (due to retinopathy of prematurity), although a higher O_2 concentration may be needed during right lung compression or retraction.

- The goal is to extubate at the end of the procedure to prevent pressure on the suture line by the endotracheal tube. However, premature babies and those with significant pulmonary disease may require postoperative mechanical ventilation.

■ Common neonatal disease and anesthetic management

Choanal Atresia

This condition involves occlusion of one or both posterior nares; it is associated with premature fusion of suture (craniosynostosis). The child is pink when screaming, cyanotic when quiet.

Neonates are obligate nasal breathers, so the mouth must be kept open with an oral airway or a plastic nipple to avoid suffocation. Unilateral choanal atresia may go undiagnosed for years; bilateral choanal atresia must have surgical correction or a tracheostomy be performed in the first few days of life.

Anesthetic Management

- Must have oral airway or large nipple secured in mouth.
- Awake intubation with oral RAE.
- Should be fully awake and meet all extubation criteria prior to extubation.

Retinopathy of Prematurity

The immature retina is deficient in a number of enzymes that make it more susceptible to the deleterious effects of oxygen. High inspired concentrations of oxygen can affect the immature vasculature in the eyes. Effects of retinopathy of prematurity (ROP) can range from mild (with no defects) to severe (with neovascularization and possible retinal detachment and blindness). Long duration of supplemental oxygen increases the risk.

Predisposing factors to ROP are as follows:

- Prematurity; the most significant risk for ROP, it is inversely related to birth weight, especially a birth weight < 1,500 Gm.
- Occurrence up to 44 weeks post-conceptual age.
- Gestational age immaturity.

In utero oxygen tension is 20–30 mm Hg; birth raises the PaO_2 to 55–85 mm Hg. The use of supplemental oxygen should be limited to that required to maintain the oxygen saturation between 85% and 95% in neonates and pediatric patients 1–3 months old.

Necrotizing Enterocolitis

Necrotizing enterocolitis (NEC) involves idiopathic death of the lining of the intestine wall. It is the most common life-threatening intestinal emergency in the newborn. The infant presents with generalized signs of sepsis, hypothermia, distended abdomen, bloody stool, and vomiting.

If possible, medically stabilize the infant before surgery with fluid resuscitation, ventilator support, and antibiotics. Surgery becomes emergent if a pneumoperitoneum occurs from intestinal wall perforation and/or clinical deterioration (persistent metabolic acidosis).

Anesthetic Management
- Maintain a warm ambient temperature in rooms, use a warming light/lamp, and use warming blankets. Keep every possible body part covered.
- Insert an orogastric tube if not already done preoperatively.
- Provide for vigorous fluid resuscitation for third-space losses and sepsis.
- Have blood products immediately available for coagulopathy.
- Inotropes may be needed for hemodynamic support.
- Antibiotics are essential.
- The use of supplemental oxygen should be limited to that required to maintain the oxygen saturation between 85% and 95% to prevent retinopathy of prematurity.
- Avoid nitrous oxide.
- The neonate will need to remain intubated postoperatively.

Persistent Pulmonary Hypertension of the Newborn

Persistent pulmonary hypertension of the newborn (PPHN) (also see "Shunting") results in the persistence or return of fetal circulation after birth from failure of pulmonary vascular resistance to decrease at birth. PPHN is caused by hypoxia and acidosis; it also occurs secondary to elevated pulmonary vascular resistance (PVR) with resultant right-to-left shunt via the ductus arteriosus and foramen ovale. It can be a primary disease, but is often secondary to other conditions, including pneumonia, congenital diaphragmatic hernia, aspiration, and sepsis.

- Signs and symptoms: respiratory distress, tachypnea, marked cyanosis, poor cardiac function and perfusion, and acidosis.

- Treatment: hyperventilation to cause alkalosis, pulmonary vasodilators (prostaglandin), correct acidosis. ECMO may be needed if endotracheal intubation and ventilation fail to maintain oxygenation and perfusion.

Anesthetic Management

- Stress should be avoided and there should be minimal handling of the baby.
- Adequate ventilation and oxygenation are key.
- Nitric oxide may be used for direct pulmonary vasodilation.
- Adequate depth of anesthesia is needed to ablate the rise in pulmonary vascular resistance associated with surgical stimuli.
- Maintain normal body temperature.
- Provide inotropic support: dopamine, dobutamine, milrinone.
- Be prepared for cardiovascular collapse associated with a pulmonary hypertensive crisis with an acute rise in pulmonary vascular resistance.

8

Pediatric Pearls, Diseases, Emergencies, and Procedures

■ Pediatric pearls

An *infant* is defined as 1–12 months of age; a *child* is defined as age 1 year to puberty.

Pediatric: Volume Status
Volume status in the child can be assessed by the following means:

- Laboratory values that include hematocrit, glucose, blood urea nitrogen, albumin, and serum electrolytes
- Skin turgor
- Skin pink and capillary refill < 3–5 seconds if well hydrated
- Eyes become sunken when dehydrated
- Heart rate increases linearly with dehydration
- Blood pressure decreases linearly with dehydration
- Weight loss: 5% with mild dehydration, 10% with moderate dehydration, and 15% with severe dehydration

Pediatric: Cardiac
- Stroke volume is relatively fixed by a noncompliant and poorly developed left ventricle in infants. Thus, cardiac output is very dependent on heart rate.

- In older children, to help meet increased oxygen requirements, cardiac output is increased 30–60% by an elevated heart rate.
- Bradycardia (HR < 80 BPM) should be treated in a child less than 12 years old.
  - Hypoxia: give 100% FiO_2.
  - Vagal stimulation: give atropine 10–20 mcg/kg IV; may repeat q 5 min to max 1.0 mg.
  - Hypotension/hypovolemia: IVF bolus LR 10–20 mL/kg.
- Atropine is typically given prior to or during induction of anesthesia to prevent bradycardia:
  - Infant: Recommended dose is 0.01–0.02 mg/kg with a minimum dose of 0.1 mg (lower doses have been associated with paradoxical bradycardia).
  - Dose may be repeated in 5 minutes to maximum dose of 1.0 mg in a child and 2.0 mg in an adolescent.
  - Dose may be administered via ETT or sublingually if there is no IV access. The ETT dose of atropine is 2–3 times the IV/IO dose.

Pediatric: Respiratory

The sniffing position is the best option for airway management in children (the child's occiput is larger in proportion to the body). Placing a rolled-up towel under the shoulders works well.

Airway

- Epiglottis is narrower, longer, stiff, and "U"-shaped; at a more acute angle, it makes it more difficult to lift out of view during laryngoscopy.
- Glottis is at C3–C4 (older children: C4; adults: C5).
- Narrowest portion of the pediatric airway is the cricoid cartilage, just below the vocal cords.
- Length of trachea is 5–9 cm.
- Tongue is relatively large and may cause obstruction.
- Loose teeth are possible in children ages 6–8. It is best to prepare parents in the preoperative area for potential dislodgement of loose tooth.
- Uncuffed tubes are more commonly used in children up to age 8.
- Tube size calculation: age + 16/4 or age/4 + 4.
- Air leakage of 20–25 cm H_2O is expected.

Lungs

- Although tidal volumes are proportionally the same as in adults (6 mL/kg), to compensate for increased oxygen consumption the child's respiratory rate needs to be faster (3 times faster than in adults), leading to a higher alveolar ventilation in relation to function residual capacity (5:1 in infants, 1.4:1 in adults). This results in a faster inhalational induction and emergence in children.

- Children's lungs are prone to collapse. Small airway closures occur because of increased closing volume, which is at or above functional residual capacity (FRC). When awake, the infant terminates the expiratory phase before reaching FRC to compensate; once the child is anesthetized, this protective mechanism is abolished. This causes collapse and VQ mismatch.

- Intrinsic PEEP keeps lungs from collapsing; therefore, +4 cm PEEP should be given to every infant or child less than 2 years old. When awake, a child will terminate expiratory phase before reaching FRC. Once anesthetized, this protective mechanism is abolished.

- Strong elastic recoil and weak intercostal muscles are present in infants. At 2 months of life, intercostal muscles have matured. However, it takes 8 months for the diaphragmatic muscles to mature. This predisposes the 3- to 4-month-old child to fatigue more readily in response to obstruction, chronic illness, and disease.
- By 3 weeks of age, hypoxia produces sustained hyperventilation.
- Oxygen requirements of infants are 6 mL/kg (adult 3 mL/kg): 2–3 times that of an adult.
- In the first three weeks of life, oxygen consumption is 120–130 mL/min/m^2 (6 mL/kg vs 3 mL/kg in adults). A warm environment will help minimize oxygen consumption.

Pediatric: Renal
- Over the first 3 months of life, the glomerular filtration rate (GFR) increases two- to three-fold.
- At 6–12 months of age, infants are able to concentrate urine as well as adults.

- A baby will produce dilute urine to the point of dehydration.
- Young infants have inadequate sodium conservation, so IV fluids must contain sodium; D5.2NS is usually given to children less than 1 year old. Children greater than 1 year old can receive IV fluids without sodium; lactated Ringer's is usually given.

Pediatric: Hepatic

- Hepatic enzymes start to mature at birth.
- By 3 months, most tasks of maturation have been accomplished and all common anesthetics can be used on a per-kilogram basis.

Pediatric: Temperature

A child's body temperature is affected by four processes: conduction, convection, evaporation, and radiation (the biggest source of heat loss).

There are two stages of heat loss: (1) body core to skin surface and (2) skin surface to environment.

The ability of infants to thermoregulate is limited and easily overwhelmed owing to the following factors:

- The infant's small size
- Increased surface area to volume ratio
- Little subcutaneous fat
- Increased thermal conductance
- Limited ability to shiver
- Nonshivering thermogenesis mediated by brown fat metabolism—brown fat is located in the mediastinum, adrenals, axilla, and scapulae

The main site of thermoregulation is the hypothalamus, a negative feedback system. Homeothermic organisms maintain a stable core temperature during changes in ambient temperature. Infants are homeotherms despite an internal temperature that varies widely. Homeostasis is accomplished by balancing heat production with heat loss.

- Hypothermia is associated with cardiac irritability, respiratory depression, altered drug responses, and delayed awakening from anesthesia.

■ Hypothermia prevention and treatment: warm ambient temperature in rooms, radiant heat lamps, warming mattress, warm IV fluids, heated and humidified gases, warm blankets, cover exposed body cavities, and wrap the top of the head in plastic.

Anesthetic Management

Hypothermia decreases MAC of inhaled agents, increases tissue solubility of inhaled agents, decreases requirements for muscle relaxants, and prolongs their duration.

■ Pediatric diseases, emergencies, procedures, and anesthetic management

Anaphylaxis

Common causes:

■ Food: peanuts, walnuts, cashews, shellfish, fish, milk, eggs
■ Insect stings: bees, wasps, hornets
■ Medications: NSAIDs, IV contrast, blood products, colloids
■ Common anesthetic agents: NDMR, latex, antibiotics, induction agents, local anesthetics

The allergic response triggers mast cells to release immunological mediators (e.g., histamine, prostaglandins, leukotrienes, etc.) into the bloodstream. This results in the following effects:

- Profound systemic vasodilation. Capillary permeability increases and arteriolar dilation occurs, leading to a decreased return of blood to the heart:
  - Decreased central venous pressure or preload
  - Decreased pulmonary capillary wedge pressure
  - Decreased systemic vascular resistance
- Edema of bronchial mucosa, bronchoconstriction, and dyspnea; angioedema.

  Signs and symptoms:
  - Respiratory distress
  - Hypotension
  - Urticaria
  - Flushed appearance
  - Angio edema: swelling of lips, face, neck, and throat
  - Anxiety
  - Tachycardia, hypotension

Treatment: anaphylactic shock can lead to death in a matter of minutes if left untreated. Treatment includes these measures:

- Stop administration or decrease absorption of the offending agent if possible.
- 100% FiO_2; airway control with endotracheal intubation or tracheostomy if unable to maintain oxygen saturations with natural airway.
- Albuterol: beta$_2$ agonist used to treat bronchoconstriction.
- H$_1$ blockers: diphenhydramine to decrease histaminic effects.
- Epinephrine IV to increase blood pressure.
- Racemic epinephrine: a sympathomimetic bronchodilator for laryngeal edema or laryngospasm.
- H$_2$ blockers: famotidine **or** ranitidine (both listed) to decrease secretion of gastric acid in parietal cells of gastric mucosa.
- Steroid: hydrocortisone or methylprednisolone (both listed) to decrease mediator release.

- Hydrocortisone to stabilize cell membrane for persistent symptoms.
- Phenylephrine: alpha$_1$-adrenergic receptor agonist to increase blood pressure if needed.

ANAPHYLAXIS

Albuterol *Ventolin/Proventil* (inhalation)	4-8 puffs q 20 min PRN with spacer weight < 20 kg: 2.5 mg/dose q 20 min in NS via nebulizer Weight > 20 kg: 5 mg/dose q 20 min in NS via nebulizer
diphenhydramine *Benadryl*	1-2 mg/kg IV/IM/IO; max: 50 mg/dose
epinephrine *Adrenalin*	0.01 mg/kg (0.01 mL/kg) 1:1,000 IM in thigh q 15 min PRN; max: 0.5 mg **Or** 0.01 mg/kg (0.1 mL/kg) 1:10,000 IV/IO q 3-5 min; max: 1 mg If hypotension persists despite fluids and IM injection: 0.1-1 µg/kg/min IV/IO infusion ETT dose of epinephrine is 10 times the IV/IO dose max ETT dose: max 2.5 mg/dose
epinephrine racemic 2.25%	<20 kg: 0.25 mL of 2.25% into 4 mL NS for nebulizer 20-40 kg: 0.5 mL of 2.25% into 4 mL NS for nebulizer >40 kg: 0.75 mL of 2.25% into 4 mL NS for nebulizer Administer over 10-15 min; may repeat q 1-2 hr
famotidine *Pepcid*	Start: 1 mg/kg/day divided BID PO/IV; max: 40 mg/day **Or** 0.5-1 mg/kg/day IV divided BID
hydrocortisone *Solu-Cortef*	2-3 mg/kg IV/IO slowly; max: 100 mg

methylprednisolone *Solumedrol* (*methylprednisolone sodium succinate*)	0.5-1.7 mg/kg/day IV/IM slowly; divided 6-12 hr
phenylephrine *Neosynephrine*	IV bolus: 5-20 mcg/kg/dose every 10-15 min PRN IM or SQ: 0.1 mg/kg every 1-2 hr; max: 5 mg
ranitidine *Zantac*	1 mg/kg/dose IV/PO
IV fluid	10-30 mL/kg 0.9% normal saline to restore intravascular volume from massive vasodilation

Asthma: Acute Exacerbation

Asthma is a common, chronic inflammatory disorder of the airway associated with airway hyperresponsiveness. The perioperative presentation of acute asthma is a potentially life-threatening event.

A focused physical is needed to assess the severity of the airway obstruction. A silent chest is an ominous sign that respiratory failure is imminent. Mental agitation, drowsiness, and confusion are signs of cerebral hypoxemia.

Assess for anaphylaxis, which can mimic a severe asthma attack; if anaphylaxis is suspected, give epinephrine immediately. *See "Anaphylaxis" for more information.*

Epinephrine in Anaphylaxis

Epinephrine:

- 0.01 mg/kg (0.01 mL/kg) 1:1,000 IM in thigh q 15 min PRN (max 0.5 mg) **or**
- 0.01 mg/kg (0.1 mL/kg) 1:10,000 IV/IO q 3–5 min (max 1 mg)
- If hypotension despite fluids and IM injection: 0.1–1 µg/kg/min IV/IO infusion

Epinephrine racemic 2.25%:

- <20 kg: 0.25 mL of 2.25% into 4 mL NS for nebulizer
- 20–40 kg: 0.5 mL of 2.25% into 4 mL NS for nebulizer
- >40 kg: 0.75 mL of 2.25% into 4 mL NS for nebulizer

Treatment

- Give oxygen by face mask or nasal cannula; intubation may be needed. Intubation should be the last resort, as up to 26% of children intubated due to acute asthma develop complications such as pneumothorax, impaired venous return, or cardiovascular collapse because of increased intrathoracic pressure. Mechanical ventilation is ultimately associated with an increased risk of death.

- Give short-acting beta$_2$ agonists: albuterol, terbutaline (metered-dose inhaler or nebulizer treatment) or salbutamol IV infusion.
  - Terbutaline *Brethine:*
    - Nebulizer: 0.01–0.03 mg/kg/dose with a minimum dose of 0.1 mg; maximum dose is 2.5 mg diluted with 1–2 mL of normal saline every 4–6 hr
    - Inhalation aerosol: 2 inhalations separated by 60 sec q 4–6 hr
    - Subcutaneous: 0.01 mg/kg SQ; max: 0.25 mg
    - Bolus IV: 10 mcg/kg IV (range 2–10 mcg/kg); max: 750 mcg
    - Infusion: 0.08–6 mcg/kg/min IV infusion; max: 3 mcg/kg/min
  - Albuterol *Ventolin, Proventil*
    - Inhaler
      - 4–8 puffs q 20 min PRN with spacer

- ▫ Nebulizer
    - ○ Weight < 20 kg: 2.5 mg/dose q 20 min in NS via nebulizer
    - ○ Weight > 20 kg: 5 mg/dose q 20 min in NS via nebulizer
- IV salbutamol infusion *Ventolin; albuterol*: can be given if no response to above treatments; *Salbutamol is also available in oral form*
    - ▫ IV infusion: drug must be diluted
        - ○ Usual bolus dose 10 mcg/kg over 2 min; max: 500 mcg
        - ○ Usual infusion range: 5–10 mcg/kg/min for 1 hr, then reduce to 1–2 mcg/kg/min
    - ▫ Inhaler: use metered-dose inhalers for intubated patients
        - ○ Respigen, Salamol, and Ventolin: 100 mcg/dose
        - ○ Combivent: salbutamol 100 mcg/dose plus ipratropium 20 mcg/dose
    - ▫ Nebulizer: 2.5–5 mg nebulizers as needed

- Give inhaled anticholinergics.
  - Ipratropium bromide *Atrovent: inhalation* 0.02%: 500 mcg/2.5 mL
    - **Neonates:**
      Nebulized solution: 25 mcg/kg 3 times daily
    - **Infants and children:**
      Nebulized solution: 125–250 mcg 3 times daily
    - **3–12 years:**
      - Inhalation aerosol: 1–2 inhalations (18–36 mcg) 3 times daily, up to 6 inhalations/day
      - CFC-free inhalation aerosol: 1–2 inhalations (17–34 mcg) 4 times daily, up to 12 inhalations/day
- Give corticosteroids (oral or IV).
  - Methylprednisolone sodium succinate *Solumedrol*
    - Start: 2 mg/kg × 1 IM/IV slowly
    - 0.5–1.0 mg/kg IV q 6 hr
- Give epinephrine SQ 0.01 mg/kg SQ (0.01 mL/kg) 1:1000 q 15 min. Same as 10 mcg/kg; max: 0.5 mg/kg.

- Magnesium sulfate has been shown to be effective in treating children with status asthmaticus: 25–50 mg/kg IV/IO slow infusion over 15–30 min; max: 2 Gm.

Bradycardia

Bradycardia should be treated in any child younger than age 12 years.

- Hypoxia is likely: Give 100% FiO_2.
- Vagal response: Give atropine 10–20 mcg/kg IV/ETT; may repeat q 5 min to max 1.0 mg. The ETT dose of atropine is 2–3 times the IV/IO dose.
- Hypotension/hypovolemia: Give IVF bolus LR 10–20 mL/kg.
- If unresponsive to above treatment: Give epinephrine 0.01 mg/kg IV/IO; ETT dose of epinephrine is 10 times the IV/IO dose with a max dose of 2.5 mg.

Cerebral Palsy

Cerebral palsy (CP) is part of a group of nonprogressive disorders characterized by motor deficits from hypoxic/anoxic cerebral damage. It may be caused by prematurity, birth trauma, hypoglycemia, intrauterine and neonatal infections, or congenital CVMs. CP presents with skeletal muscle spasticity and contractures.

- Cerebral palsy patients are prone to aspiration due to gastroesophageal reflux disease (GERD) and impairment of laryngeal and pharyngeal reflexes.
- Drug therapy for spasticity includes dantrolene and baclofen.
- Approximately 50% of all children with CP have seizures and are on phenobarbital, phenytoin, or carbamazepine; they should take these medications on the day of surgery. Some seizure medications stimulate hepatic microsomal enzymatic activity, which may lead to altered responses to drugs that are metabolized in the liver; these responses are referred to as being "enzyme induced." In such cases, other drugs metabolized through the liver will be metabolized more quickly and repeated doses will need to be given more often.

Anesthetic Management

- Administration of an antisialagogue will help to decrease secretions.
- Succinylcholine does **not** produce an exaggerated potassium release (unless the patient is in a wheelchair).
- The response to nondepolarizing muscle relaxants is normal.
- Opioids may impair airway reflexes.
- Caudal epidurals would be appropriate to cover postoperative pain for lower abdominal/extremity surgeries.
- Emergence from general anesthesia may be delayed because of cerebral damage from cerebral palsy.

Cleft Lip/Palate

Infants with cleft lip or palate have difficulty feeding and are at risk for aspiration with increased incidence of URIs and otitis media.

Cleft lips are usually repaired at 2–3 months of age, while a cleft palate is repaired at approximately 18 months of age.

These children often have associated anomalies including congenital heart disease.

Anesthetic Management

- All bubbles must be meticulously removed from IV fluids due to the possibility of atrial or septal defects.

- The method of induction depends on the degree of airway abnormality. An inhalation induction can often be done while the child maintains spontaneous respirations; however, an awake induction may be necessary.

- Use of an oral Rae endotracheal tube (taped to the bottom lip) may be used to minimize distortion of the facial anatomy. A reinforced endotracheal tube can be used to prevent compression from the Dingman gag (i.e., the instrument that the surgeon uses to open the child's mouth).

- In an infant with a large defect of the palate, intubation may be difficult if the laryngoscope blade slips into the cleft. To help prevent this from happening, pack the cleft with gauze or wrap the laryngoscope blade in gauze.

- Breath sounds and chest compliance must be continually monitored while using the Dingman gag.

- Children with cleft lip or palate are at risk for unrecognized blood loss.
- Eye injury is possible during surgery about the face; lubrication, tape, and eye pads should be considered.
- The child should be fully awake and meet all extubation criteria prior to extubation.
- Laryngospasm is a big concern after extubation. Have all emergency drugs and equipment available.
- Postoperatively, airway obstruction from edema of the mouth and throat is a major concern. A suture can be placed through the tongue and taped to the cheek so that if obstruction occurs, pulling the suture will move the tongue forward, thereby reestablishing the airway.

Clubfoot

Clubfoot can occur in healthy infants or children with cerebral palsy or muscular dystrophy. With this structural deformity, the child has shortened, medial tendons of the lower leg and a shortened Achilles tendon. The foot is pointed downward and rotated inward.

Treatment consists of manipulation and casting. The infant may need surgical correction and casting at 3–6 months.

Anesthetic Management

- Anesthesia: general and regional.
  - Inhalation induction
  - Caudal: bupivacaine 0.25% 1 mL/kg gives analgesia for 4–6 hours and decreases inhalational requirement
- If caudal anesthesia is not done, give IV opioids: fentanyl 2–5 mcg/kg or morphine 0.1 mg/kg. This repair is *very* painful.
- Once intubated, move the baby to the bottom of the table. Know where the IVs and ETT are to prevent inadvertent removal of these lines/tubes.
- Tourniquets are used during the surgical procedure. When the tourniquet is let down, cold blood perfuses the child and body temperature will drop; $ETCO_2$ also increases.

Craniofacial Syndromes

Mandibular hypoplasia (micrognathia) is a common feature in craniofacial abnormalities. The affected child's small mandible leaves little room for the tongue, makes the larynx seem anterior, and usually causes upper airway obstruction and difficult intubations.

Goldenhar: this facial deformity has unilateral mandibular hypoplasia. Eye, ear, and vertebral abnormalities occur on the affected side. **Pierre-Robin triad** and **Treacher-Collins** syndromes are characterized by bilateral facial defects.

- **Pierre-Robin triad:** micrognathia, glossoptosis, and a cleft palate.
  - These structural abnormalities may lead to feeding problems, failure to thrive, and cyanotic episodes.
  - Examine from the side as well as facing the child; structures may appear normal from the frontal view.
  - If upper airway obstruction occurs, the tongue may need to be sutured down and forward.
  - These children often have associated congenital heart disease.

- **Treacher-Collins syndrome:** the most common of the mandibular–facial syndromes.
  - Manifests bilaterally involving the eyes, cheek bones, external ears, and lower jaw
  - A downward slant of the lateral (outer) eyes
  - Deficiencies of the cheek bones
  - Absent or malformed external ears; ear tags
  - Associated with cleft palate, congenital heart disease, and gross deformities of the external auditory canal and ossicular chain

Anesthetic Management

- Many children with craniofacial syndromes pose challenges to airway management, intubation, and extubation. The anesthetic evaluation in patients with craniofacial syndromes should begin with a thorough airway evaluation and formulation of a plan for intubation. An emergency intubation situation should always be considered as a possibility, with all necessary equipment available.

- The inclusion of an anticholinergic drug in the preoperative area will help avoid anesthetic-associated bradycardic events as well as reduce upper airway secretions.
- Oral or IV administration of a histamine receptor antagonist should be part of any preoperative regimen in infants with craniofacial syndromes at risk for aspiration.
- Avoid ventilatory depressants preoperatively.
- Intubation should be preceded by 100% O_2 and atropine. Maintain spontaneous respirations during inhalation induction.
- No muscle relaxation should be given until ETT placement is confirmed.
- Extubate only when the child is fully awake and meets all criteria for extubation. Emergency airway equipment must be available in case reintubation is needed.

Craniosynostosis
- Craniosynostosis refers to early closing or fusion of one or more of sutures of infant's head; it causes the skull to expand in the direction of the open sutures. When the

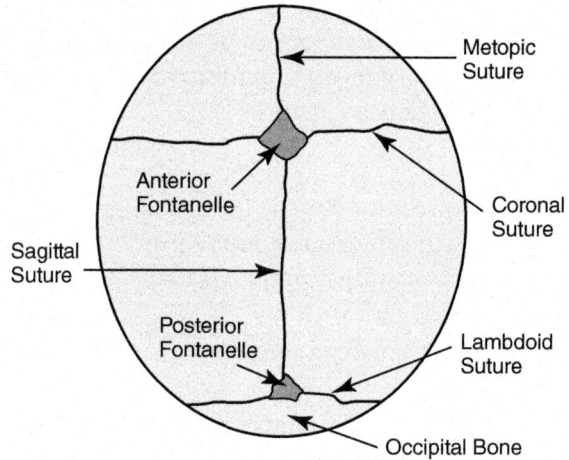

FIGURE 8-1

skull cannot compensate, the brain can become pressed, increasing intracranial pressures (ICP) and causing vision changes. Involved sutures may be sagittal, coronal, metopic, and/or lambdoid.

Two types are distinguished:

- Nonsyndromic: usually affects only one suture and is not associated with other congenital abnormalities

- Syndromic: affects more than one suture and is often accompanied by other abnormalities (e.g., obstructive sleep apnea, neurobehavioral impairment, Apert's syndrome, Crouzon syndrome, and others)

Surgery may be done for cosmetic reasons or to relieve elevated ICP and hydrocephalus. Calvarial vault remodeling (surgical remodeling) may be performed, usually before the child reaches 1 year of age. Alternatively, in endoscopic surgery, the surgeon opens one suture. The child is then required to wear a molding helmet postoperatively to re-shape the skull.

Anesthetic Management
- Concerns include the child's face shape changes and difficulty with mask ventilation and intubation.
- Securing the endotracheal tube carefully prevents loss of airway patency during potential head movement by the surgeon. These surgeries can be quite long.
- Standard inhalation induction is often utilized.
- The child's body position may be supine, prone, or both, depending on the sutures involved.

- Large blood loss is possible and can be significant. Have very good IV access in case fluid resuscitation and blood products are required. Blood products should be in the operating room before the surgery starts.

- Venous air embolism (VAE) is a risk with the surgery. A central venous line (air aspiration) and precordial Doppler are recommended. Close attention to vital signs is crucial: Watch for hypotension, bradycardia, and rhythm changes. An abrupt drop and sustained decrease in $ETCO_2$ indicates a VAE.

- Disseminated intravascular coagulation (DIC) is a possible consequence of massive blood loss and replacement.

- Hypothermia is an issue with the head being exposed. Warm the room, bed, IV fluids, and patient.

- An arterial line may be needed for larger cases.

- If ICP is elevated, be prepared to administer mannitol and/or furosemide.

- Place a nasopharyngeal airway (trumpet) before the child's emergence from anesthesia.

- Assess for facial and neck swelling before considering extubation.
- The majority of patients can be extubated but should be fully awake and meet all extubation criteria prior to extubation. Be prepared for reintubation if needed.

Croup (Acute Laryngotracheobronchitis)

Croup is an upper respiratory infection that spreads to the larynx, vocal cords, and subglottic structures; it progresses to a hoarse cry or barking cough due to glottic or tracheal edema.

Causes may include any of the following:

- Viral infection (85%)
- Oversized endotracheal tube
- Bucking on endotracheal tube
- Traumatic intubation
- Upper respiratory infection
- Manipulation of head/neck when intubated

Symptoms include: respiratory compromise from progressive swelling of subglottic tracheal mucosa, which leads to hacking, a barking cough, low fever (<39°C), and inspiratory stridor. Croup has a gradual onset, with progression of symptoms over 24–72 hours.

If croup is caused by post-extubation laryngeal edema, it usually presents within 4 hours after extubation, but sooner in severe cases. The greatest incidence occurs in children 1–4 years old. Causes of this type include mechanical trauma to the airway and placement of a tube that produces a tight fit.

Anesthetic Management
- Cool, humidified O_2.
- Racemic epinephrine: administer over 10–15 min; may repeat q 1–2 hr.
  - <20 kg: 0.25 mL of 2.25% into 4 mL NS
  - 20–40 kg: 0.5 mL of 2.25% into 4 mL NS
  - >40 kg: 0.75 mL of 2.25% into 4 mL NS

- Dexamethasone IV: 0.6 mg/kg slow IM/IV; max: 20 mg/dose.
- Antipyretics for fever.
- Intubation is rarely needed unless exhaustion occurs. If there is a need to reintubate the child, use ½ to 1 full size smaller than calculated size of ETT; tracheostomy may be considered.

Cystic Fibrosis

Cystic fibrosis is a disease of the exocrine glands: It affects the lungs, pancreas, gastrointestinal tract, and hepatobiliary systems. These glands produce thickened mucus, which obstructs the respiratory system and causes subsequent infections. Pancreatic insufficiency can lead to malabsorption and glucose intolerance.

Perioperative implications include increased risks for the following complications:

- Pneumothorax
- Atelectasis
- VQ mismatch
- Hemoptysis

- Hypoxemia
- Hypercarbia
- Cor pulmonale

Anesthetic Management
- Check serum blood glucose frequently.
- Use smaller tidal volumes and higher respiratory rates to maintain $ETCO_2$.
- Warm and humidify gases.
- Ensure conservative opioid administration to prevent respiratory depression postoperatively.
- Use of bronchodilators and suctioning the lungs are helpful.

Diabetes Insipidus
Signs of diabetes insipidus (DI) include dilute polyuria:
- Output > 2 mL/kg/hr
- Urine osmolality < 250 mOsm/L
- Serum hyperosmolality > 300 mOsm/L

- Sodium > 145 mEq/L

Treatment for DI consists of desmopressin (DDAVP 4 mcg/mL = 16 IU); 1 mcg of DDAVP is equivalent to 4 IU (international units).

- 3 mo–12 y:
  - Intranasal: 5–30 mcg/day
  - Slow IV/SQ: 0.1–1 mcg/day
- >12 y: 2–4 mcg/day divided q 12 hr slow IV/SQ

Down Syndrome (Trisomy 21)

Patients with Down syndrome tend to have the following abnormalities:

- Subglottic stenosis
- Large tonsils and adenoids
- Cervical instability (subluxation of C1–C2 from joint laxity)
- Large tongue
- Midface hypoplasia
- Narrow nasopharynx
- Pharyngeal hypotonia

- Cardiac abnormalities: 50% of patients with Down syndrome have a high incidence of atrial and ventricular septal defects (most often with mitral regurgitation)
- High pulmonary vascular resistance related to chronic hypoxemia
- Other issues: obesity, hypothyroidism, bowel obstructions from congenital duodenal atresia, frequent otitis media, strabismus, mental retardation, and obstructive sleep apnea

Anesthetic Management

- Obtain IV access prior to induction; children can become bradycardic on induction.
- Avoid heavy or unsupervised sedation due to the predisposition to upper airway obstruction.
- Anticipate the need for an oral airway. Effective mask ventilation often requires manual forward displacement of the mandible and placement of an oral airway.
- Patency of the airway may be difficult to maintain during induction of anesthesia; obstruction and desaturation may occur during normal sleep (OSA common).

- Use smaller ETT than calculated due to subglottic stenosis.
- Measure the leak pressure after placement of the ETT to confirm use of proper size of ETT (avoid additional subglottic pressure).
- Avoid neck hyperextension or flexion (intubate with manual in-line stabilization) due to atlantoaxial joint laxity.
- Remove all air bubbles in IV fluid and tubing carefully due to the potential for septal defects.
- Patients need antibiotic (SBE) prophylaxis if they have congenital heart disease.
- Use less narcotics.
- Extubate only when the patient is wide awake.
- Perioperative pulse oximeter monitoring is essential due to the predisposition for airway obstruction.

Duchenne's Muscular Dystrophy

Duchenne's muscular dystrophy (DMD) is a rapid and progressive form of muscular dystrophy characterized by symmetric and degenerative atrophy and weakness of skeletal muscles, while sensation and reflexes remain intact. It occurs primarily in boys; they become wheelchair bound by 8–11 years old.

- These patients have myocardial dysfunction due to infiltration of their muscles with fat—a condition associated with dilated cardiomyopathy. Death is often due to cardiopulmonary causes in later stages. Resting tachycardia is common.

- Most patients die from pneumonia by age 15–25 years due to the affected muscles of respiration, decreased pulmonary reserve, retention of secretions, and weak upper airway dilator muscles.

- Patients have delayed gastric emptying and macroglossia.

- Patients have kyphoscoliosis (with restrictive lung disease) and long bone fractures, skeletal muscle necrosis, and increased permeability of muscle cell membranes.

Anesthetic Management

The medical literature details poor anesthetic outcomes with DMD patients related to loss of airway secondary to medication-induced respiratory depression, aspiration of stomach contents, and sudden death secondary to cardiac conduction delays and dysrhythmias.

Patients with DMD are especially sensitive to the respiratory depressive effects of sedation and general anesthesia. General anesthesia decreases functional residual capacity (FRC).

- Perform thorough pulmonary testing and cardiovascular evaluation preoperatively.
- Have a defibrillator and external pacer in the operating room due to the risk of sudden death.
- Consider preoperative metoclopramide, sodium bicitrate and/or a histamine-2 blocker to reduce the risk of acidic aspiration pneumonia.
- Be very cautious when administering any preoperative sedation.
- Rapid-sequence induction with cricoid pressure is recommended.
- Patients with DMD should not receive volatile anesthetics (they exacerbate myocardial depression and can cause a malignant hyperthermia-type response) or succinyl-

choline (because of an increased incidence of malignant hyperthermia).

- Propofol or etomidate induction and minimal IV opioids (TIVA with remifentanil and propofol infusions have been used safely).
- Patients with muscular dystrophy often have scoliosis, which may present problems with positioning.
- Postoperative pain control should be managed with NSAIDs, regional techniques using local anesthetics, and acetaminophen when possible. If opioids are employed (systemic or neuraxial), then ICU care and continuous pulse oximetry must be considered given the high risk for respiratory depression and aspiration.
- Avoid nondepolarizing muscle relaxants, very sensitive; if needed, use only short-acting agents. Train of four monitoring can elicit a myotonic response.
- Hypercapnia and hypoxemia can worsen chronic cardio-pulmonary abnormalities found in some patients with DMD, such as pulmonary hypertension or conduction defects.

- Hypothermia and shivering can induce a myotonic contracture. Maintain a warm operating room, and use warmed IV fluids and forced-air blankets during surgery.
- Patients with DMD have an increased incidence of malignant hyperthermia: $ETCO_2$ and temperature monitoring is essential.
- Postoperative mechanical ventilation with continued intubation should be strongly considered. Extubation should occur only in optimal circumstances when strict extubation criteria are met.
- Consider extubating directly to BIPAP and/or CPAP. Be prepared for reintubation. Monitor the EKG along with pulse oximetry and capnography postoperatively.

Epiglottitis (*Haemophilus influenzae*)

Epiglottitis may be caused by bacterial infection; *Haemophilus influenzae* is most often the pathogen involved.

Presentation differs somewhat for children and adults:

- Child: Cellulitis at base of tongue, which spreads to epiglottis. Airway obstruction is possible.

- Adult: Same as child but with less risk of airway obstruction.

Signs and symptoms include rapid progression of sore throat to severe airway obstruction, muffled voice, high fever, and drooling. Child is distressed and sits erect.

Management:

- Preventive: Vaccine for children (*Haemophilus influenzae*).
- Emergency: Transport to ED; observe. Child may require artificial airway and steroids; antibiotics are crucial.

Anesthetic Management

If intubation is needed, go to the operating room. The child may need a surgical airway if the intubation attempt fails.

- Keep the child calm; allow the parents to stay at all times. Let the child get in his or her position of choice: Don't force child to do anything!
- Ensure that an ENT surgeon is present and ready for emergency cricothyrotomy or tracheostomy, if needed.

- Take the child to the operating room with the parents; allow the parents to stay during induction to decrease the child's emotional stress. The child can sit on the parent's lap.
- Perform mask induction with humidified oxygen via CPAP in the OR while maintaining spontaneous ventilation. The parent should leave immediately after the child anesthetized.
- Apply standard monitors and insert an IV once the child is asleep.
- Give atropine or robinul 0.01 mg/kg to prevent bradycardia and as an antisialagogue.
- Intubate with a stiletted oral ETT—one size smaller than calculated.
- Once the child is stable, change the oral ETT to a nasotracheal ETT and secure it very well.
- Epiglottitis usually resolves within 48–96 hours.
- Extubate only after complete resolution of epiglottic edema; confirm this resolution by direct visual laryngoscopy. Be prepared to reintubate the child if necessary.

Foreign Body Obstruction or Foreign Body Aspiration

Airway obstruction from foreign body aspiration into the airway can produce a wide range of responses. These range from cough, dyspnea, wheezing, and decreased breath sounds on the affected side, to complete obstruction and death from asphyxiation.

The most frequent site of foreign body obstruction (FBO) is the right bronchus because of the less acute angle in which it comes off the trachea.

Radiographic evidence of the foreign body can be obtained if the aspirated object is radiopaque. If the object is radio-lucent, indirect evidence can be obtained by demonstrating hyperinflation of the affected lung due to air trapping, with possible shifting of the mediastinum toward the opposite side. Atelectasis distal to the obstruction is a late finding.

To remove the object, perform direct laryngoscopy and bronchoscopy, using either a flexible or rigid scope.

Anesthetic Management

- Rigid bronchoscopy is the gold standard for FBO, although flexible bronchoscopy can also be done.

- Preoperative administration of anticholinergics is undertaken to reduce airway secretions and to attenuate the vagal response with induction/intubation. Anticholinergics also help to block reflex bronchoconstriction.
- The induction technique depends on the severity of the obstruction.
  - Without significant airway obstruction, proceed with IV induction.
  - With airway obstruction, maintain spontaneous respiratory effort during inhalation induction. Use a mask to deliver sevoflurane, 70% N_2O, and 30% O_2. This is done despite the possibility of a full stomach.
- Administer a topical local anesthetic to the vocal cords prior to intubation.
- Avoid muscle relaxation; the child should maintain a spontaneous respiratory effort. It may be necessary to paralyze the patient if the aspirated object is too large to pass through the moving cords or if there is a risk of patient movement when the rigid bronchoscope is in the airway.

- Insert an orogastric tube to suction the stomach before emergence.
- Giving corticosteroids helps to limit/decrease bronchus/airway inflammation.
- Postoperatively, give a racemic epinephrine nebulizer.
- Complications may include fragmentation of the foreign body, bronchospasm, hypoxemia, hypercarbia, subglottic edema, and severe laryngeal edema. Hypoxic cardiac arrest during retrieval of the object, pneumothorax, pneumomediastinum, and bronchial rupture are a few more serious complications that can occur.

Hip Dislocation, Congenital

Severity of hip dislocation ranges from joint laxity (ligaments stretched) to irreducible displacement (which needs a spica cast).

Treatment consists of a Pavlick harness; fluoroscopy-guided closed reduction, and spica casting. The short operative procedure is not considered very painful.

Anesthetic Management

- **The greatest concern is LOSS OF AIRWAY** because the child must be lifted from the OR table to the spica casting table, and then back to the OR table. Secure the LMA/ETT so it does not become dislodged with movement.
- Keep the child in stage III so that movement does not induce laryngospasm if the patient is intubated with an LMA.
- Need 100% O_2 prior to circuit disconnections with patient positioning.
- Use the esophageal stethoscope continuously!
- Make sure the infant is kept warm during procedure and is at least 36°C before extubation.

Hirschsprung's Disease

Hirschsprung's disease is a congenital condition in which there is an absence of ganglion cells in all or part of the colon, which affects muscle movement along the large intestine and results in a functional obstruction. Most cases affect the most distal portion of the colon, although the entire colon can be affected in some patients—even the stomach and esophagus (i.e., antecedent parts of the gastrointestinal tract can be affected). Although usually diagnosed shortly after birth, Hirschsprung's disease can also develop later in life.

Hirschsprung's disease is associated with neurologic, cardiovascular, other gastrointestinal, and urologic abnormalities. Down syndrome is seen in 9% of patients with this condition.

In mild cases, most affected infants present in the first few months of life with constipation, progressive abdominal distention, and poor feeding. In severe disease, enterocolitis, peritonitis from perforation, and toxic megacolon are found.

Greatest risks to the child are vomiting that leads to electrolyte imbalance, intestinal obstruction with regurgitation/aspiration, and intestinal perforation and sepsis.

Medical treatment includes placement of an orogastric or gastric tube for stomach decompression, volume resuscitation, antibiotics, and correction of electrolyte abnormalities.

Surgical treatment involves removal of the diseased portion of the colon. A colostomy may need to be placed before a definitive ileal–anal pull-through (AKA J-pouch) procedure is done.

Anesthetic Management
- Ensure volume resuscitation is done prior to induction to prevent hypotension.
- Perform rapid-sequence induction.
- Muscle relaxation is needed.
- Avoid nitrous oxide.
- Ensure normothermia.
- The child should be fully awake and meet all extubation criteria prior to extubation at the end of surgery.

Hyperkalemia
If a child suffers cardiac arrest after receiving succinylcholine, immediately treat him or her for hyperkalemia.

Usually a potassium level of greater than 5.5 mEq/L is considered hyperkalemia, although the range in infants and children is age dependent and can be higher than in adults. Levels higher than 7 mEq/L can lead to significant hemodynamic and neurologic consequences, whereas levels exceeding 8.5 mEq/L can cause respiratory paralysis or cardiac arrest and can quickly be fatal.

EKG changes include the following:

- Tall, peaked (tenting of) T waves with a narrow base
- Lengthening and eventual disappearance of the P wave
- Widening of the QRS complex
- Heart block, ventricular fibrillation, or asystole

Treatment for hyperkalemia:

- Calcium chloride 20 mg/kg IV
- Insulin 0.1 unit/kg IV SQ
- Dextrose 0.25–1 g/kg IV
- Sodium bicarbonate 1–2 mEq/kg IV
- Furosemide 0.1 mg/kg IV
- Dialysis if refractory to pharmacologic intervention

Hypoglycemia (Pediatric Blood Glucose Normal and Goals)

After 3 days of life, glucose levels should be > 40 mg/dL. Hypoglycemia is diagnosed in the following cases:

- Glucose < 25 mg/dL for premature infant
- Glucose < 30 mg/dL for full-term infant

Signs of hypoglycemia in the neonate include irritability, hypotension, bradycardia, seizures, and apnea.

- Consequences of decreased glucose are too great! Keep this level at 50 mg/dL or higher.
- Consequences include hypoxia, bradycardia, hypotension, and brain damage.

To treat hypoglycemia, give glucose 0.5–1 **Gm**/kg IV slowly:

- D_5NS: 10–20 mL/kg
- $D_{10}W$: 5–10 mL/kg IV slowly
- $D_{25}W$: 2–4 mL/kg IV slowly
- $D_{50}W$: 1 mL/kg IV slowly

Check levels and administer glucose intraoperatively for patients younger than 1 year of age if procedure is longer than 1 hour or the child has a prolonged NPO time.

Especially avoid hypoglycemia in patients at risk for cerebral ischemia (e.g., heart and neurologic surgery).

Notes:

- *You can convert a 500 mL bag of D_5W to $D_{10}W$ by adding 25 g of dextrose.*
- *A 250 mL bag of $D_{5.22}NS$ contains 12.5 g dextrose.*

Hypotension in Pediatric Patient

Causes of hypotension in pediatric patients include the following conditions:

- Anemia
- Hypovolemia
- Hypoglycemia
- Hypocalcemia

Treatment includes the following measures:

- Oxygen 6–10 L/min via mask
- IVF bolus normal saline or lactated Ringer's 20 mL/kg IV over 5–10 min

- Legs elevated; Trendelenburg position

If the child is bradycardic:

- Give atropine 0.02 mg/kg IV; minimal initial dose is 0.1 mg
- Can repeat with a double dose

If child is unresponsive to fluid resuscitation:

- Give epinephrine 0.1–1 mcg/kg IV/IO.
- Give vasopressin 0.0003–0.002 unit/kg/min infusion **or** 0.3–2 milliunits/kg/min infusion. Vasopressin can be given via ETT but human studies regarding dosing are limited.
- Consider dopamine infusion.
- Check blood glucose.
- Give 5% albumin only if shock persists after 40–60 mL/kg of crystalloid has been administered; this drug can produce significant pulmonary edema.

Laryngospasm

Laryngospasm is caused by stimulation of the superior laryngeal nerve and subsequent contraction of the adductor muscles (cricoarytenoids) in response to fluid, foreign bodies, mucous, noxious gases, painful stimuli, and/or airway manipulation. It can usually be avoided by extubating the patient while he or she is deeply anesthetized (stage 3 and spontaneously breathing) or when the patient is wide awake and meets all extubation criteria. Extubation during the interval between these two times is generally recognized as hazardous.

Anesthetic Management
- Treat by removing the irritating stimulus, and deepen anesthetic if appropriate.
- Maintain sustained positive pressure with 100% O_2.
- Perform manual forward displacement of the mandible.
- If unable to break spasm, give succinylcholine 0.5 mg/kg IV with atropine 0.02 mg/kg IV.

Malignant Hyperthermia
In this clinical syndrome, the child experiences a self-perpetuating hypermetabolic state involving the skeletal

muscles. Hyperthermia results from an acute uncontrolled increase in skeletal muscle metabolism from a pathological release of stored muscle calcium. Malignant hyperthermia may be caused by succinylcholine or any inhaled agent.

Signs include increased $ETCO_2$, tachycardia, arrhythmias, acidosis, shock, trunk or limb rigidity, masseter spasm, and cyanosis. Increased temperature may be a late sign. The differential diagnosis includes thyroid storm, pheochromocytoma, and sepsis.

Treatment is to **get help**, **get dantrolene**, and notify the surgeon.

- Discontinue volatile agents and succinylcholine.
- Hyperventilate with a 10 L flow of 100% oxygen; hyperventilate to decrease $ETCO_2$.
- Halt the procedure as soon as possible.
- **Dantrolene**: Start at **2.5 mg/kg q 5 min; max: 30 mg/kg.**
  - Dantrolene 20 mg with 3 Gm mannitol mixed in 60 mL sterile water: 1 mg/3 mL
  - *Example: 70 kg patient: initial 2.5 mg/kg = 175 mg or 525 mL (9 vials)*

- Cool patient if temperature $> 38.5°C$.
- Sodium bicarbonate 1–2 mEq/kg IV for pH < 7.2.
- Treat hyperkalemia. *See treatment under "Hyperkalemia."*
- Dantrolene acts on the sarcoplasmic reticulum of skeletal muscle by reducing the release of calcium or by inhibiting excitation–contracture coupling at the transverse tubule.
- MH Hotline: 1-800-644-9737.

Myringotomy

Myringotomy is a surgical incision into the eardrum to relieve pressure or drain fluid. It is usually performed for an ear infection referred to as otitis media.

Anesthetic Management

- Preoperative PO *Tylenol*, IM ketorolac, transnasal butorphanol 25 mcg/kg, **or** intraoperative *Tylenol* per rectum (PR) can be given for anticipated postoperative discomfort.
- Inhalation induction consists of 70% N_2O and 30% O_2 with 8% sevoflurane.

- Use a mask for general anesthesia; an oral airway is usually helpful to maintain a patent airway.
- A peripheral IV is not usually started unless there are coexisting comorbid conditions and potentially a need for intravenous medication.
- Get the child back breathing spontaneously; it may be necessary to support this respiratory effort.
- Inhalation agent is discontinued during the second ear portion of the procedure so the child has time to breathe off the volatile agent for wakeup.
- Provide gentle oropharyngeal suction at the end of the case.
- Transport while giving blow-by oxygen to the child in the lateral decubitus, head-down position.

Osteogenesis Imperfecta

Osteogenesis imperfecta (OI) is caused by a defect in collagen production, leading to abnormal bones (bowing of long bones, kyphoscoliosis), ligaments, teeth, and sclera of the eyes. OI is associated with platelet abnormalities and decreased factor VIII in 30% of patients. Cardiac defects, hypermetabolic syndromes, basilar invagination (occurs when the top of the C2 vertebrae migrates upward into the intracranial vault and potentially presses on the lower portion of the brain stem), otosclerosis, and deafness are also seen.

In treatment of OI, the goals are to prevent bone deformity with prompt surgical treatment of fractures and to reduce the possible negative sequelae from scoliosis, if present.

Anesthetic Management
- A difficult airway must be assumed.
- Gentle manipulation of the cervical spine and airway is essential.
- Be aware that spinal deformities can cause decreased functional residual capacity (FRC) and hypoxemia due to ventilation–perfusion mismatch. Preinduction oxygenation for 3–5 minutes may help to prevent rapid desaturation during intubation. *See "Scoliosis" for more information.*

- Tidal volumes should be smaller than normally calculated (decreased to 3–4 mL/kg instead of 6–7 mL/kg) with increased respiratory rates to maintain $ETCO_2$ and prevent barotrauma.
- Meticulous attention to padding and positioning is necessary to avoid fractures or nerve damage.
- Avoid aggressive heat conservation; occasionally patients with OI have developed malignant hyperthermia. Use standard precautions against malignant hyperthermia.
- OI patients have been found to have a multitude of metabolic defects. Cooling blankets should be available.
- Avoid anticholinergics (atropine, scopolamine, and glycopyrrolate), as they have been shown to cause hyperthermia.
- Fresh frozen plasma, platelets, and cryoprecipitate should be available for patients with factor deficiencies or low preoperative platelet levels.
- Regional anesthesia techniques will help to avoid pulmonary complications associated with general anesthesia.

- Succinylcholine-induced fasciculations may cause fractures.
- Antiemetics should be given to prevent possible fractures from vomiting and retching.

Scoliosis

Scoliosis is a lateral and rotational deformity of the thoracolumbar spine. The progression and severity of systemic manifestations advance with the severity of the curve.

Scoliosis can lead to restrictive lung disease, manifested as decreased chest wall compliance, vital capacity (VC), functional vital capacity (FVC), total lung capacity (TLC), and forced expiratory volume in 1 second (FEV_1), with increased dead space resulting from lung compression. There is alveolar hypoventilation with VQ mismatch—that is, increased alveolar–arterial O_2 difference and increased dead space to tidal volume ratio. The child may also demonstrate pulmonary hypertension—that is, increased pulmonary vascular resistance, which may progress to right ventricular hypertension and cor pulmonale.

Approximately 25% of patients with scoliosis have mitral valve prolapse.

Treatment may consist of instrumentation and spinal fusion with Harrington rods or segmental spinal fusion.

Anesthetic Management

- A balanced technique with O_2/N_2O/low-dose volatile/ narcotic and muscle relaxation is best.
- Aggressive temperature conservation is needed.
- There is a potential for large blood loss: Do hourly checks of hemoglobin levels; prepare for autologous, direct donor, and/or cell saver blood.
- Deliberate hypotension may be enforced, while keeping MAP at 50–60 mm Hg.
- Problems with the prone position may include compression of the lungs, increased intra-abdominal pressure, compression of the inferior vena cava, decreased venous return, and decreased cardiac output. Epidural vein engorgement can lead to increased bleeding.
- SSEPs neurophysiologic monitoring is likely to be used.

Shunting

Left-to-right shunt (acyanotic shunt): recirculation of pulmonary venous blood	Right-to-left shunt (cyanotic shunt): recirculation of systemic venous blood; no contact with lungs and oxygenation
■ PDA patent ductus arteriosus ■ ASD atrial septum defect ■ VSD ventricle septum defect ■ Atrioventricular septal defects	■ Tetralogy of Fallot ■ Pulmonary valve atresia ■ Tricuspid atresia ■ Total anomalous pulmonary venous return ■ Persistent truncus arteriosus

Strabismus

Strabismus is caused by weakened extraocular muscles.

Patients with strabismus have an increased predisposition to malignant hyperthermia, and succinylcholine is contraindicated (because of the potential risk of succinylcholine triggering malignant hyperthermia in patients with localized muscle weakness such as strabismus). Succinylcholine is also contraindicated when a forced duction test is considered, because it produces a prolonged increase in extraocular muscle tone).

Three major concerns arise with this surgery:

- Bradycardia from oculocardiac reflex (greater risk in pediatric patients, as they have higher vagal tone) occurs with:
  - Traction on the extraocular muscles between the ophthalmic branch of the trigeminal cranial nerve and the vagus nerve
  - Direct pressure on the eyeball
  - Ocular manipulation
  - Retrobulbar block and hemorrhage
- Postoperative nausea and vomiting
- Risk of malignant hyperthermia

Anesthetic Management

- Preoperative atropine or glycopyrrolate can decrease the incidence of the oculocardiac reflex.
- If bradycardia occurs, notify the surgeon immediately. Removal of traction on extraocular muscles or pressure on the eyeball should cause an increase in heart rate; if no increase occurs, atropine or glycopyrrolate should be given.

- Aggressive postoperative antiemetic prophylaxis should be given to prevent vomiting, which is associated with increased face and eye pressure. One regimen is to use weight-specific dosing of dexamethasone 0.25 mg/kg (immediately after induction) and ondansetron 0.05–0.15 mg/kg IV with a maximum dose of 8 mg (within 15 minutes of emergence).

- Temperature monitoring, along with avoidance of succinylcholine, helps minimize the risk of malignant hyperthermia.

- Smooth emergence is important to prevent bucking, which places increased pressure on the eyes.

Tet Spell

In tetralogy of Fallot (TOF), patients have right outflow tract (RVOT) obstruction, an overriding aorta, ventricular septal defect, and pulmonary stenosis or atresia. They may or may not have cyanosis at rest.

Hypercyanotic episodes, called "tet spells," are a hallmark of unrepaired TOF and can be life threatening due to a rapid drop in the amount of oxygen in the blood.

Tet spell events occur most often after the child wakes up but can also be due to crying, fever, defecation, and feeding.

Anesthetic Management
Non-anesthetized children:

- 100 FiO_2
- Knee–chest position to increase pulmonary blood flow
- Morphine 0.05–0.1 mg/kg IM or IV to relieve air hunger
- Crystalloid or colloid IV fluids given to increase preload
- Neosynephrine to increase the systemic vascular resistance
- Beta blockers (propranolol or esmolol) to slow the heart rate
- Sodium bicarbonate to correct metabolic acidosis

If the spell persists, general anesthesia and intubation should be initiated.

Tonsillectomy and/or Adenoidectomy
Tonsillectomy and/or adenoidectomy (T&A) may be required for hypertrophy of throat lymphoid tissue in

children who have developed obstructive sleep apnea and airway obstruction. If left untreated, pulmonary hypertension or cor pulmonale can result in hypoxia from the chronic obstruction.

Anesthetic Management

- Minimize preoperative sedation to prevent respiratory depression.
- Decrease oral secretions with an antisialagogue.
- Children with obstructive sleep apnea may have an increased sensitivity to opioids. Assess for opioid sensitivity during anesthesia, with a spontaneously breathing child, by titrating small doses of opioids (e.g., 0.1 mg/kg IV of morphine or 0.25 mcg/kg of fentanyl). Any evidence of apnea after receiving small doses of narcotics indicates increased sensitivity to opioids, and smaller overall doses should be given.
- An oral Rae or reinforced endotracheal tube can be used to prevent compression from the Dingman gag.

- The head of the bed often turned 90 degrees from anesthetist, so tape the ETT securely.
- Decrease FiO_2 to 30% with any cautery use in the airway; good communication with the surgeon is essential. Have a bottle of sterile water available in case of airway fire.
- Careful suctioning of the stomach is performed before emergence (remove any blood/fluid that has drained down the throat into the stomach).
- Softly suction the back of the throat before extubating the child; do so carefully to prevent trauma to the fresh surgical stasis.
- Watch for facial grimacing and hip flexion; safely extubate the patient when awake and with intact protective airway reflexes.
- Transfer the patient to the PACU in lateral, head-down position to facilitate drainage of mouth or throat secretions.

Post-tonsillectomy bleeding presents with frequent swallowing, tachycardia, hypotension, pallor, and restlessness.

- Early: Usual presentation occurs in the first 6–24 hours postoperatively.

- Delayed: Peak occurs at 7 days postoperatively when the eschar falls off, leaving the exposed tonsillar bed.

Anesthetic Management of Post-Tonsillectomy Bleeding

- Provide fluid resuscitation before induction of anesthesia.
- Establish an IV before induction.
- Perform rapid-sequence induction. Make sure to have suction available for intubation.
- Ketamine may be the induction agent of choice due to the risk of hypovolemia.
- Carefully suction the stomach contents after induction.
- Use a soft catheter to suction the throat to prevent more bleeding.

Trauma

Shock in a child is a late manifestation of hypovolemia/hemorrhage due to enormous reserve and compensatory mechanisms. Treat it aggressively.

Spinal Cord Injury Without Radiographic Abnormality (SCIWORA)

Spinal cord injury without radiographic abnormality (SCIWORA) is the occurrence of a spinal cord injury despite normal cervical and thoracic spine films and CT scans. Due to the inherent elasticity in the pediatric spine, severe spinal cord injury can occur without radiologic evidence of injury.

SCIWORA occurs in conjunction with approximately 20% of all pediatric spinal cord injuries in children younger than 8 years. The areas of the spine most often affected are both the cervical and thoracic spine; the lumbar spine is rarely involved.

■ Abbreviations

BP blood pressure

CDH congenital diaphragmatic hernia

CNS central nervous system

CV cardiovascular

ETT endotracheal tube

FEV forced expiratory volume (during first second of forced exhalation)

FVC forced vital capacity

GA general anesthetic

GERD gastroesophageal reflux disease

GFR glomerular filtration rate

HCT hematocrit

HR heart rate

IM intramuscular

IVF intravenous fluids

LMA laryngeal mask airway

LOC level of consciousness

LR lactated ringers

MAC minimal alveolar concentration
MR muscle relaxant
NDMR nondepolarizing muscle relaxant
NPO nothing by mouth
NS normal saline
PDA patent ductus arteriosus
Ped/pedi pediatric
PEEP positive end-expiratory pressure
RR respiratory rate
SBP systolic blood pressure
SC subcutaneous
SQ subcutaneous
TB tuberculin
TEF tracheoesophageal fistula
TLC total lung capacity
UOP urinary output
WNL within normal limits
yo year(s) old

■ References

Duke J. *Anesthesia Secrets*. 2nd ed. Philadelphia: Hanley & Belfus; 2000.

Motoyama EK, Davis PJ, eds. *Smith's Anesthesia for Infants and Children*. 5th ed. St. Louis, MO: Mosby; 2005.

The PeriAnesthesia CheckMate—Critical Care CheckMate Series. Lancaster, KY: www.nncusa.com; 2000.

Hazinski MF, ed. *PALS Provider Manual*. Dallas, TX: American Heart Association; 2002.